Investigation & Management of Eye Disease in Primary Care

This handbook offers concise, evidence-based guidance for clinicians who diagnose and manage ocular disease outside tertiary centres. Written for general practitioners, optometrists, ophthalmic nurses and primary care eye professionals, it translates core science into practical steps for assessment, urgent decision making and initial therapy.

The book covers common sight-threatening conditions, including glaucoma, age-related macular degeneration, diabetic and hypertensive retinopathies, uveitis, cataracts and inflammatory and immune-mediated eye disease. It provides clear, illustrated pathways for history taking, focused examination and red-flag recognition, with pragmatic advice on when to treat, when to refer and how to arrange safe follow-up.

KEY PRACTICAL FEATURES

- Clinical diagnostic aids and annotated images to support decision making
- Management algorithms and treatment pearls for emergencies and routine care
- Practical procedures such as corneal scraping, microscopy and basic microbiology with guidance on appropriate antimicrobial therapy
- Therapeutic rationale covering ocular pharmacology, prescribing considerations and when to use immunomodulatory agents
- Public health and tropical perspectives on ocular infections, epidemiology and prevention of cross-infection in practice

This book bridges the gap between specialist ophthalmology texts and everyday primary care needs, equipping clinicians with the knowledge to protect vision, reduce avoidable harm and coordinate care effectively within diverse global health settings.

Investigation & Management of Eye Disease in Primary Care

Infection, Inflammation and Immune Response

David V. Seal, Uwe Pleyer, Michelle L. Hennelly,
John G. Lawrenson and Bhavina Patel

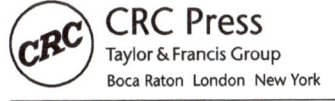

CRC Press
Taylor & Francis Group
Boca Raton London New York

CRC Press is an imprint of the
Taylor & Francis Group, an **informa** business

Designed cover image: David V. Seal, Uwe Pleyer, Michelle L. Hennelly, John G. Lawrenson, Bhavina Patel, and Soumyava Basu

First edition published 2026
by CRC Press
2385 NW Executive Center Drive, Suite 320, Boca Raton FL 33431

and by CRC Press
4 Park Square, Milton Park, Abingdon, Oxon, OX14 4RN

CRC Press is an imprint of Taylor & Francis Group, LLC

For Product Safety Concerns and Information please contact our EU representative GPSR@taylorandfrancis.com. Taylor & Francis Verlag GmbH, Kaufingerstraße 24, 80331 München, Germany.

ISBN: 978-1-032-99937-1 (hbk)
ISBN: 978-1-032-99936-4 (pbk)
ISBN: 978-1-003-60678-9 (ebk)

DOI: 10.1201/9781003606789

Typeset in Minion Semibold
by Apex CoVantage, LLC

Access the Support Materials: https://resourcecentre.routledge.com/books/9781032999364

Contents

Part 3   Appendices

Acknowledgement

We wish to acknowledge Mr. J.Z. Ong and Mrs. Elaine Lucas for their contributions to Chapters 8 and 9, respectively.

Preface

This book has been produced to enhance recognition and early management of sight-threatening and other ocular diseases in primary care. There are excellent books available in both optometry and ophthalmology, for both student and practitioner, but they do not fulfill the role for early disease recognition and management in primary care nor provide basic science in immunology and pharmacokinetics.

Primary care is offered in very different ways between the USA and Canada, UK, EU, Middle East, Africa and Asia by family doctors, optometrists, ophthalmologists, opticians and ophthalmic nurses. They may use basic or advanced equipment, in community or private practice, in hospitals or remote facilities. We have tried to cover all circumstances with text, photographs, drug formularies and appendices for basic laboratory work and infection control.

We have written the book for both print and electronic versions with multiple links to give more detailed clinical advice and therapeutic options. Prevention of sight-threatening infectious diseases, especially in tropical Africa and Asia, is equally important. We have reviewed the ongoing extensive eradication campaigns for trachoma, onchocerciasis, *Loa loa* and neglected tropical diseases, including microbial keratitis due to mixed fungal and bacterial aetiology, which responds well to appropriate antibiotics, saving vision in the eye.

The new developments of good quality fundus photography and OCT (optical coherence tomography) are an extraordinary advancement that allows for investigation of retinal disease at the cellular level to make an early diagnosis for management and therapy. Equally exciting is the development of 'telemedicine' using the mobile telephone camera to take photographs of both anterior and posterior segments and transmit them for diagnostic and therapeutic advice. This technology provides advanced patient care to ophthalmic nurses in remote areas with limited facilities in a remarkable way. We have tried to cover both these very different situations to enable diagnosis of early disease.

We are grateful to our colleagues, both in the UK and overseas, for advice and assistance with this book, especially to Dr. L. Cordoves, Universitario de Canarias, Tenerife, Spain, and Mr. W. Leslie Alexander, UK. We thank colleagues for their help in providing educational photographs as follows: Dr. S. Radhakrishnan, Glaucoma Center of San Francisco, California, USA; Drs. F. Mesa-Lugo, M. Crespo-Rodriguez and M. Acosta-Darias, Hospital Universitario de Canarias, Tenerife, Spain; and Dr. S. Basu, LV Prasad Eye Institute, Hyderabad, India. We also thank Dr. G. Johnson, International Centre of Eye Health, London; and Drs. R. Bansal and V. Gupta, Post-Graduate Institute of Medical Education and Research (PGIMER), Sector-12, Chandigarh, India, for allowing us to present their photographs. In addition, we thank the following for their excellent drawings:

Dr. Samantha Armstrong, Aston University, Birmingham (Figures 1.2, 2.3 and 3.19) and Mr. J.Z. Ong, RCSI/UCD Malaysia Campus (RUMC), Penang, Malaysia (Figures 1.6, 3.1, 3.18, 9.1, 9.2, 9.3, 9.4, 10.1, 10.2 (S2.1, S3.19, S3.21, S11.1, S11.2 & S11.3)). We especially thank Miss Jill Bloom, Moorfields Eye Hospital, London for her many helpful discussions.

Author Biographies

Dr. David V. Seal, MD, FRCOphth, FRCPath, Dip. Bact. (LSHTM), holds fellowships in both ophthalmology and pathology (medical microbiology) and has practised in both. He was Senior Lecturer in the Tennent Institute of Ophthalmology, Glasgow University, and NHS Consultant in Microbiology for the Public Health Laboratory, Maternal and Paediatric services for Glasgow. Previously, he worked with the Medical Research Council for microbiology and infectious diseases at the Clinical Research Centre and Northwick Park Hospital, Harrow. Prior to that, he was Consultant Medical Microbiologist at Southampton General (University) Hospital and Public Health Laboratory. He studied medicine at St. George's Hospital, London, where he started his career. He has published over 100 scientific papers and four books.

Professor Uwe Pleyer is Professor of Ophthalmology at Charité Hospital, Humbolt University, Berlin, Germany. He was awarded his medical degree from the RWTH Aachen, Germany, and Cornell University, New York, USA. Dr. Pleyer did a fellowship at the Jules Stein Institute, UCLA, Los Angeles. He is involved with both research aspects and clinical treatment of infectious and immune-mediated ocular diseases. He is a founding member of the International Ocular Inflammation Society, IOIS, and past president of the European Association for Vision and Eye Research (EVER).

Dr. Michelle L. Hennelly BSc (Hons) FCOptom PhD SFHEA is Associate Professor and Head of Optometry and Visual Science at City St George's, University of London, with over 30 years' experience in clinical optometry, academic leadership, and global eye health. A registered optometrist, she holds a PhD in psychophysics and is both Senior Fellow of the Higher Education Academy and Fellow of the College of Optometrists. She has led on postgraduate and undergraduate program development, including Independent Prescribing and MOptom pathways, and represents UK optometry on national and international panels. Michelle serves as a reviewer, editor, and advisor for journals, funding bodies, and global education boards, contributing to research and policy in clinical education and public eye care. Her leadership is defined by a commitment to inclusive teaching, global collaboration, and innovation in optometric education.

Professor John G. Lawrenson, MSc (Oxon), PhD, FCOptom, is Clinical Scientist and Professor of Clinical Visual Science at City St George's, University of London. His primary research interests are in the field of ophthalmic public health, including global causes of visual impairment—e.g. myopia, diabetic retinopathy, glaucoma, and age-related macular degeneration. He has edited the eye and orbit sections in the last four editions of *Gray's Anatomy*. He is an advocate for evidence-based clinical practice, holds a master's degree in Evidence-based Healthcare from the University of Oxford, and is a senior editor for Cochrane and authored a number of high-profile Cochrane systematic reviews in eyes and vision.

Bhavina Patel, BSc (Hons), DipTp (IP), DipGlauc, Prof Cert MR, LV, is a postgraduate lecturer specialising in independent prescribing. With over two decades of experience across both the multiple and independent sectors, she combines academic expertise with active clinical practice. Bhavina is currently Clinical Lead and Senior Triager for South-East London's Primary Ophthalmic Solutions, where she oversees ophthalmic triage pathways and referral refinement across primary and secondary care interfaces, including services into King's College Hospital and St Thomas' Hospital. She holds senior roles within independent optometric practices, serving as clinical lead, information governance lead, and part of the senior management team. Her extensive portfolio includes specialist optometrist work in glaucoma at St Thomas' Hospital and active involvement with the Lambeth, Southwark, and Lewisham Local Optical Committee.

Contributors

Michelle L. Hennelly
City St George's, University of London

John G. Lawrenson
City St George's, University of London

Elaine Lucas
Private Practice, London

J.Z. Ong
RCSI & UCD Malaysia Campus, Penang

Bhavina Patel
City St George's, University of London

Uwe Pleyer
Charité, Universitätsmedizin Berlin

David V. Seal
London

PART 1
Main Chapters

1: How to Assess and Examine the Eye for Disease

CORE MESSAGES

Assessment of the eye for disease requires a structured and holistic approach that integrates knowledge of anatomy, physiology, immunology, history, observation, measurement and imaging. Early detection depends on attention to subtle signs, the use of appropriate technology (where available) and an understanding of the systemic context of ocular findings.

A systematic, thorough assessment of the eye is essential for detecting ocular disease, monitoring progression and making informed decisions about management. Eye care practitioners (ECPs) must be proficient in both history taking and clinical examination to identify pathology at an early stage and distinguish between benign and sight-threatening conditions. The following outlines the core principles and key techniques for the examination of the eye for disease in adults and children.

a) Anatomy of the Eye

Figure 1.1 illustrates the anatomical structure of the globe. Figure 1.2 is a schematic diagram of the 'open angle' between the cornea and iris to drain the aqueous humour, produced by the ciliary body, out of the anterior chamber through the trabecular meshwork and the canal of Schlemm into the episcleral veins.

b) Essential Clinical Skills

A comfortable patient who is at ease is more likely to provide complete and true information. With a practised holistic approach, patients' symptoms and signs should be considered as a whole and not just for the eye. It is essential to listen to the patient carefully to detect possible disease. For example, concern about walking in dimly lit areas may be indicative of a visual field defect (Chapter 2), early retinopathy or even subtle manifestation of neurodegeneration such as Alzheimer's disease or dementia (Chapter 3) [1, 2].

History Taking and Recording Observations

Evaluating a patient's history and symptoms is a fundamental part of any comprehensive eye examination. This initial step offers crucial insights that direct the examination and additionally standardises disease understanding for coordinated multidisciplinary care. Ultimately, a thorough history and symptoms assessment serves as the foundation of clinical reasoning, enhancing diagnostic accuracy and ensuring the best possible patient outcomes.

DOI: 10.1201/9781003606789-2

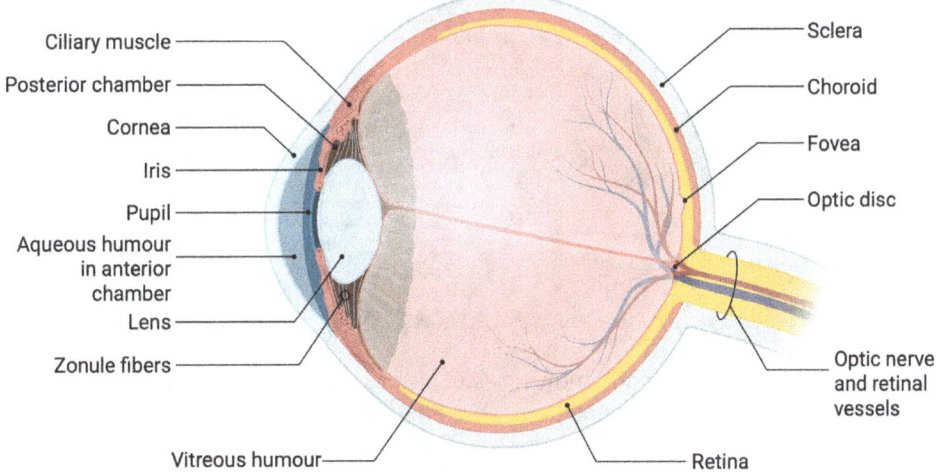

FIGURE 1.1 Structure of the eye.

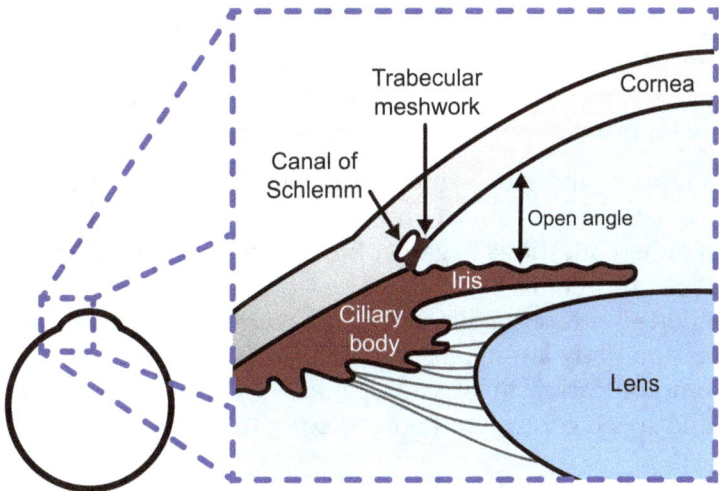

FIGURE 1.2 Structure of the 'open angle'.

Source: (Courtesy of Dr. Samantha Armstrong, Aston University, Birmingham)

Having a structured set protocol ensures a systematic, thorough and efficient process to diagnosis and management. In particular, this protocol:

1) Safeguards that no key information is missed
2) Allows for a more logical investigative approach
3) Assists with symptom-disease correlation
4) Facilitates a focused and efficient consultation
5) Can highlight benign from potentially sight or life-threatening conditions
6) Enables tracking of disease progression and assessment of treatment effectivity

Beginning with presenting complaints and problems with their eyes, it is useful to consider them systematically before exploring external factors that may

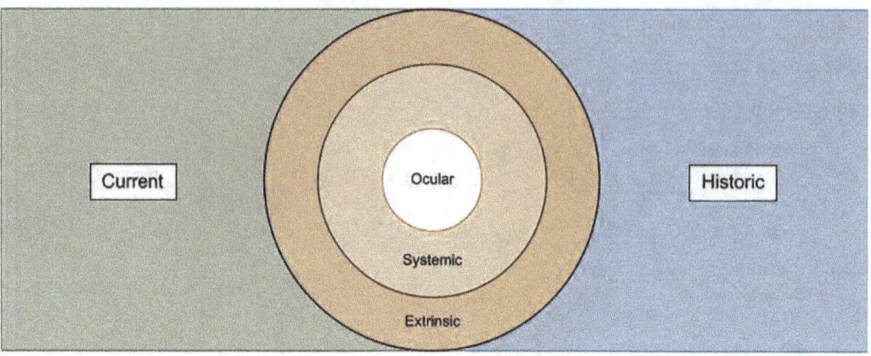

FIGURE 1.3 A conceptual schematic showing how history and symptoms can be approached for current and historic ocular, systemic and extrinsic elements.

be influential. Both relevant current and historic information can be elucidated through effective verbal and non-verbal communication (Figure 1.3).

Effective Communication
Key strategies in history-taking, which builds affinity with patients, ensuring accurate and complete information gathering, should be followed, with additional considerations for those with complex or additional needs [1].

Fundamental principles include the following:

- Establish rapport and trust—introduce yourself and greet the patient warmly; maintain a level of eye contact and calm, reassuring tone [2].
- Use open-ended questions to gather broad information and closed-ended questions for specific details.
- Pay attention—with active listening and awareness of non-verbal cues such as facial cues and body language [3].
- Adapt communication to fit your patient—verbally through language, tone, volume and speed control and non-verbally through body language [4].

History and Symptoms Framework

The history and symptoms framework is a structured approach used to systematically gather relevant information. It helps guarantee that no key details are missed and guides the clinician in identifying the cause, context and impact of a patient's given symptoms. There are several key elements which can be categorised as follows:

1) Presenting Complaint (PC)
2) History of Present Complaint (HPC)
3) Previous Ocular History (POH)
4) Systemic Medical Health and History (MHx)
5) Medication and Allergy History (Rx and Ax)
6) Review of Systems (ROS)
7) Family History (FHx)
8) Social History (SHx)

Presenting Complaint

The primary reason for their attendance should be documented using the patient's own description. Providing a benchmark for current disease impact, it

TABLE 1.1 Table Showing Typical Symptoms that Can Be Categorised into Three Broad Aspects

See	Look	Feel
• Decreased vision	• Eye alignment	• Pain
• Distorted vision	• Redness	• Itch
• Night blindness	• Swelling	• Burning
• Double/multiple vision	• Twitching	• Discomfort
• Flashes of light	• Oscillopsia	• Irritation
• Floaters	• Proptosis	• Foreign body sensation
• Haloes	• Discharge and/or tearing	• Photophobia
• Hallucinations	• Ptosis	• Headaches
• Glare	• Hair loss or change	• Desensitisation

also informs any future communication—i.e. supplementary questions regarding the presenting complaint between clinician and patient especially regarding management response in time.

Ocular symptoms can be thought of in three broad ways—how the eyes see, how the eyes look and how the eyes feel (Table 1.1). Though not mutually exclusive, these three parameters are typically what drives patients' concerns about their eyes.

There is a great deal of overlap with patients experiencing features of all three—for example, a patient reporting a red, painful, blurry eye that is light sensitive will be troubled by how the eyes see, look and feel. Understanding how the symptoms arose would be the next natural step.

Detailed Recording of Presenting Complaint

There are a number of useful mnemonics to ensure a structured, patient-centred approach is adopted to explore the nature, duration and progression of symptoms (Table 1.2). Applying these with a mixture of open-ended and closed questions, followed by focused questions to clarify, helps identify red flags and potential triggers and contextualises the impact so as to govern the urgency and diagnosis.

Any mnemonic would provide a detailed history, but each vary slightly in their focus and application. Clinicians may choose to stick with one particular system for all examinations or switch depending on the presenting complaint. In practice, these mnemonics are complementary and can be used in combination.

A detailed History of Presenting Complaint (HPC) provides insight into the onset, nature and progression of current ocular symptoms, while the Previous Ocular History (POH) helps contextualise these symptoms by identifying any past eye conditions, treatments or surgeries that may be relevant. Integrating HPC with POH ensures that clinicians can distinguish between new and recurring issues, assess risk factors for disease progression and avoid overlooking chronic or previously treated conditions that may influence the current presentation.

Many systemic conditions can have an effect on the eyes either directly or indirectly. Understanding a patient's medical history (MHx) helps identify risk factors for ocular disease, guides clinical decision making and ensures that eye care is safely integrated with their general health management.

Medication and Allergy History (Rx and Ax) is highly relevant to ocular examination as many systemic and ocular medications can affect health, contribute to visual symptoms or interact with treatments.

A structured overview of other body systems (ROS) can uncover systemic links to the eye. It should be concise but cover the major systems relevant to eye care.

TABLE 1.2 A List of Mnemonics Commonly Used in Medical Examinations

SOCRATES

• Site	Best for:
• Onset	Pain or discomfort
• Character	Strengths:
• Radiation	Deep pain analysis, systemic
• Associations	relevance
• Timing	
• Exacerbating/relieving factors	
• Severity	

OLDCARTS

• Onset	Best for:
• Location	Any general or systemic symptom
• Duration	Strengths:
• Character	Chronological overview, systemic
• Aggravating/alleviating	links
factors	
• Radiation	
• Timing	
• Severity	

LOFTSEA

• Location	Best for:
• Onset	Vision symptoms
• Frequency	Strengths:
• Type	Vision-specific, detailed and targeted
• Severity	
• Exacerbating/relieving factors	
• Associated symptoms	

TASTER

• Timing	Best for:
• Associated symptoms	Ocular surface/non-visual symptoms
• Site	Strengths:
• Type	Discomfort profiling, trigger-focused
• Exacerbating/relieving factors	
• Radiation	

It is important to explore the possibility of systemic inflammatory or infectious associations when symptoms are suggestive of particular eye conditions, e.g. uveitis.

Many eye conditions and systemic diseases with an ocular involvement have a genetic or hereditary component and so understanding a patient's family history (FHx) can identify those at higher risk of developing certain diseases. It can inform on early detection, monitoring and preventative care strategies.

Social history (SHx) refers to aspects of a patient's lifestyle including occupation and visual demands (e.g. screen use, driving, precision work). Their daily environment may influence their health, exposure to transmissible pathogens and noxious substances and access to care.

Clinical Reasoning to Determine a Diagnosis

Clinical reasoning can be defined as the process by which clinicians collect and analyse patient information, make judgments regarding diagnosis and management and reflect upon their decisions. For ECPs, this process encompasses interpreting both subjective symptoms and objective findings to make informed clinical decisions. A working diagnosis based on just history and symptoms is the most effective and logical way to move through a systematic patient examination.

Practitioners frequently move between different types of reasoning; Type 1 is fast, intuitive and performed preconsciously—i.e. one has awareness of the outcome but not of the steps taken to make a clinical decision—whereas Type 2 is analytical, reflective and a conscious process testing hypotheses and gathering data to justify decision making. Ainge [5] promotes awareness of Type 1 and 2 reasoning to enhance patient care by reducing cognitive bias and misdiagnosis in clinical settings.

For equipment needed to assess vision both in domiciliary and practice accommodation, refer to Supplementary Chapter S1.

c) Functional Testing

These assessments evaluate ocular function:

1. *Visual Acuity Testing*
   - Assesses clarity or sharpness of vision (e.g. Snellen chart, LogMAR)
2. *Pinhole Test*
   - Helps differentiate between refractive error and other causes of vision loss
3. *Refraction*
   - Evaluation of the refractive ability of the eyes
4. *Accommodation Assessment*
   - Evaluates the eye's ability to focus on near objects
5. *Binocular Vision Assessment*
   - Assesses how well both eyes work together and whether they are able to maintain single, clear and comfortable vision
6. *Eye Movement (Extraocular Muscle) Testing*
   - Assesses cranial nerves III, IV and VI for eye movement disorders.
7. *Pupillary Reflex Assessment*
   - Tests direct and consensual light reflexes; assesses optic and oculomotor nerve function.
8. *Visual Field Testing* (kinetic versus static, peripheral versus central)
   - Level and extent of testing can be varied using different strategies from Amsler, central standard automated perimetry to confrontation
9. *Colour Vision Testing*
   - Commonly done with Ishihara plates; identifies red-green colour deficiencies
10. *Reflex Assessment*
    - Includes corneal, light, near, accommodative, dazzle and menace

d) Health Assessment

New advances in technology and knowledge broaden the scope of health assessment from viewing structural features to testing key characteristics.

1. *External Eye*—can be grossly observed unaided, carried out using a torch/penlight with or without loupes or with the aid of a slit lamp
2. *Internal Eye*—can be viewed directly using an ophthalmoscope, or indirectly using a head-mounted biomicroscope or slit lamp with condensing lenses

Anterior Segment Devices—meibography systems, tear film osmolarity system, ocular surface analyser, topographer, keratometer, ophthalmometer, pachymeter,

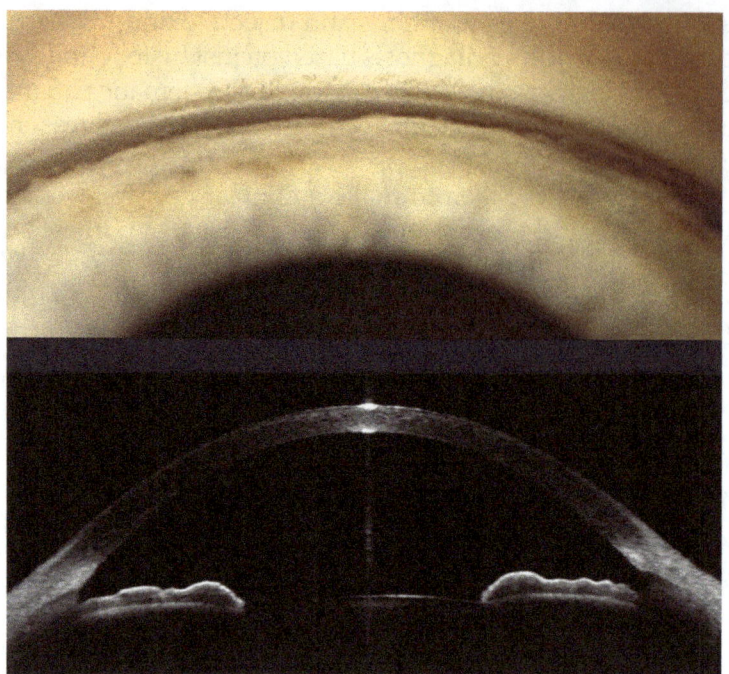

FIGURE 1.4 Gonioscopy (top) versus AS-OCT (bottom) for angle assessment.

Source: (Courtesy of Dr. S. Radhakrishnan, San Francisco)

specular microscope, anterior segment optical coherence tomography (OCT), gonioscopy [6].

Anterior-segment (AS)-OCT, using light at a different wavelength, is more effective for angle assessment, but gonioscopy remains the gold standard for diagnosing angle closure; there are some advantages and disadvantages between both techniques (Figure 1.4).

Posterior Segment Devices—e.g. direct or indirect ophthalmoscope, fundus camera, wide-field fundus camera, OCT, OCT-A, scanning laser ophthalmoscope.

Fundus photographs are used to document abnormalities of the disease process and to follow up conditions including diabetes mellitus, age-related macular degeneration (AMD), glaucoma and multiple sclerosis (Chapter 3). A normal fundus is shown later (Figure 1.5).

For diabetic patients, regular fundus screening examinations are important to check for retinopathy as vision loss can be prevented with laser treatment or intravitreal injections if retinal lesions are detected early (Chapter 3) [7].

RETINAL OPTICAL COHERENCE TOMOGRAPHY (OCT)

This non-invasive imaging technique uses parallel light waves to capture high-resolution, cross-sectional images of the retina and other ocular structures (Figure 1.6).

It is possible to establish in which layer abnormalities, such as fluid or exudate, are present as well as measure and monitor changes in tissue thickness. Increases may be due to age-related macular degeneration (AMD), diabetic maculopathy or

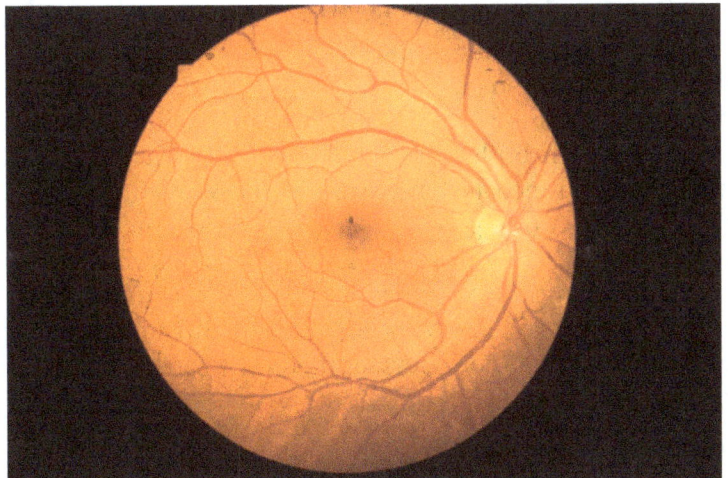

FIGURE 1.5 Photograph of a normal fundus showing the optic nerve cup and disc, macular and fovea areas of the retina, with healthy vessels within the nerve fibre and ganglion cell layer, easily visualised through an ophthalmoscope; veins are more prominent than arteries and have a larger diameter. Near the fovea, where central vision is concentrated, capillaries terminate and join a single-layer macular capillary ring to form a capillary-free region.

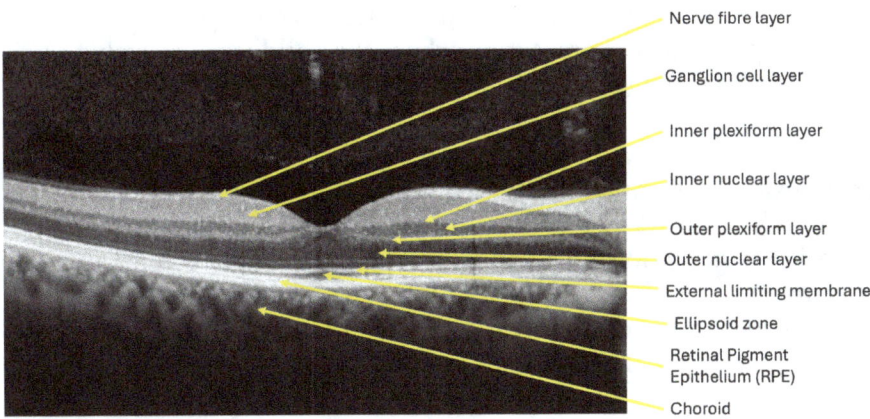

Nerve fibre layer
Ganglion cell layer
Inner plexiform layer
Inner nuclear layer
Outer plexiform layer
Outer nuclear layer
External limiting membrane
Ellipsoid zone
Retinal Pigment Epithelium (RPE)
Choroid

FIGURE 1.6 OCT of the macular region of a normal retina with the fovea in the centre.

Source: Courtesy of Dr. L Cordoves, Hospital Universitario de Canarias, Canary Islands, Spain and Mr. J.Z. Ong, RUMC, Penang, Malaysia

macula oedema (related to any other vascular or inflammatory disease) whilst decreases may be an indication of atrophy. Being non-invasive, such bio-imaging has become essential in clinical practice [8].

3. *Intraocular Pressure*—measured using tonometry devices such as applanation tonometers, noncontact tonometers, rebound tonometers and ocular response analysers.

e) Examination of Children

Although the core principles of eye examination are consistent across all age groups, assessing children's eyes often necessitates adaptations in communication, technique and equipment. Building a strong rapport with the child is crucial for an effective examination, as it fosters cooperation, reduces anxiety and improves the accuracy of the assessment. In these consultations, while the child is the primary patient, clinicians must remain mindful of the need for dual communication, engaging with both the child and the parent or guardian to ensure understanding, reassurance and effective information gathering. Furthermore, a comprehensive understanding of both structural and functional aspects of ocular development, combined with knowledge of age-appropriate testing methods, is crucial for accurate clinical interpretation and effective management.

To accommodate these considerations, it is useful to account for differences in communication, cooperation, developmental stage and physical examination techniques to ensure an effective and accurate assessment.

Communication
Language: use simple, age-appropriate language and tone
Engagement: turn instructions into games or challenges
Reassurance: constantly reassure and encourage the child
Duality: speak both to the child and the parent or guardian

Environment/Equipment
Child-friendly setting: decorated rooms, smaller furniture, availability of toys
Portable or modified equipment: puppet or light fixation targets
Flexible setup: to allow examination where the child is comfortable, such as parent's lap or on the floor

Examination Technique
Shorter, flexible sessions: be ready to pause and resume based on child's attention and mood
Observations prior to formal testing: initial assessment of behaviour, fixation, eye movements can be inferred through play or casual interaction
Prioritise key assessments: focus first on critical elements and only explore detailed tests if the child remains cooperative.

Behavioural Management
Positive reinforcement: consider verbal praise or small prizes such as stickers
Distraction techniques: animated fixation targets, singing, storytelling
Parental involvement: having parents hold or position the child, or role-playing to model cooperation

Clinical Mindset
Patience and flexibility: expect variability in cooperation and be able to adjust order or method of tests accordingly
Prioritise based on clinical need: sometimes a full examination is not possible in one visit so plan for staged assessments if needed.

History Taking
During history taking, it is important to ensure the child remains actively involved, as it can be easy to overlook them due to assumptions about their level of understanding. Directing questions initially to the child, before turning to the

parent or guardian, can help foster rapport and build trust. Key areas to cover include the following:

- Birth history—gestational disease, prematurity, birth complications
- Developmental milestones—gross and fine motor, language, cognitive, socio-emotional
- General health—presence of systemic or neurological conditions
- Family history—hereditary systemic or ocular disease including strabismus, congenital cataract, glaucoma and retinal disease
- Specific symptoms—squint, poor vision, photophobia, eye rubbing, clumsiness

Vision Assessment

Using age-appropriate techniques and having a clear understanding of expected normal findings at different developmental stages are essential for accurate assessment. The approach to vision testing varies according to the child's age:

Infants: assessment of fixation, following behaviour and preferential looking tests
Toddlers: use of picture-based acuity charts
Older children: use of letter-based acuity charts

It is important to obtain both monocular and binocular measurements, as each provides valuable independent information for clinical interpretation.

Binocular Vision Assessment

Clinical significance of findings must be interpreted in the context of the child's developmental stage, given the rapid change in ocular anatomy that takes place during the early years of life. Behavioural observations can offer valuable diagnostic clues, and where possible, both distance and near assessments should be performed to obtain a comprehensive evaluation.

Ocular Alignment

Assessment of ocular alignment includes the following:

- Cover tests: cover-uncover test, alternate cover test and prism cover test
- Hirschberg corneal reflex test: observing the position of the light reflex to detect misalignment
- Krimsky test: quantifying ocular deviation using prisms if a deviation is present

Ocular Motility

Ocular motility testing evaluates the coordinated movement of both eyes across all gaze positions, with attention to the following:

- Fullness of the range of movement
- Smoothness, accuracy and speed of saccades and pursuits
- Presence of any movement restrictions, underactions or overactions

Fusion

Fusion testing assesses the brain's ability to combine images from both eyes into a single percept.

- Motor fusion can be evaluated using a penlight with red/green glasses to see if the child maintains single vision while the target is moved.
- Sensory fusion can be assessed with newer tablet-based or gamified tests that present fusion tasks in an engaging way for children.

Stereopsis

Various stereopsis tests are available, often presented in a playful, game-like format.

- It is useful to begin with gross stereopsis tests before progressing to fine stereoacuity.
- Clinicians should be mindful that some tests may allow monocular cues, so careful interpretation of the child's behaviour—such as hesitation, reaching into space or searching movements—provides valuable diagnostic information.

Accommodation and Vergence

- Accommodation can be assessed by the following:
  - Dynamic retinoscopy to measure accommodative response
  - Amplitude of accommodation testing to evaluate maximum focusing ability
  - Accommodative facility testing using ±2.00D flipper lenses
- Vergence in older children can be assessed by measuring vergence amplitudes using prism bars or similar tools.

Colour Vision Testing

Colour vision testing assesses the ability to perceive and differentiate colours, helping detect congenital or acquired colour vision deficiencies (CVD). In children, early identification is important for educational support, career advice and detecting underlying ocular or neurological issues.

Peripheral Vision Testing

Assessing peripheral vision in children is crucial for identifying conditions such as optic nerve disorders, glaucoma, neurological abnormalities and retinal diseases. Since young children often lack the ability to reliably perform formal visual field tests, examination techniques must be adapted according to the child's age, developmental stage and level of cooperation such as using toys or lights for confrontation or kinetic field screening.

Anterior Segment Examination

Using portable equipment is often helpful in the very young, though accessing the table-based slit lamp is possible with cooperative children and parental assistance. Distraction techniques can assist with maintaining fixation. Prioritising essential structures and the detection of significant anomalies may be required if cooperation is limited. Key areas include the following:

1. *Eyelids and Periorbital Area*—inspect for:
   - Ptosis (drooping eyelid)
   - Eyelid malposition (entropion, ectropion)
   - Swelling, masses, or signs of infection (e.g. chalazion, preseptal cellulitis)
   - Signs of trauma or congenital anomalies (e.g. coloboma)
2. *Conjunctiva and Sclera*—inspect for the following:
   - Redness or injection (suggesting infection, allergy, or inflammation)
   - Discharge (type and quantity)
   - Conjunctival lesions or subconjunctival haemorrhage
   - Systemic signs (e.g. blue sclera in osteogenesis imperfecta)
3. *Cornea*—assess for the following:
   - Clarity (detecting opacities or scarring)
   - Size (e.g. megalocornea, microcornea)

- Surface irregularities, oedema or vascularization
- Signs of congenital glaucoma (e.g. enlarged cornea, Haab's striae)

4. *Anterior Chamber*—evaluate the following:
- Depth and clarity
- Presence of cells, flare, hyphema (blood) or hypopyon (pus cells)
- Signs of inflammation (uveitis)

5. *Iris*—inspect for the following:
- Colour and texture abnormalities
- Corectopia (displaced pupil) or aniridia (absence of the iris)
- Colobomas, neovascularization or synechiae (iris adhesions)

6. *Lens*—assess for the following:
- Clarity (look for congenital or developmental cataracts)
- Position (checking for lens subluxation or dislocation)

7. *Pupils and Pupil Reflexes*—examine the following:
- Size, shape and symmetry of pupils
- Direct and consensual light reflexes (assess for prompt constriction)
- Relative afferent pupillary defect (RAPD)—use the swinging flashlight test (Chapter 3)
- Presence of any abnormal responses suggesting optic nerve or retinal pathology

Posterior Segment Examination

Examining posterior segment structures is crucial for detecting conditions that can threaten vision or indicate systemic disease. However, adaptations are required based on the child's age, cooperation and clinical context. Breaking the exam into quick, manageable parts and examining with parental assistance and distraction may be necessary.

Refraction

In the very young, objective measures using retinoscopy dominate with subjective measures becoming more useful as the child's ability to cooperate advances. Utilising the option to use cycloplegia can add to the clinical picture. It is important to have an awareness of expected normal findings, the significance of abnormal findings, as well as an understanding of the impact and need of any intervention.

Interpretation and Clinical Significance of Findings

Interpreting clinical findings in paediatric eye examinations requires a nuanced understanding of both normal ocular development and the wide variability in children's cooperation and communication. It is essential to contextualise all findings within the child's age, developmental stage and general health status.

Developmental variations in ocular anatomy and visual function mean that what is considered normal in a newborn or toddler may be abnormal in an older child. For example, intermittent ocular misalignment can be normal in the first few months of life but may indicate pathology if persistent beyond this period. Similarly, a high hyperopic refractive error may be physiological in infancy but warrants closer monitoring or intervention if it persists or is associated with strabismus or amblyopia risk.

Behavioural observations during testing—such as a child's fixation preference, response to peripheral targets, ability to maintain fusion or hesitancy during stereopsis tasks—provide vital supplementary information that supports clinical findings and enhances diagnostic accuracy.

Functional tests such as vision assessment, ocular alignment, motility, fusion, stereopsis, accommodation and colour vision should be interpreted both individually and collectively. Inconsistent or incomplete results should not be dismissed but rather explored further, often requiring repeat testing or referral for more specialised evaluation.

Findings from anterior and posterior segment examinations must also be carefully integrated into the clinical picture. Incomplete examinations due to poor cooperation should be documented clearly, and clinicians should maintain a low threshold for further investigation, especially when visual behaviour or parental concerns suggest underlying pathology.

Objective assessments, such as dynamic retinoscopy and cycloplegic refraction, provide critical quantitative information, particularly in cases where subjective testing is unreliable. Here, interpretation must consider the child's age-appropriate refractive norms, risk factors for amblyopia and potential need for optical correction or amblyopia treatment.

Ultimately, a holistic approach combining clinical findings, behavioural cues, developmental expectations and parental observations forms the foundation of accurate diagnosis and appropriate management planning. Where uncertainty remains, or if key components of the examination could not be completed, clinicians should consider follow-up assessments, interdisciplinary collaboration or early referral to specialist paediatric ophthalmology services.

Management of Ocular Examination Findings in Children

The management of ocular findings in children must be individualised, developmentally appropriate and timely, recognising the critical periods of visual development during which early intervention can significantly improve long-term outcomes.

1. *General Principles*
   - Early identification and intervention are key to preventing long-term visual impairment.
   - Age-appropriate treatment strategies should be used, balancing the child's cooperation, developmental needs, and family context.
   - Parental education and involvement are vital to ensure understanding of the condition, treatment adherence, and realistic expectations.
   - Multidisciplinary collaboration with paediatricians, orthoptists, optometrists, or neurologists may be necessary for systemic or complex cases.

2. *Condition-Specific Management Approaches*

   Refractive Errors
   - Hypermetropia, myopia, astigmatism: Prescribe glasses based on clinical significance and risk to visual development (e.g. amblyopia, strabismus). For myopia control, refer to Chapters 3 and 9.
   - Cycloplegic refraction often guides prescription decisions in younger children.
   - Regular follow-up: Monitor for changes in refractive error as the child grows.

   Strabismus (Ocular misalignment)
   - Urgent referral if strabismus is constant, new onset or associated with systemic symptoms.

- Management options:
  - Glasses (especially if significant hypermetropia is found)
  - Occlusion therapy (patching) if amblyopia is present
  - Orthoptic exercises (selected cases)
  - Surgical correction where necessary

Amblyopia
- Occlusion therapy (patching the better-seeing eye) remains the standard treatment.
- Pharmacologic penalization (using atropine drops) is an alternative in certain cases.
- Early intervention provides the best outcomes; treatment effectiveness diminishes with age.

Cataract
- Prompt referral to paediatric ophthalmology.
- Surgical intervention may be needed early (within the first few months of life in dense bilateral cataracts).
- Postoperative visual rehabilitation with glasses or contact lenses and amblyopia management is essential.

Glaucoma
- Urgent referral for specialist care if congenital or juvenile glaucoma is suspected.
- Management usually requires surgical intervention, with medical therapy as an adjunct.

Retinal Disease
- Urgent management if retinal detachment, tumours (e.g. retinoblastoma) or vascular abnormalities (e.g. retinopathy of prematurity are detected)
  (https://www.aao.org/education/clinical-video/how-to-take-retinal-images-with-smartphone).
  Treatment may involve surgery, laser therapy or systemic treatment depending on the diagnosis.

Optic Nerve Abnormalities
- Further imaging and neurology referral if optic nerve swelling, pallor or hypoplasia is observed.
- Visual support services may be indicated for long-term visual impairment.

3. *Management of Functional Findings*
- Poor fusion or stereopsis: Address underlying causes (e.g. strabismus, anisometropia), and initiate therapy early.
- Reduced accommodation: Prescribe near vision support (e.g. reading glasses), and consider vision therapy in selected cases.
- Colour vision deficiency: No treatment but it is important to document, counsel families and liaise with educators.

4. *Practical Management Strategies*
- Scheduling: Break up long examinations and treatments into shorter, child-friendly visits.
- Use of child-friendly materials: Coloured patches, fun glasses frames, rewards for treatment compliance.
- Continuous reassessment: Children's visual needs change with growth, so regular follow-up is necessary to adapt management.

5. *When to Refer*
- Any suspicion of serious or progressive ocular disease (e.g. cataract, glaucoma, retinal pathology).
- Persistent abnormal findings without clear cause.
- Complex refractive, strabismic or neurological cases.
- Lack of expected improvement with initial management.

6. *Conclusion*

Effective management of ocular findings in children relies on early, accurate diagnosis and a dynamic, child-centred approach to treatment. Clear communication with families and coordinated multidisciplinary care where necessary underpin the best visual and developmental outcomes.

Advice for examining and managing children is given by the UK College of Optometrists *https://www.college-optometrists.org/category-landing-pages/chil dren*. Provision of suitable facilities include a play area with toys and toilet access.

For a detailed examination of the normal eye and refraction, including children, refer to Elliott D, 2020 (https://www.asia.elsevierhealth.com/clinical-proce dures-in-primary-eye-care–9780702077890.html).

For assisting eye care practitioners, refer to *PRIMARY EYE CARE A Guide to Diagnosis and Management* by Anthony Chigwell of World Sight Foundation 2025 (available in English, French, Spanish and Portuguese) (https://www.world sightfoundation.com/eye-care-guide/).

For examination of the diseased eye, refer to *Ophthalmology: Lecture Notes* by James B, Bron A and Parulekar M. 2024 (https://www.wiley.com/en-au/ Ophthalmology%3A+Lecture+Notes%2C+13th+Edition-p-9781119905).

REFERENCES

1. Hennelly M. et al. How to assess refractive error in adults with additional or complex needs. Comm Eye Health J 2024. PMID: 38827965 (https://pubmed.ncbi.nlm.nih.gov/38827965/).
2. Elliott D. Clinical Procedures in Primary Eye Care. 5th ed. Elsevier 14/04/2020. ISBN: 9780702077890 (https:// www.asia.elsevierhealth.com/clinical-procedures-in-primary-eye-care-9780702077890.html).
3. Murphy K. You're Not Listening, 1st ed. Celadon Books 2020. ISBN: 9781250297204.
4. Berman A et al. Korean J Med Educ 2016. PMID: 26913771 (https://doi.org/10.3946/kjme.2016.21).
5. Ainge LE, Edgar AK, Kirkman JM et al. Developing Clinical Reasoning Along the Cognitive Continuum: A Mixed Methods Evaluation of A Novel Clinical Diagnosis Assessment. BMC Med Educ 25(31) 2025 (https:// doi.org/10.1186/s12909-024-06613-6).
6. Radhakrishnan S. Review of Ophthalmology 05/2019. Accessed 28/05/2025 (https://www.reviewofophthal-mology.com/article/diagnosing-angle-closure-gonioscopy-vs-oct).
7. NHS. Diabetic Eye Screening 2024. Accessed 18/08/25 (https://www.nhs.uk/tests-and-treatments/diabetic-eye-screening/).
8. Yorston D. Comm Eye Health J 2025. PMID: 40151367 (https://cehjournal.org/articles/833).

2: Clinical Pearls for Diagnosis—Signs and Symptoms (Anterior and Posterior)

CORE MESSAGES

Identifying red flags through the patient's history and symptoms helps triage and prioritise urgency and guide management. It allows for the early detection of serious conditions such as retinal detachment, stroke and intracranial masses. It guides diagnostic prioritisation and prevents delay in care. Equally important, knowing which red flags are absent helps reassure patients when their symptoms are likely to be benign and assists in issuing advice.

Targeted Approach to Red Eyes

Initial priority should be in distinguishing between benign and sight-or life-threatening conditions. Some aspects (red flags) determined through history and symptoms should raise the level of concern (Figure 2.1 and Table 2.1).

Differential causes could be ocular, adnexal or even systemic and have origins that are based in allergies, infections, inflammation, injury or a combination of these. For example:

Corneal—dry eye disease (Chapter 4), foreign body, recurrent corneal erosion, corneal injury, medicamentosa, contact lens related, neurotrophic keratopathy, keratitis, pterygium

Conjunctival—infective conjunctivitis (Chapter 6), allergic conjunctivitis, subconjunctival haemorrhage, pingueculitis, giant papillary conjunctivitis, superior limbic keratoconjunctivitis, foreign body, symblepharon, neoplasia

Adnexal—blepharitis, trichiasis, distichiasis, entropion, ectropion, lagophthalmos, floppy eyelid syndrome, dacryocystitis, canaliculitis

Other—trauma, endophthalmitis, uveitis, episcleritis, scleritis, cavernous fistula, cluster headaches, angle closure glaucoma

A useful way to discriminate between potential causes is to establish whether vision has been affected.

Where vision remains unaffected, a red eye may be painful or painless, and the level of redness (inflammation) suggests the following:

Painful

Diffuse superficial—infective, allergic or chemical
Diffuse deep—anterior scleritis
Circum-limbal—keratitis, uveitis, corneal foreign body
Sectoral—episcleritis, pingueculitis, marginal keratitis

17

DOI: 10.1201/9781003606789-3

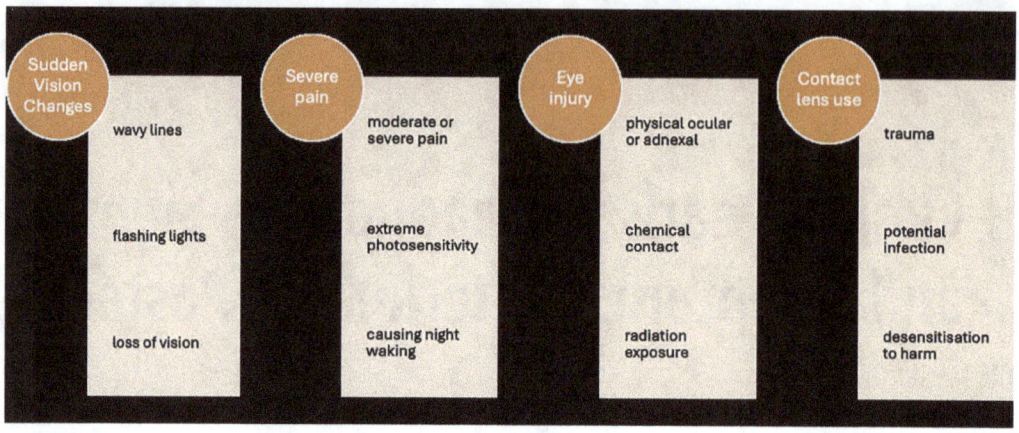

FIGURE 2.1 Red flag considerations when examining a patient presenting with a red eye.

TABLE 2.1 Common Conditions Associated with a Red Eye

Condition	Pain	Discharge	Vision Affected	Photophobia	Onset	Other Key Features
Viral Conjunctivitis	Mild	Watery	No	Sometimes	Sudden	Often bilateral, recent URTI, *contagious*
Bacterial conjunctivitis	Mild	Purulent	No	No	Sudden	Stuck lids on waking, unilateral or bilateral
Allergic conjunctivitis	Mild— itchy	Watery/mucoid	No	No	Sudden or seasonal	Bilateral, itchy
Subconjunctival haemorrhage	None	None	No	No	Sudden	Painless, often after straining
Episcleritis	Mild ache	None	No	No	Gradual	Localised, self-limiting
Scleritis	Severe, deep	None	Sometimes	Yes	Gradual	Pain worse on eye movements
Keratitis	Moderate to severe	Watery or mucopurulent	Yes	Yes	Variable	Photophobia, FB sensation, CL use
Uveitis	Dull aching	None	Yes	Yes	Gradual	Abnormal pupil shape and response
Acute angle closure	Severe, throbbing	None	Yes	Yes	Sudden	Haloes, mid-dilated pupil, cloudy cornea

URTI - upper respiratory tract infection
FB - foreign body
CL - contact lens

Painless

Even redness—subconjunctival haemorrhage

Where the vision is affected, determining IOP involvement is essential:

Normal IOP

Abnormal cornea/sclera—corneal abrasion, infiltrate, keratitis
Abnormal uvea—uveitis, endophthalmitis

TABLE 2.2 Key Features to Assess

Question	Purpose
Onset: Sudden or gradual?	**Sudden** implies vascular **Gradual** implies form or function such as cataract or macular degeneration
Duration: Persistent or transient?	**Persistent**—causation is still present **Transient**—may be amaurosis fugax or migraine
Laterality: One eye or both?	**Monocular**—ocular or optic nerve **Binocular**—often neurological or systemic
Degree: Is it total or partial vision loss?	**Central**—macular or optic nerve related **Peripheral**—retinal damage/detachment or glaucoma
Pain: Associated eye pain or headache?	**Painful**—neuritis, angle closure, uveitis **Painless**—retinal or vascular cause
Visual phenomena: Flashes, floaters, shadows, haloes?	**Flashes/floaters**—posterior vitreous detachment or retinal detachment **Haloes**—angle closure
Any other symptoms? Nausea, weakness, speech problems?	May suggest stroke, transient ischemic attack or other neurological cause
History of trauma or surgery	Retinal tear, traumatic optic neuropathy or lens dislocation
Past ocular history: Any known eye conditions	Glaucoma, AMD, diabetic retinopathy can predispose to acute events
Medical history: Diabetes, hypertension, multiple sclerosis, autoimmune disease?	Vascular or inflammatory cause of vision loss
Medication use: Corticosteroids, hydroxychloroquine?	Some drugs may cause optic or retinal toxicity

Elevated IOP

Angle closure
Hypertensive uveitis

Vision Loss (Sudden Versus Gradual)

Understanding the onset, nature and course of this symptom helps delineate potential causes and again identifies between urgent and non-urgent cases.

Red Flags Include

- Sudden *painless* vision loss
- Severe *painful* vision loss
- Vision loss associated with flashes and/or floaters

Other key features should be determined (Table 2.2).

Discharge

The type, colour and consistency of discharge can provide important diagnostic clues (Table 2.3).

TABLE 2.3 Types of Infective Discharge

Type of Discharge	Likely Cause	Associated Symptoms
Watery	Viral conjunctivitis Allergic conjunctivitis	Redness, irritation, foreign body sensation, often bilateral
Mucous	Allergic conjunctivitis	Intense itching, lid swelling, environmental triggers
Purulent	Bacterial conjunctivitis	Sticky lids, redness, lid swelling, often unilateral but may spread
Serous	Irritative conjunctivitis Viral conjunctivitis	Mild discomfort or burning, history of exposure
Crusting on lashes	Blepharitis	Grittiness, burning, red lid margins, worse in the morning

Red Flags Include

- Associated pain and vision loss—consider keratitis or endophthalmitis
- Contact lens use—always assess for microbial keratitis (Chapter 6)
- Newborn with purulent discharge—rule out ophthalmia neonatorum (conjunctivitis in newborn, refer to Chapter 6), urgent antimicrobial therapy needed

Diplopia

Distinguishing between monocular and binocular diplopia is imperative.

Monocular diplopia persists when one eye is covered and is suggestive of a corneal, lenticular or retinal issue that is refractive or structural in origin.

Binocular diplopia, which resolves when one eye is covered, suggests ocular misalignment due to either extraocular muscle imbalance or cranial nerve dysfunction. This may be linked to serious neurological or systemic disease and should be investigated as a priority.

Gradual onset may be due to muscle weakness whilst sudden onset may indicate an ocular motor palsy due to stroke, aneurysm or trauma. While the nature of image separation—e.g. horizontal, vertical or oblique separation—may help localise the affected muscle or cranial nerve, it is important to remember that myasthenia gravis can mimic most forms, although often shows worsening with fatigue.

Associated symptoms are worth noting:

- Ptosis and limb weakness suggests neurological cause.
- Headaches or ocular pain may be due to optic neuritis or even aneurysm.
- Proptosis is typically caused by increasing volume of orbital contents due to thyroid eye disease or orbital mass.

Headaches

According to the International Classification of Headache Disorders ICHD-3 [1], headaches can be considered as primary, secondary or other. In eyecare, headaches may be related to refractive error, ocular misalignment or visual fatigue, but they can also be a sign of a neurological, vascular or inflammatory condition.

Red flags for headaches that warrant urgent investigation include the following:

- Sudden, severe "thunderclap" headache reaching peak intensity within seconds, which may indicate a subarachnoid haemorrhage or other serious vascular event.
- New-onset headache in individuals over 50, raising concern for giant cell arteritis or a space-occupying lesion.
- Progressive, persistent headache, especially with neurological signs, may suggest a brain tumour or subdural haematoma.
- Fever accompanying headache could signal infection, with differentials including meningitis or encephalitis.
- Neurological deficits such as weakness, numbness, speech difficulty or vision changes could point to a stroke or neurological disease.
- Swollen optic discs may indicate raised intracranial pressure, anterior ischaemic optic neuropathy or accelerated hypertension (refer to Chapter 5).
- Neck stiffness with fever may be a sign of meningitis.
- Headaches that wake the patient from sleep or are present upon waking may suggest a serious intracranial issue.
- Headaches triggered by coughing, sneezing or bending could be linked to raised intracranial pressure.
- When accompanied by transient vision loss in one eye, it may indicate a stroke or vascular occlusion.

These features should prompt urgent referral or investigation to rule out life- or sight-threatening conditions.

Non-urgent headaches are typically benign and self-limiting, and, though not life-threatening, they can be significantly impactful and are often related to visual demands, lifestyle or underlying refractive issues.

Tension type headaches can be linked to stress, posture or fatigue and can mimic ocular strain.

Visual strain headaches are often described as frontal ache that is worse after reading or concentrated work. Poor lighting and prolonged duration of task are exacerbating factors.

Sinus headaches may cause a pressure around the eyes, cheeks or forehead that worsens when bending forward. It can cause referred ocular pain mimicking ocular pathology.

Cervicogenic headaches with neck pain or stiffness that radiates to the head can be triggered by neck movements or poor posture.

These types of headaches are often managed conservatively with refractive correction, visual hygiene advice and lifestyle modification.

Flashes and Floaters

Vitreous floaters are common in myopes, especially with increasing age. They appear as black flecks floating in their vision and are most obvious in bright light conditions; they often begin on waking and last several days to four weeks. With ageing, liquefaction and shrinking (syneresis) of the vitreous occurs, which can lead to posterior vitreous detachment, usually asymptomatic, but people become aware of a cobweb-like 'floater' (Figure 2.2) that can be intrusive at first. It is commonly found in people over 70.

There are a number of reasons why a patient may experience flashes or floaters in their vision, many of which are harmless. However, there are some red flags

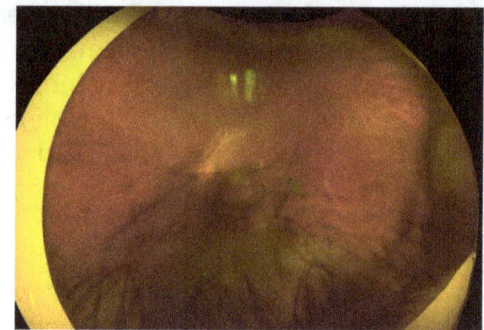

FIGURE 2.2 View of floaters.

Source: (Courtesy of Dr. S. Basu, LV Prasad Eye Institute, Hyderabad, India)

that indicate a more serious pathology that requires urgent attention. Symptoms that warrant immediate investigation include the following:

- A sudden increase in floaters or flashes
- Repeated flashes of light, especially in the peripheral vision
- A sudden bunch or shower of floaters
- A shadow, veil or curtain partially coming over vision
- Loss of peripheral vision
- Floaters with persistent blurred or distorted vision
- Those following head or eye trauma

Flashes may be true flashes, such as those caused by retinal traction, or pseudo-flashes caused by glare from environmental or even corneal and lenticular opacities.

Causes of floaters include tear film debris, vitritis, asteroid hyalosis, amyloidosis, posterior vitreous detachment and vitreous condensation.

In combination, posterior vitreous detachment, retinal tear, retinal detachment and ocular tumours should be considered.

Anisocoria

Unequal pupil sizes (anisocoria) may be physiological and so totally benign. However, it may be a sign of a more serious condition [2] (refer to College of Optometrists' Clinical Management Guidelines (CMGs) for—Abnormalities of the pupil). The red flags to be aware of include the following:

- Sudden onset
- Associated eye or head pain
- Blurred or double vision
- Ptosis
- Eye movement abnormalities
- Light response differences between the eyes
- Recent trauma or eye surgery
- History of neurological symptoms

It is important to evaluate eyelid position, globe position and extraocular motility whenever anisocoria is noted.

The main conditions to rule out are as follows:

- Third nerve palsy—The III cranial nerve supplies four of the six ocular muscles, the levator palpebrae superioris and sphincter pupillae [3]

- Horner's syndrome (oculosympathetic palsy)—Symptoms include miosis (constricted pupil), partial ptosis (drooping eyelid), anhidrosis (decreased sweating) and enophthalmos (sunken eyeball)
- Acute glaucoma
- Pharmacological causes

Identifying which is the malfunctioning iris can be determined by assessing pupil responses in dark and light conditions.

If the smaller pupil is abnormal:
It may be due to iris structural damage, such as posterior synechiae and iritis, or due to functional impediment—either extrinsically, through pharmacological agents, or intrinsically, such as those found in Horner's syndrome, Argyll-Robertson (syphilis, Chapter 6) or chronic Adie's pupil.
If the larger pupil is abnormal:
It may be due to structural damage, such as from trauma or surgery, pharmacological causes or may be an early Adie's pupil. Third nerve palsies are associated with an enlarged pupil, extraocular muscle palsies (four out of six) and/or ptosis with blurred vision.
Use the swinging light test for abnormalities of the afferent nerve pathway, in particular, to investigate the symmetric pupils of optic neuritis when there is a relative afferent pupillary defect; refer to Chapter 3.

Nystagmus

Early onset is segregated into those with a stable head position, in which there may be a sensory deprivation or fusion maldevelopment, or with an unstable head position, which requires careful examination to rule out serious pathology.

Late onset can be conjugate or disconjugate, but there may be some causes that require urgent investigation. Symptoms that should raise a level of concern include the following:

- Sudden onset, especially in adults, suggest stroke, vestibular disorders or brainstem issues.
- Vertical nystagmus is almost always brain-related and can be caused by brainstem lesions, multiple sclerosis, cerebellar stroke and Chiari malformation.
- Direction-changing nystagmus, dependent on the direction of gaze, is also almost always central in origin.
- Associated neurological symptoms, such as ataxia, weakness, numbness, dysarthria or diplopia.
- New nystagmus in a child needs investigation for congenital issues, tumours or metabolic/genetic conditions.
- Recent head trauma could indicate concussion, skull fracture or brain injury.

The main conditions to rule out are as follows: stroke, multiple sclerosis, vestibular neuritis, Wernicke's encephalopathy, Chiari malformation or brainstem tumour.

Visual Field Defects

Both retinal and neurological disease can manifest as a visual field defect and can be subtle or obvious in nature. While changes may occur unilaterally, it is often by considering the visual fields of both eyes that inferences can be made (Figure 2.3) [4]. Some features, however, increase the level of concern.

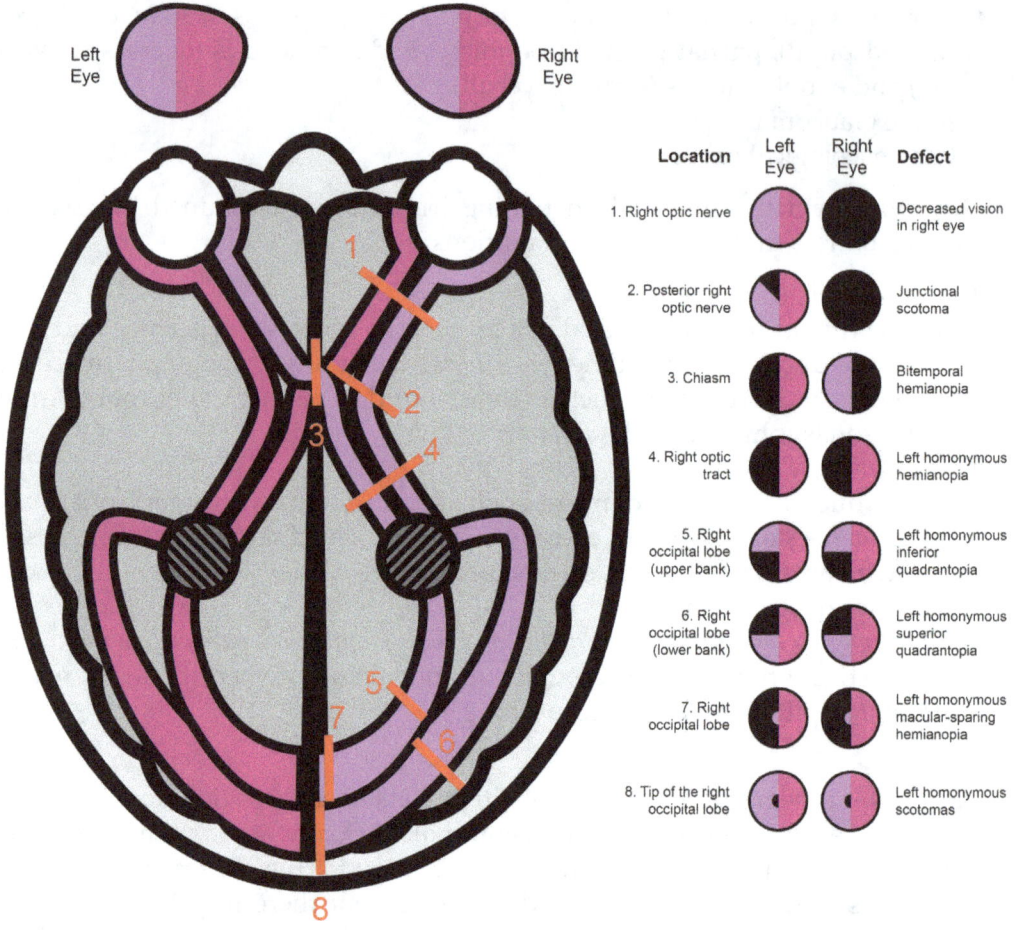

FIGURE 2.3 Guide to visual pathways and scotomas.

Source: (Courtesy of Dr. Samantha Armstrong, Aston University, Birmingham)

- Sudden onset of vision loss, especially if it is painless, could indicate a retinal artery occlusion, optic neuritis, stroke or pituitary apoplexy.
- Bitemporal hemianopia is characteristic of optic chiasm compression, and this is typically due to a pituitary tumour.
- Homonymous hemianopia is often a sign of a stroke, brain tumour or occipital lesion.
- Altitudinal field defects may suggest ischemic optic neuropathy or retinal disease.
- Field loss with accompanying headaches or neurological signs or symptoms may be indicative of mass lesions, meningitis or idiopathic intracranial hypertension (check for papilloedema).
- Unilateral field loss with eye pain is found in optic neuritis and is a common symptom of multiple sclerosis (Chapter 3).
- Peripheral field loss is characteristic of glaucoma—(Chapter 3).
- Central field loss is characteristic of wet AMD (Chapter 3).

For detailed visual pathways, and clinical examples, refer to [4, 5]:

REFERENCES

1. Classification Committee. The International Classification of Headache Disorders. 3rd ed. 2018. PMID: 29368949 (https://ichd-3.org/).
2. College of Optometrists. Clinical Management Guidelines (Abnormalities of the Pupil) 2025. Accessed 03/09/25.
3. Mayo Clinic. The Causes of Acquired 3rd Nerve Palsy 2025. Accessed 18/08/2025 (https://www.mayoclinic.org/medical-professionals/ophthalmology/news/the-causes-of-acquired-third-nerve-palsy/mac-20431238).
4. Ruia S et al. Humphrey Visual Field. StatPearls Publishing 2025. PMID: 36256759 (https://www.ncbi.nlm.nih.gov/books/NBK585112/).
5. Tsuchitani C. NeuroScience Online 2020. Accessed 28/05/2025 (https://nba.uth.tmc.edu/neuroscience/m/s2/chapter15.html).

3: Sight-Threatening Conditions in Primary Care—Clinical Presentation and Management

CORE MESSAGES

This chapter covers the sight-threatening diseases commonly found in the population, which may be repeatedly encountered in practice, such as glaucoma, age-related macular degeneration (AMD), diabetic retinopathy, central retinal artery occlusion (CRAO), branch retinal artery occlusion (BRAO), retinal detachment, macula and neurodegenerative conditions. Each of the important diseases are reviewed with full details given in the online links.

The chapter identifies signs and symptoms to enable early detection where possible. In addition, recommendations are suggested, aided in some cases by grading schemes, viz. the NHS diabetic eye screening. Grading definitions for referable disease (diabetic retinopathy—UK National Screening Committee [UK NSC]—GOV.UK) helps ECPs manage cases locally and identify when patients need referral for specialist care.

As usual, early recognition is paramount to help manage sight-threatening conditions in primary eye care and reduce the chance of further reduction or loss in vision.

Glaucoma

In 2020, 3.61 million people were blind and nearly 4.14 million were visually impaired by glaucoma. The contribution of glaucoma to blindness and moderate-to-severe vision impairment by region, and the change in this distribution between 2000–2020, were recorded in a meta-analysis with differences by sex and region [1].

Chronic (or primary) open-angle glaucoma occurs even though the drainage of aqueous humour through the trabecular meshwork is physically unimpaired through an open angle between the iris and the cornea. Initially, it is asymptomatic until pathological optic disc cupping and optic nerve damage lead to awareness of visual field defect and irreversible vision loss [2] (refer to College of Optometrists' CMGs for—Glaucoma (chronic open angle [COAG])).

Visual Field Loss

Visual field (VF) defects in glaucoma are characterised by specific patterns that reflect the anatomical arrangement of the retinal nerve fibres. These defects include arcuate scotomas, paracentral scotomas and nasal steps, which correspond to the arcuate-like arrangement of the axons emerging from the optic

DOI: 10.1201/9781003606789-4

disc (Figure 3.1). In glaucoma, the superior and inferior poles of the optic nerve head are most vulnerable to damage, leading to localised scotomas that conform to the nerve fibre bundle patterns. Thus, superior or inferior arcuate defects are the most commonly detected (30%) VF loss in early to mid-stage glaucoma. They represent the corresponding loss of nerve bundles radiating from the optic nerve head. For instance, damage to the superior or inferior poles results in arcuate scotomas in the corresponding visual field areas, which are inverted.

Respect of the horizontal meridian is anatomically attributable to the horizontal raphe, an imaginary line dividing the upper and lower hemispheres of the retina.

Paracentral scotomas are an early sign of localised glaucomatous damage and can be detected through visual field testing. As the disease progresses, more extensive visual field defects may develop. Visual field testing is critical for detecting and evaluating these defects to diagnose and monitor glaucoma progression. Commonly used tests include the Humphrey visual field (HVF) test, which maps the patient's visual field using stimuli of varying intensity and provides a graphical representation of central, paracentral and peripheral field defects [3].

The HVF 24-2 and 30-2 test patterns are frequently used in glaucoma monitoring, with the 24-2 test being useful for older adults due to its reduced test duration and lower risk of false negatives from patient fatigue. Since central vision is usually spared, with peripheral field loss, visual acuity may be (6/6) 20/20 until the optic nerve fibres are substantially affected late in the disease when patients

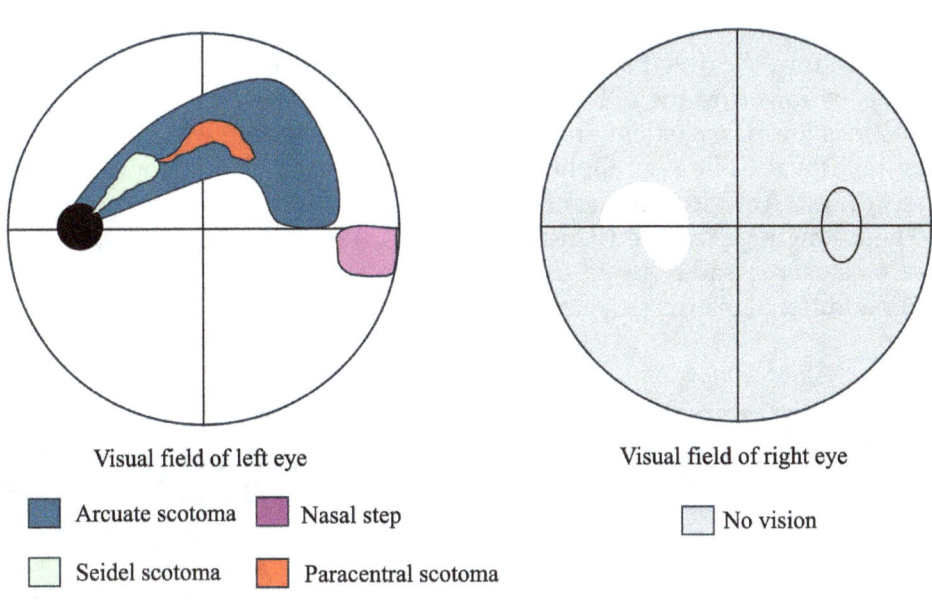

Visual field of left eye   Visual field of right eye

■ Arcuate scotoma   ■ Nasal step   ▢ No vision

▢ Seidel scotoma   ■ Paracentral scotoma

FIGURE 3.1 Visual field defects in glaucoma: left eye early scotoma; right eye end-stage glaucoma with residual island of central vision only (tunnel vision).

will notice the vision loss and seek help with a reduction in their field of vision. In advanced disease, HVF 10-2 may be utilised when only a central island of vision remains. This protocol is also beneficial in macular disease such as dry (atrophic) or wet (neovascular) age-related macular degeneration (AMD).

Blind spot enlargement can be seen not only in glaucoma but also in other disc pathology such as disc oedema, e.g. from papilloedema or idiopathic intracranial hypertension [4], as well as in eyes with peripapillary atrophy, e.g. myopic eyes.

Damage to the Optic Nerve

The vertical cup-to-disc ratio can be measured to track the extent of axonal (nerve fibre) loss. Calculated by dividing the maximal vertical diameter of the optic cup by the vertical diameter of the optic nerve head (disc), expected healthy findings are often dependent on the overall disc size, with larger discs having larger cups due to the spatial distribution of nerve fibres. Regardless, a vertical CD ratio > 0.8 is highly suspicious with an increase in cupping or nerve fibre loss indicative of progressive glaucoma. Other anatomical changes, such as formation of optic disc pits, blood vessel baring, bayonetting and nasalisation, can become visible in the optic nerve head as disease progresses. Disc ischaemia, evidenced by disc margin haemorrhages, can be prognostic of further glaucomatous decline.

Raised Intraocular (IOP) Pressure

Exact aetiology of glaucomatous damage is largely unknown. Traditionally considered to be a disease caused by raised intraocular pressure, paradoxically, damage can still occur within normative ranges (10–21 mmHg). Many believe pathological axonal apoptosis stems from a complex process where perfusion pressure (difference between intraocular pressure and arterial pressure) also plays an important role.

At this time, the only proven intervention for preventing and controlling glaucoma is by lowering the IOP (Appendices 1 and 6). Refer to appropriate clinical guidelines for management and therapy advice, including when to refer for surgery [5], Royal College of Ophthalmologists guidance [6], European Glaucoma Society [7] or American Glaucoma Society.

The following example (Figures 3.2 and 3.3) is from a patient with bilateral severe glaucoma and a cup-to-disc (C/D) ratio of 0.8.

For additional examples, refer to Supplementary Chapter S3.

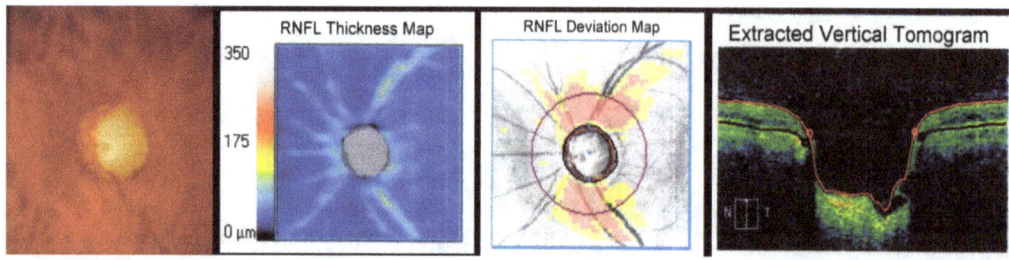

FIGURE 3.2 Retinal nerve fibre layer (RNFL) thickness map and RNFL deviation map of a patient with advanced glaucoma.

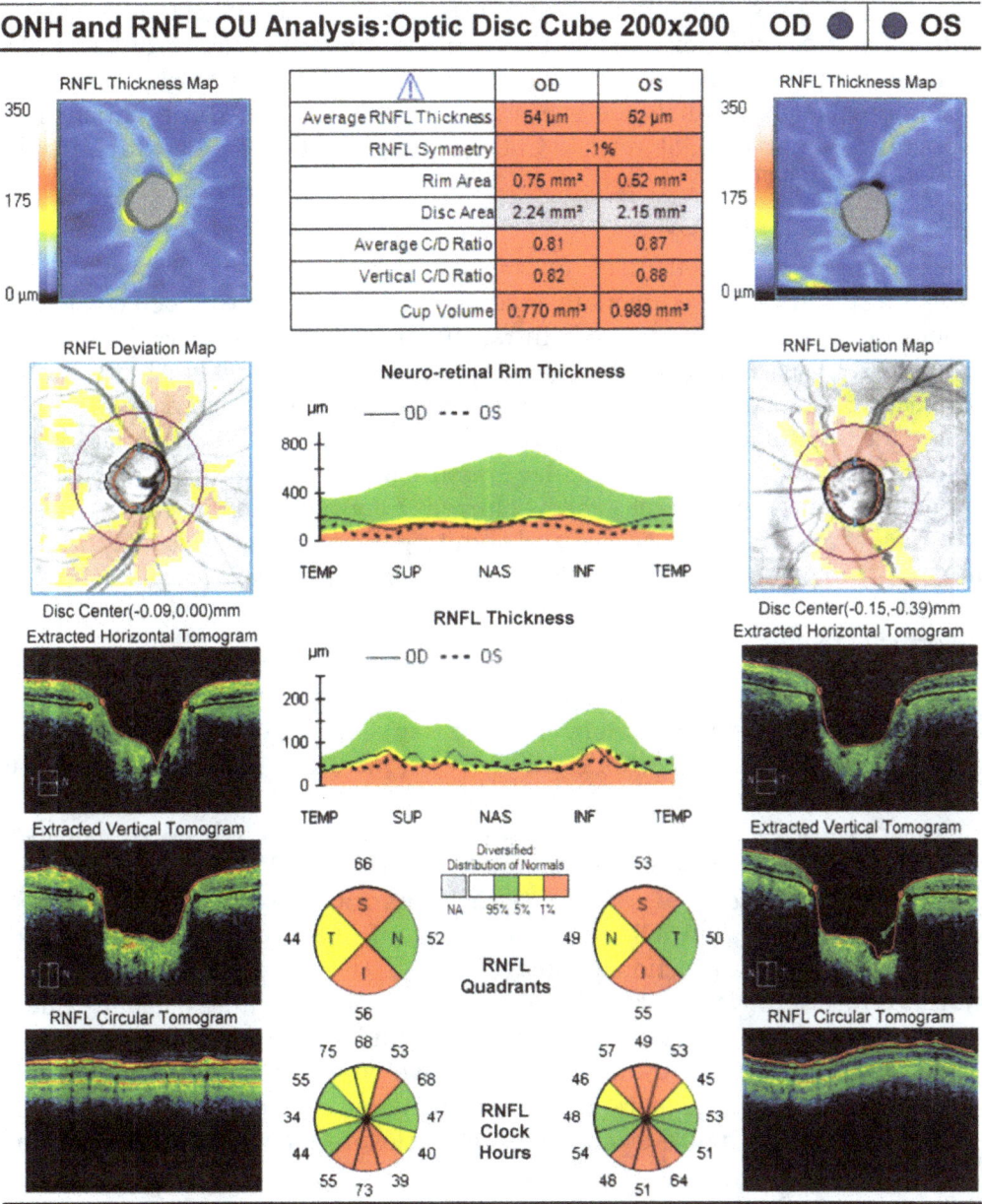

FIGURE 3.3 Scans and tomography with severe bilateral glaucoma.

Source: (Courtesy of Dr. S. Radhakrishnan, San Francisco) (https://eyesoneyecare.com/resources/utilizing-oct-for-glaucoma-diagnosis-and-management/)

Ocular Hypertension

Patients with ocular hypertension (an intraocular pressure [IOP] greater than 21 mmHg without glaucomatous optic nerve damage) are considered to have a higher risk of developing chronic open-angle glaucoma. A number of landmark studies have provided strong evidence on which patient factors carry an increased risk of progression to glaucoma, what levels of IOP control are optimal and the comparative safety and efficacy of various treatments. In the UK,

NICE guidance suggests offering 360 degree selective laser trabeculoplasty (SLT) as first-line treatment for patients newly diagnosed with an IOP of 24 mmHg or more and who are at risk. In those not suitable for or who do not want SLT, a topical prostaglandin analogue eye drop is the first-line medical management (Appendices 1 and 6(S)) [8] (refer to College of Optometrists' CMGs for—Ocular hypertension [OHT]).

Angle Closure Disease

This encompasses a spectrum of conditions under the glaucoma umbrella, where there is a structural impediment to aqueous humour drainage, which can lead to either a rapid or gradual increase in intraocular pressure, optic nerve damage and vision loss. In susceptible individuals, the iris either pulls or is pushed forward, obstructing access to the trabecular meshwork within the anterior chamber angle. Where the buildup of aqueous occurs gradually, patients are often asymptomatic despite extremely elevated intraocular pressure findings. Rapid uncontrolled rise in pressure causes symptoms such as blurred vision, severe pain, redness, headache, haloes around lights, nausea and vomiting (Primary angle closure/primary angle closure glaucoma [9]) (refer to College of Optometrists' CMGs for—(PAC/PACG)).

Forms of the disease are as follows:

1) *Primary Angle Closure Suspects (PACS)*—narrow anterior chamber angles are seen, but there is no elevated IOP or optic nerve damage. Patients with PACS-plus criteria (extra risk factors) may have an increased risk of progression to primary angle closure.
2) *Primary Angle Closure (PAC)*—narrow anterior chamber angles with increased IOP and/or presence of peripheral anterior synechiae (PAS).
3) *Primary Angle Closure Glaucoma (PACG)*—narrow/closed anterior chamber angles with increased IOP and/or presence of PAS and glaucomatous optic nerve structural or functional damage.
4) *Acute Primary Angle Closure (APAC)*—sudden, severe rise in IOP usually due to abrupt angle closure. Classic presentation includes a severely painful, blurred eye that is red, with mid-dilated non-reactive pupil and corneal oedema, in a patient who may also experience nausea and vomiting. Refer to Supplementary Chapter S3 for a figure of an acute angle closure glaucoma following graft surgery.
5) *Secondary Angle Closure Glaucoma*—narrow/closed anterior chamber angle due to an identifiable cause with increased IOP and/or presence of PAS and glaucomatous optic nerve structural or functional damage

As with open-angle forms, management of IOP is the mainstay of treatment when needed. Patients with PACS-plus criteria may be offered prophylactic laser peripheral iridotomy (LPI) or lens extraction/replacement if deemed high risk. PAC and PACG patients may require medical management preferentially with aqueous suppressants and/or surgical intervention.

APAC is considered an ophthalmic emergency and, depending on the level of IOP rise, needs immediate topical and systemic medical reduction of IOP, followed by acute management of pupillary block, such as topical pilocarpine and LPI (Appendices 1 and 6[S]). Once control is achieved, ongoing care often parallels that of PAC or PACG. The mainstay of treatment for secondary forms is to manage the underlying cause in addition to controlling IOP.

Age-Related Macular Degeneration

In 2020, 1.85 million (95% UI: 1.35 to 2.43 million) people were blind due to AMD, and another 6.23 million (95% UI: 5.04 to 7.58 million) presented with moderately severe vision impairment globally [10].

A progressive condition of the macular that typically affects people aged 50 and older, symptoms in mild to moderate disease are often reported in terms of blurred or distorted central vision with difficulty with tasks such as reading or recognising faces. Progression to advanced stages ultimately leads to significant central vision loss, though peripheral vision may be preserved. Risk factors for both development and progression include ageing, family history, smoking and potentially hypertension, dyslipidaemia, obesity and particular dietary habits. Multiple methods of grading exist worldwide with differing foci depending on setting. In the UK, NICE guidance NG82 provides guidance for monitoring and referral from primary care [5]. Different international AMD classification and staging systems are given in Table 3.1.

Accumulation of subretinal drusen and RPE dysfunction, indicative of oxidative stress and mitochondrial damage, along with impaired metabolic exchange across an ageing Bruch's membrane, contributes to the local hypoxia and inflammation (Figures 3.4 and 3.5). In some patients, this leads to areas of retinal atrophy (advanced dry AMD), whilst in others, this stimulates the release of vascular endothelial growth factors (VEGF) promoting the growth of fragile, abnormal choroidal neovascular membranes through Bruch's membrane.

Currently, there is no medical treatment for dry AMD, and though research is ongoing, management is based on support and guidance. Smokers are recommended to stop smoking, as it is thought to exacerbate the condition. Supplements with antioxidants and zinc may delay progression, as seen in the age-related eye disease (AREDS/AREDS 2) studies (age-related eye disease studies [AREDS/AREDS2] | National Eye Institute). Recently developed complement-cascade-inhibiting intravitreal drugs (pegcetacoplan and avacincaptad pegol) have been

TABLE 3.1 Different International AMD Classification and Staging Systems

System	Scope	Stages
AREDS (USA)	Clinical trials	No AMD: < 63 micron drusen Early: small/intermediate drusen Intermediate: large drusen +/− pigment changes Late: GA or CNV
ICO/AMD Alliance (Global)	Global clinical practice	Early: medium drusen only Intermediate: large drusen +/− pigment changes Late Dry: geographic atrophy Late Wet: CNV or scarring
NICE (UK)	UK clinical practice	No AMD: < 63 micron drusen Early: categorised as low, medium and high risk depending on size and type of drusen and absence or presence of pigmentary changes or vitelliform lesion Late indeterminate: RPE degeneration with SRF or IRF without CNV Late wet active: CNV, RAP, PCV Late dry: GA or significant vision loss with confluent drusen or advanced pigment changes or vitelliform lesion Late wet inactive: fibrous scar

(GA—geographic atrophy; CNV—choroidal neovascular membrane; SRF—subretinal fluid; IRF—intraretinal fluid; RAP—retinal angiomatous proliferation; PCV—polypoidal choroidal vasculopathy)

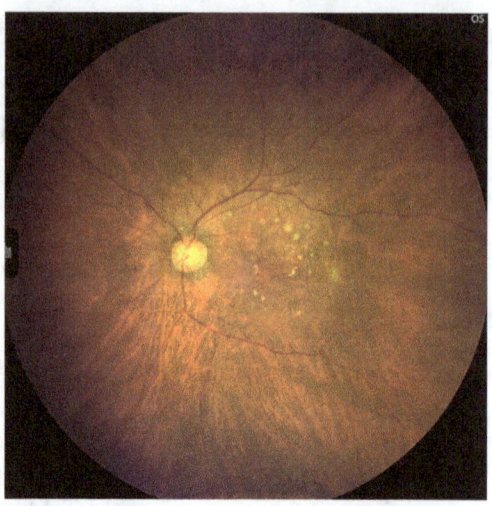

FIGURE 3.4 Dry AMD showing drusen. There is a slightly depigmented patch near the macula; on the angiogram (Figure 3.5), the choroid faintly lights up because of the window defect in the RPE.

Source: (Courtesy of Dr. S. Basu, LV Prasad Eye Institute, Hyderabad, India)

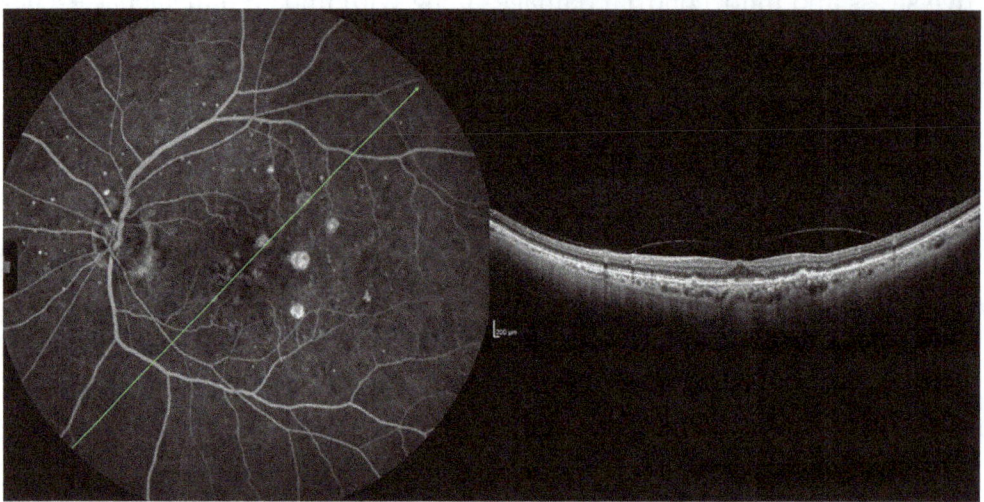

FIGURE 3.5 Angiogram (in venous phase) with bright 'spots' due to RPE detachments. On the OCT, there are tiny elevations of the RPE due to small pigment epithelium detachments (PEDs). Plan to observe with Amsler grid* and see in six to twelve months unless new symptoms develop before the next appointment.

Source: (Courtesy of Dr. S. Basu, LV Prasad Eye Institute, Hyderabad, India) * (https://www.aop.org. uk/advice-and-support/for-patients/sight-tests/amsler-chart)

shown to slow down geographic atrophy progression by targeting and regulating the overactive immune response that damages retinal cells and are being investigated in clinical trials at this time. Likewise, stem cell therapy and gene therapy are both still in early-phase clinical trials. Though no treatment is available, active monitoring is recommended, as the progression of the disease with soft drusen (Figure 3.6) may result in conversion to wet AMD.

Though less common, the wet form can lead to rapid vision loss due to the growth of abnormal, fragile blood vessels (Figures 3.7 and 3.8). Vascular endothelial growth factor (VEGF) is produced by multiple retinal cell types and is a key

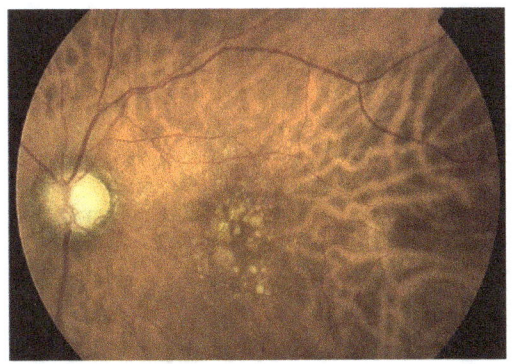

FIGURE 3.6 Soft drusen as precursors to wet AMD.

Source: (Courtesy of Dr. Fatima Mesa-Lugo, Hospital Universitario de Canarias, Spain)

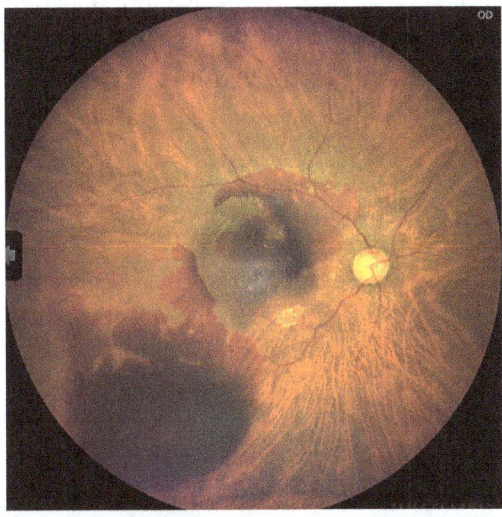

FIGURE 3.7 Wet, exudative AMD showing subretinal haemorrhage (note the vessels lying within the retina). There is a central darker circle due to blood beneath the pigment epithelial layer.

Source: (Courtesy of Dr. S. Basu, LV Prasad Eye Institute, Hyderabad, India)

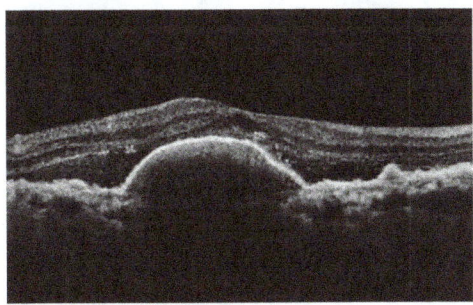

FIGURE 3.8 Exudative AMD. There is subretinal fluid, with the retinal pigment epithelium elevated and irregular, and fluid beneath it. The hyper-reflective white spots are exudates.

Source: (Courtesy of Dr. S. Basu, LV Prasad Eye Institute, Hyderabad, India)

regulator of retinal angiogenesis. In a healthy retina, it supports retinal function. However, in diseased eyes, it can stimulate neovascularisation and a breakdown of the blood-retinal barrier through increased vascular permeability.

Preferential therapy in wet AMD involves intravitreal injections of recombinant humanized monoclonal antibodies or antibody fragments that bind to and inhibit VEGF (anti-VEGF). Bevacizumab and ranibizumab are examples of anti-VEGF antibodies, given intravitreally, used to manage wet AMD. Therapeutic dosage is achieved following a course of loading successive treatments spread over a number weeks to months. Though not curative, by regulating blood vessel growth [11, 12], progression of vision loss may be slowed, and in some, the improvement to retinal homeostasis can result in subtle vision improvement. Photodynamic therapy (PDT) is an earlier but less effective treatment that is used nowadays combined with anti-VEGF injections. PDT can also be used if anti-VEGF therapy fails.

Diabetic Retinopathy

In 2020, 1.07 million people were blind and 3.25 million were visually impaired by diabetic retinopathy [13].

Persistent elevations in blood glucose levels associated with diabetes mellitus leads to damage of the retinal microvasculature, including pericyte loss, thickening of the basement membrane and endothelial dysfunction. Subsequent microvascular system breakdown is apparent through microaneurysms, capillary leakage, haemorrhages, ischaemia and, in advanced stages, neovascularisation. Despite these changes, most are asymptomatic in early stages, only becoming more aware of blurred or fluctuating vision, impaired colour and night vision and vision loss as disease progresses. Screening programs are founded on the principles of early detection, timely referral and regular monitoring, aiming to prevent irreversible visual impairment. Given its status as a leading cause of preventable blindness among the working age population globally, many countries have implemented national or large-scale regional screening initiatives with specific staging (Tables 3.2 and 3.3).

Chronic hyperglycaemia leads to early damage of the neurovascular structure with neurodegeneration, reactive gliosis, microvascular damage and choroiditis (Figure 3.9). Early neuronal dysfunction occurs before the onset of clinically visible microvascular changes [15].

TABLE 3.2 Variation in Global Grading Systems for Diabetic Retinopathy

Grading System	Country/Region	Main Stages	Notable Scope
ETDRS (Early Treatment Diabetic Retinopathy Study)	USA/International research	13 detailed levels	Gold standard for research; complex and detailed
ICDRS (International Clinical Diabetic Retinopathy Severity Scale)	International	Five stages: • No DR • Mild NPDR • Moderate NPDR • Severe NPDR • PDR	Simpler and widely used; correlates with ETDRS
NSC (UK National Screening Committee)	England/Wales	R0-R3S/R3A retinopathy grading M0-M1 maculopathy grading P1 photocoagulation U unassessable	Used in NHS diabetic eye screening program
Scottish Diabetic Retinopathy Grading Scheme [14]	Scotland	R0-R4—retinopathy grading M0-M2 maculopathy grading P photocoagulation U ungradable	Used in Scotland
Australian Grading Protocol	Australia	Aligned with ICDRS	Often simplified for remote screening
Canadian Diabetic Retinopathy Grading system	Canada	Based on ICDRS with national adaptations	Often used in teleophthalmology

DR—diabetic retinopathy; NPDR—non-proliferative diabetic retinopathy; PDR—proliferative diabetic retinopathy

TABLE 3.3 Grading Stages of Diabetic Retinopathy Found within the UK National Screening Committee (NSC) Scale

Grading	Features
R0 (None)	No retinopathy
R1 (Background)	Microaneurysms Retinal haemorrhage Venous loop Exudates Cotton wool spots
R2 (low-risk non-proliferative)	< 10 multiple blot haemorrhages non-obvious/isolated IRMA < 5 cotton wool spots Longstanding unchanging R2
R2 (high-risk non-proliferative)	> 10 multiple blot haemorrhages Multiple IRMA < 5 cotton wool spots Significant change in R2 appearance
R3A (active proliferative)	New vessel on disc (NVD) New vessel elsewhere (NVE) Preretinal or vitreous haemorrhage Preretinal fibrosis +/− tractional RD
R3S (stable proliferative)	Evidence of peripheral retinal treatment and inactive NVD/NVE
M0 (no maculopathy)	Absence of an M1 features
M1 (maculopathy)	Single exudate within 1DD of fovea or multiple exudates where at least ½ are within macular region Retinal thickening within 1DD of foveal centre Any microaneurysm/haemorrhage within 1DD of foveal centre with best VA < 6/12

IRMA—intraretinal microvascular abnormalities; RD—retinal detachment; DD—disc diameter

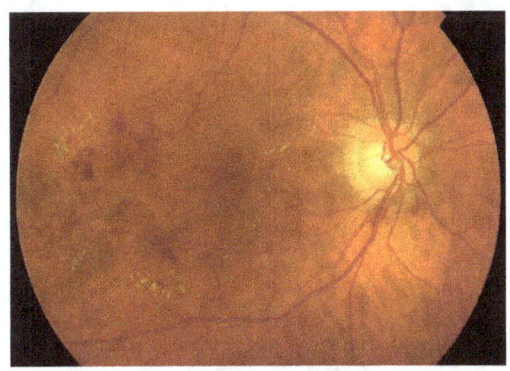

FIGURE 3.9 R3AM1—Diabetic macular oedema and hard exudates [R].

Source: (Courtesy of Dr. Fatima Mesa-Lugo, Hospital Universitario de Canarias, Spain)

Medical management of diabetic retinopathy primarily focuses on controlling blood sugar and HbA1c levels and monitoring other risk factors, such as high blood pressure, dyslipidemia and cholesterol, assisted by diet and exercise. Controlling blood sugar levels is crucial, as it helps prevent the onset and progression of diabetic retinopathy. At a retinal level, treatment options include laser photocoagulation, anti-VEGF intravitreal injections and vitrectomy as a way to reduce the bodies' natural drive to counteract resultant pathological ischaemia.

Diabetic Macular Oedema

This is caused by vessels leaking fluid in the macular region—a complication of diabetic retinopathy. When blood vessels in or close to the macula become damaged, or there is sudden bleeding or fluid leaking into the macula, vision is severely altered (Figures 3.10 and 3.11):

- Dark spots appear in central vision as 'smudges', especially in the early morning.
- Objects may change shape, size or colour or seem to move or disappear.
- Colours can fade.
- Bright light or glare cause problems with vision.
- Reading may be difficult.
- Straight lines, such as door frames and lamp posts, may appear distorted or bent.

Hyper-reflective retinal 'spots', shown in Figure 3.11, are aggregates of inflammatory-activated microglial cells. Such an increase in these 'spots' also occurs with retinal vein occlusion, AMD, multiple sclerosis and retinal ischaemic disease. In diabetic macular oedema, there is a positive correlation between the number of these 'spots' and the aqueous humour concentration of soluble CD14—a cytokine associated with the immune response given in microglia cells, monocytes and macrophages [15].

Both intravitreal anti-VEGF and corticosteroids have the ability to reduce macular oedema and treat proliferative retinopathy, though the latter is often used as second-line therapy due to a less satisfactory safety profile with adverse events of cataract formation and ocular hypertension. Extensive laser photocoagulation

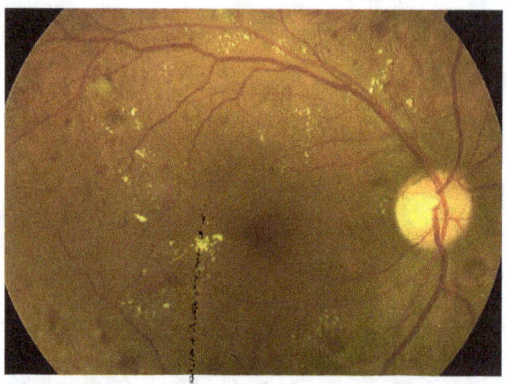

FIGURE 3.10 Severe diabetic retinopathy with macular oedema.

Source: (Courtesy of Dr. Fatima Mesa-Lugo, Hospital Universitario de Canarias, Spain)

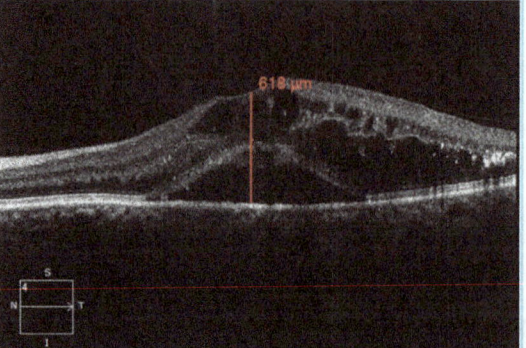

FIGURE 3.11 An OCT showing typical retinal oedema of diabetic retinopathy, exudates (hyper-reflective spots) and elevated ellipsoid zone.

Source: (Courtesy of Dr. S. Basu, LV Prasad Eye Institute, Hyderabad, India)

remains an important modality for treating proliferative diabetic retinopathy; helping to prevent new blood vessel growth and preserve vision. These two different types of treatment can be complementary. Vitrectomy, removing the vitreous gel from the eye, and replacement with a saline solution, may be required if there is significant bleeding or retinal detachment.

Hypertensive Retinopathy

Ocular signs of hypertension appear as progressive microvascular changes. In early cases, examination reveals mild arteriolar narrowing and thickening, reducing blood flow to the retina, with arteriovenous nipping at A/V crossings. As the disease progresses, there may be evidence of microaneurysms, haemorrhages, cotton-wool spots and papilloedema (Figure 3.12); grading is given later.

Retinal signs of systemic hypertension (diastolic pressure > 110) can be graded as follows [16]:

Grade I: Slight or modest narrowing of the retinal arterioles, with an arterial-to-venous ratio of ≥ 1:2.
Grade II: Modest to severe narrowing of retinal arterioles with an arterial-to-venous ratio < 1:2 or arteriovenous nicking.
Grade III: Soft exudates and flame-shaped hemorrhages.
Grade IV: Grade III changes with bilateral optic nerve oedema.

Hypertensive ocular fundus abnormalities are associated with an increased risk for cognitive impairment, cerebral atrophy and subclinical infarction. Recent advances in fundus photography allow for improved accuracy and consistency in interpretation, and are valuable for screening at-risk patient populations (age > 65). Severe hypertension (grades III and IV) needs referring for specialist medical care, as there is a risk of a stroke occurring; the systemic blood pressure must be reduced.

Some ophthalmic practices are now equipped with an automated blood pressure monitor to take systolic and diastolic blood pressures when needed. In addition, *routine* blood pressure checks are advised for all patients over 40 years. In arterial hypertension, changes in the retina closely mimic those in the brain and may predict strokes [16, 17].

Retinal imaging is useful in patients with constant headaches, diastolic blood pressure greater than 110 mmHg and with sudden vision loss. *In patients with headaches, the finding of bilateral swollen optic discs is a key sign.* It may be due to papilloedema (from raised intracranial pressure), hydrocephalus, benign intracranial

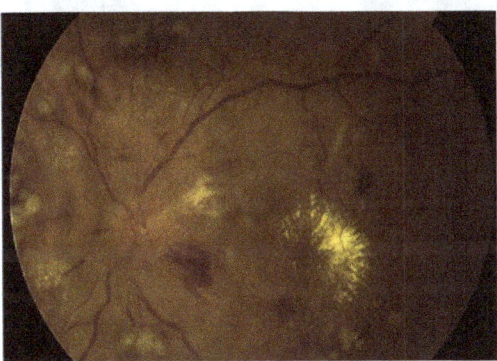

FIGURE 3.12 Severe hypertensive retinopathy grade IV.

Source: (Courtesy of Dr. Fatima Mesa-Lugo, Hospital Universitario de Canarias, Spain)

hypertension, brain tumour or intracranial bleeding (refer later). *The patient needs immediate referral to hospital.*

Papilloedema

Papilloedema refers to swelling of the optic disc. It usually occurs in both eyes and is due to raised intracranial pressure from any cause, including haemorrhage, neoplasms and infection (Figures 3.13–3.16). In children, investigation should be made for hydrocephalus. Papilloedema arises over a period from hours to weeks. Symptoms may not be obvious at first; initially, 6/6 vision can be maintained, and vision loss is not an early manifestation.

The first sign on ophthalmoscopy is venous engorgement around the disc followed by loss of venous pulsation, haemorrhages on or near the disc, blurring of optic margins and elevation of the disc. Visual field examination may find an enlarged blind spot, but the visual acuity stays relatively intact, even when severe papilloedema is prolonged.

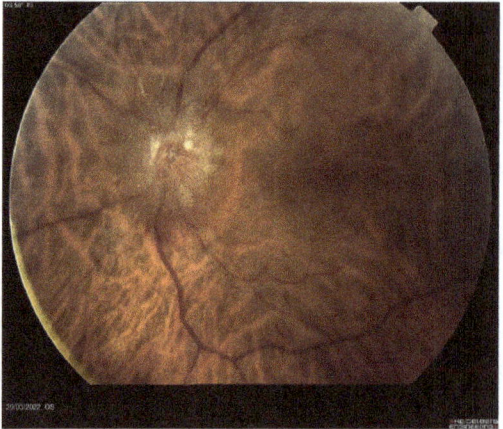

FIGURE 3.13 Papilloedema (L eye) due to an intracranial mass, modified Frisén Grading Scale 4 (https://www.uptodate.com/contents/image?imageKey=NEURO/73887&topicKey=NEURO/5253).

Source: (Courtesy of Drs. Marta Crespo-Rodriguez and Miguel Acosta-Darias, Hospital Universitario de Canarias, Spain)

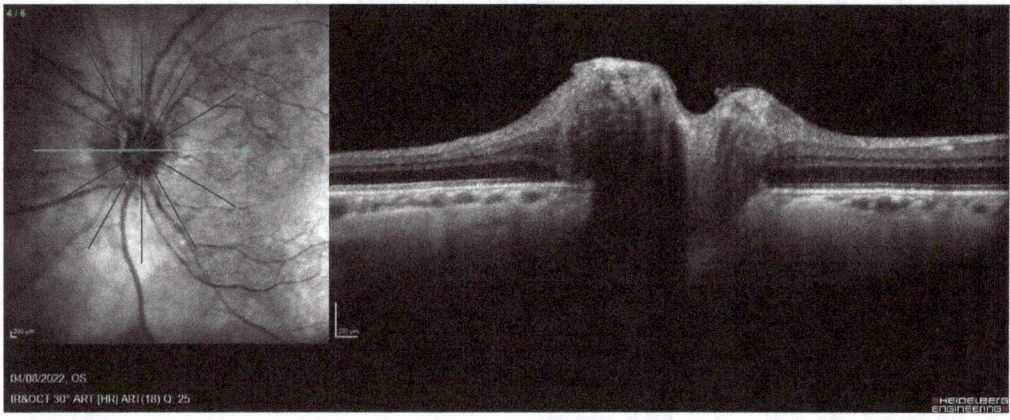

FIGURE 3.14 OCT of papilloedema (L eye) due to an intracranial mass, showing retinal nerve fibre layer (RNFL) oedema. (https://www.uptodate.com/contents/image?imageKey=NEURO/73887&topicKey=NEURO/5253)

Source: (Courtesy of Drs. Marta Crespo-Rodriguez and Miguel Acosta-Darias, Hospital Universitario de Canarias, Spain)

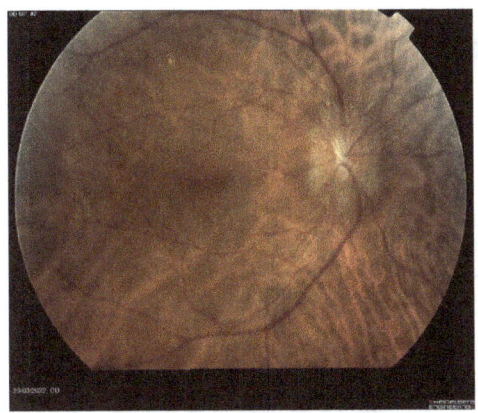

FIGURE 3.15 Papilloedema (R eye) due to an intra-cranial mass, modified Frisén Grading Scale 4.

Source: (Courtesy of Drs. Marta Crespo-Rodriguez and Miguel Acosta-Darias, Hospital Universitario de Canarias, Spain)

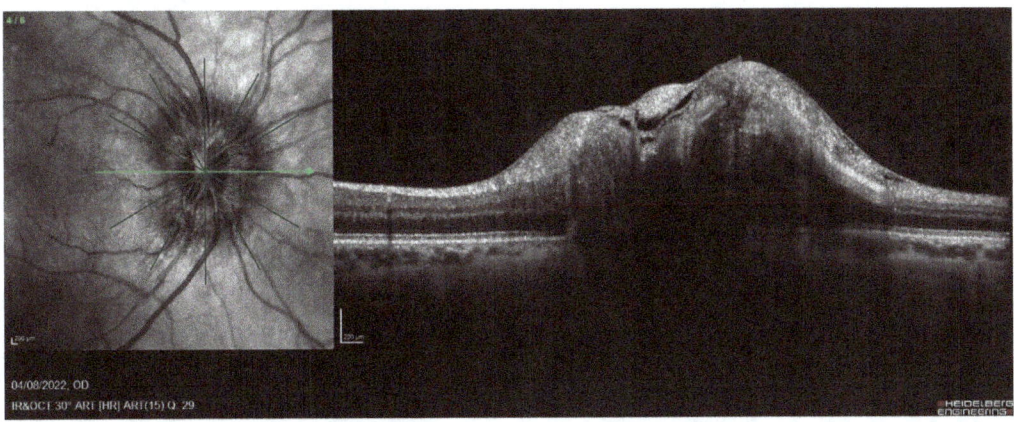

FIGURE 3.16 OCT of papilloedema (R eye) due to an intracranial mass, showing RNFL oedema.

Source: (Courtesy of Drs. Marta Crespo-Rodriguez and Miguel Acosta-Darias, Hospital Universitario de Canarias, Spain)

For lower Frisén grade abnormalities, OCT compares favourably with clinical staging of optic nerve head fundus photography [18]. With higher Frisén grades, OCT RNFL thickness processing algorithms often fail, while OCT total retinal thickness performs more favourably [18].

Optic Neuritis

Optic neuritis gives reduced acuity and impaired colour vision (Ishihara plate testing). It has various causes, including multiple sclerosis, secondary syphilis, cytomegalovirus, Lyme's disease and herpes simplex infection. Additionally, it is associated with autoimmune diseases, such as lupus, neuromyelitis optica, metastases and toxins. Disc swelling (Figure 3.17) also occurs in ischaemic optic neuropathy in the elderly either non-arteritic or due to temporal arteritis (giant cell arteritis).

A problem in the afferent half of the pupillary light reflex (viz. optic neuropathy) produces symmetric pupils. *Only the swinging flashlight test uncovers the afferent abnormality in these patients to show a relative afferent pupillary defect.* The integrity of the pupil depends on the iris, cranial nerves II and III and the sympathetic nerves innervating the eye. The examination of pupils is fundamental in the evaluation

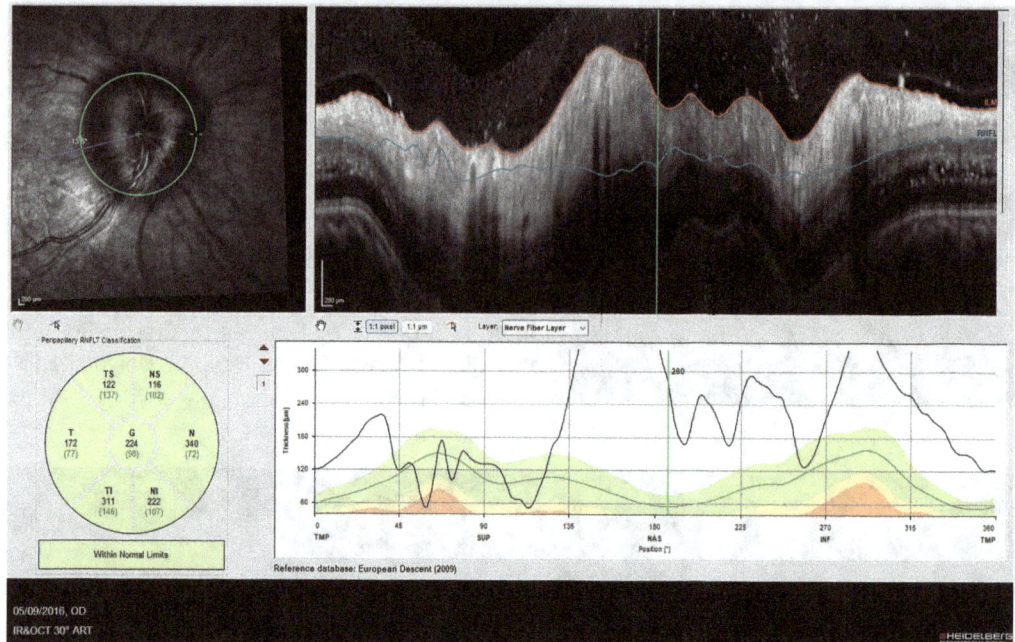

FIGURE 3.17 OCT of early optic neuritis. The segmentation map shows frank 360 degree increased nerve fibre thickness. Note that system errors in mapping translates to the TSNIT plot, so it should always be checked before interpretation.

Source: (Courtesy of Drs. M. Crespo-Rodriguez and M. Acosta-Darias, Hospital Universitario de Canarias, Tenerife)

of patients with visual blurring, visual field defects, coma, stroke, third cranial nerve palsy, red eye, supraclavicular or lung apex masses or neck pain [19].

The nerve pathway involved in the *swinging flashlight test* is shown later. Note that the efferent pathway is crossed bilaterally, from the pretectal nuclei to the Edinger-Westphal nuclei, and is then conducted via the third cranial nerve to the ciliary ganglion and ciliary nerves to the iris (Figure 3.18).

The swinging flashlight test is illustrated later (Figure 3.19) with optic neuritis in the *right* eye. This is performed by shining a light in one eye (left) and observing the pupillary response; the iris of both eyes constricts, demonstrating an intact afferent pathway. The light is then moved to the other (right) eye; both eyes remain dilated because the afferent pathway of the *right* eye is non-functioning (viz. optic neuritis). The test is then repeated for the other eye.

Central Retinal Artery Occlusion (CRAO)

The central retinal artery is an end artery—i.e. there is no collateral backup. Its occlusion presents with sudden, painless monocular vision loss requiring emergency treatment. Individuals with carotid artery disease and atherosclerotic plaque are at highest risk; emboli are the commonest aetiology of CRAO. On examination, there is a cherry-red spot (90%), retinal greyness in the posterior pole (60%), optic disk pallor (40%), retinal arterial attenuation (30%), optic disc oedema (20%) and intra-arterial emboli (20%) (Figure 3.20) (https://www.aao.

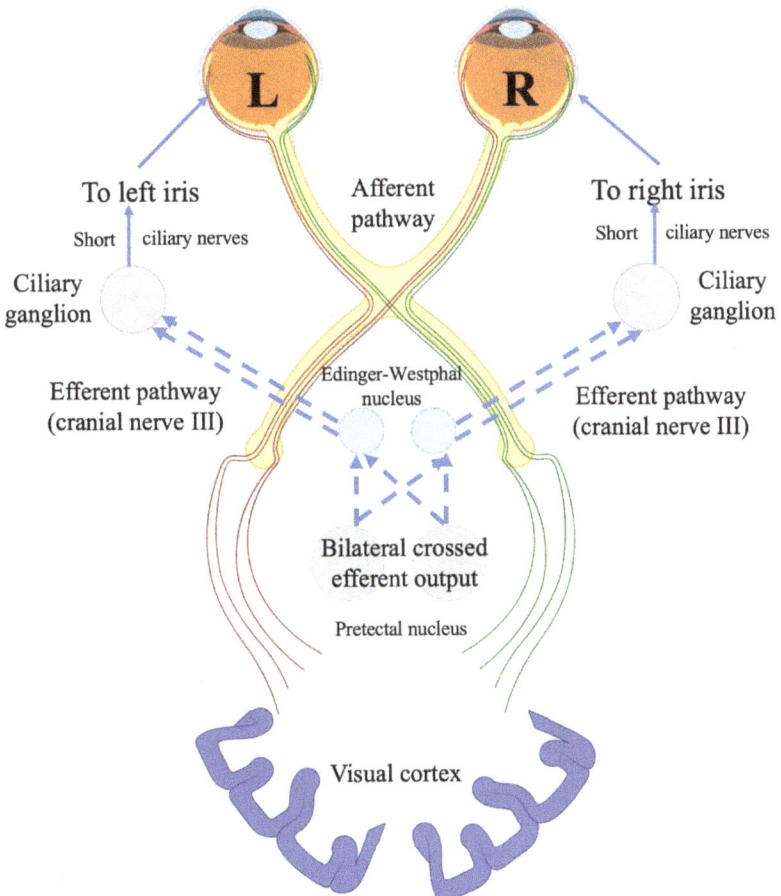

FIGURE 3.18 Pathway to test the RAPD.

org/eyenet/article/diagnosis-and-management-of-crao). On fluorescein angiography, delayed filling time of the affected vessel may be present. Treatment aims to restore perfusion of the central retinal artery. It is managed as a cerebrovascular ischemic episode; systemic or local fibrinolysis are indicated if detected promptly [21].

Although the fovea is not affected because of its alternative perfusion from the choroid, there is still complete loss of vision. The central fovea appears red because the choroid shows through, hence the 'cherry red spot' seen on examination.

Branch Retinal Vein Occlusion (BRVO)

BRVO is a common retinal vascular disease that typically affects older individuals. It occurs when a branch of the central retinal vein becomes blocked, leading to sudden or gradual blurred vision or a visual field defect. The blockage results in blood and other fluids leaking into the retina, causing superficial hemorrhages, retinal oedema and cotton-wool spots in the sector drained by the affected vein (Figure 3.21). The supero-temporal quadrant is most commonly affected, with BRVO occurring in about 0.1% of the population over 65. Complications include

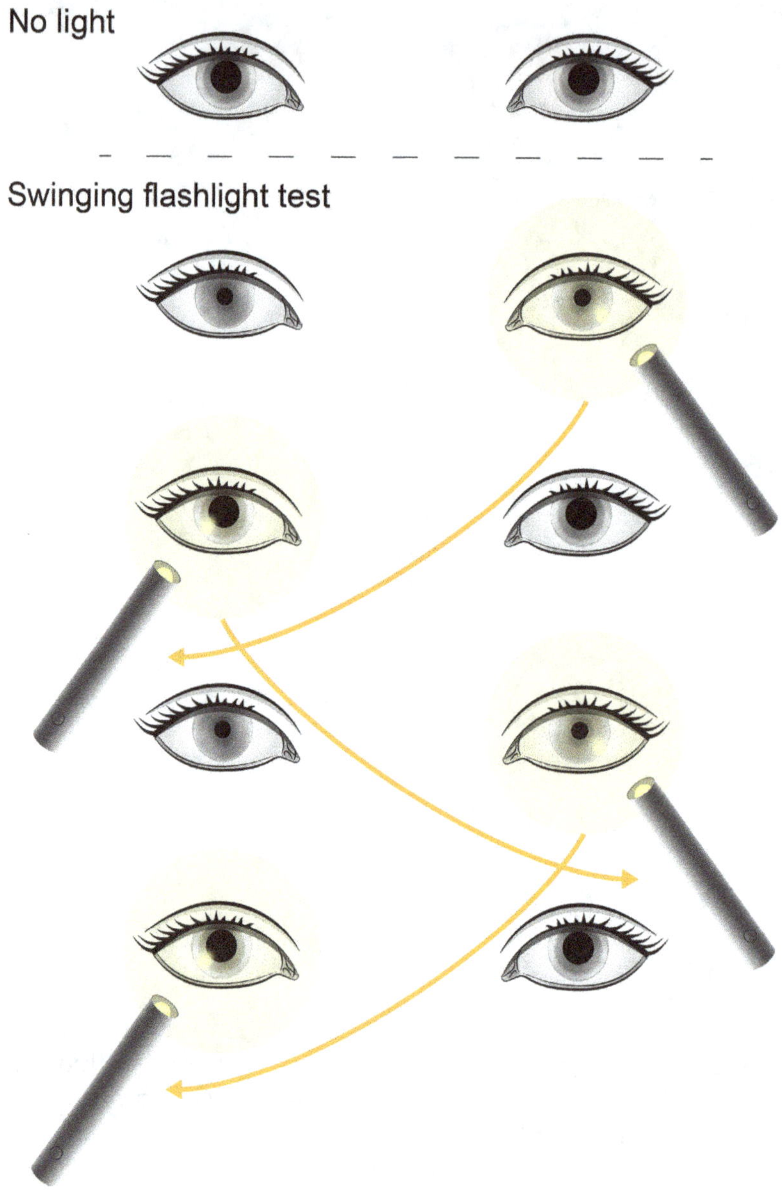

No light

Swinging flashlight test

FIGURE 3.19 How to test for a RAPD in the 'normal appearing' right and left pupils [20].

Source: (Courtesy of Dr. Samantha Armstrong, Aston University, Birmingham)

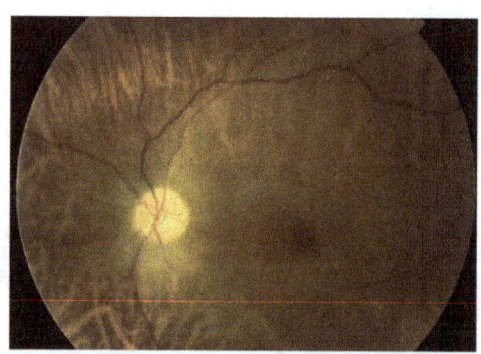

FIGURE 3.20 Central retinal artery occlusion with 'cherry red' spot.

Source: (Courtesy of Dr. Fatima Mesa-Lugo, Hospital Universitario de Canarias, Spain)

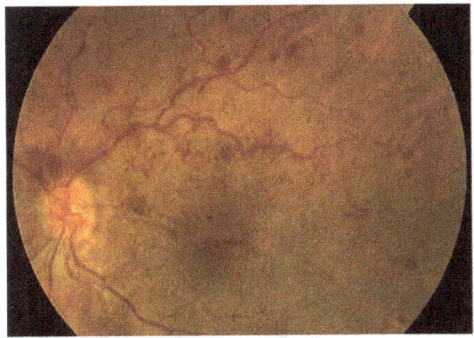

FIGURE 3.21 Branch retinal vein occlusion.

Source: (Courtesy of Dr. Fatima Mesa-Lugo, Hospital Universitario de Canarias, Spain)

retinal neovascularization in about 20% of cases within six to twelve months of occlusion [22].

Acute BRVO presents with superficial haemorrhages, retinal oedema and often cotton-wool spots in the retinal sector drained by the affected vein. The obstructed vein appears dilated and tortuous. It often occurs at the site of arteriovenous nicking due to hypertensive atherosclerosis.

Risk factors for BRVO include high blood pressure, high cholesterol, history of heart attacks, strokes, diabetes and glaucoma. Early diagnosis and management are crucial to prevent vision loss.

Amaurosis Fugax

Amaurosis fugax involves monocular, painless, transient vision loss. The pathophysiology is similar to that of CRAO: occlusion or stenosis within the internal carotid circulation. On retinal examination, there may be microemboli of cholesterol plaques (Hollenhorst plaques) in the arteries. Hollenhorst plaques are associated with systemic vascular diseases, viz. atherosclerosis, and their presence is significant. Identifying these plaques during a retinal examination is crucial, as it is an indicator of underlying cardiovascular pathology needing referral for investigation. Amaurosis fugax is a manifestation of carotid artery insufficiency; patients with these symptoms may have similar cerebral carotid ischaemic episodes.

Retinal Detachment

Retinal detachment is usually due to a hole or tear in the retina (rhegmatogenous) with fluid from the vitreous cavity leaking underneath, but this does not always happen. The vitreous separating from the retina is a normal physiological event accompanied by flashing lights and floaters. In a few people, the separation also leads to a tear in the retina, which can lead to a retinal detachment.

Initial symptoms of a retinal tear include a sudden increase in floaters with flashes of light in the peripheral vision. A visual field defect occurs as the detachment progresses. There will be a sudden and severe loss of vision, usually to less than 6/60, if the macula detaches.

The detachment is visible as a grey, floppy membrane (Figure 3.22). Intraocular pressure may be reduced. The red reflex is usually pale or grey compared to the usual orange colour.

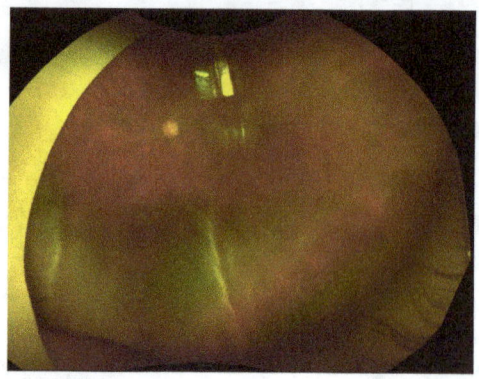

FIGURE 3.22 Severe inferior bullous retinal detachment appearing as a translucent grey membrane; there is normal retina above and retinal folds below.

Source: (Courtesy of Dr. S. Basu, LV Prasad Eye Institute, Hyderabad, India. Further photos in Supplementary Chapter S3.)

Retinal detachment is managed with surgery to close the break; this stops fluid from leaking under the retina and allows it to reattach. *The patient needs urgent referral to hospital care.* A vitrectomy is performed, filling the eye with a bubble of gas to hold the retina in place. Alternatively, a piece of plastic is stitched to the sclera (a scleral buckle), which pushes the outer layers of the eye against the retinal tear to allow functional attachment. The majority of retinal detachments can be reattached with a single operation, but surgery must be performed quickly to gain best outcomes [23].

Macular Holes

A macular hole is a small defect that develops in the central part of the retina, the macula, responsible for visualising fine details [24]. It can cause blurred and distorted vision, giving difficulty in reading, recognizing faces or driving a car. It often occurs from shrinking and separation of the vitreous jelly from the retina after the age of 50, which can pull on the macula (vitreomacular traction). It occasionally results from trauma and in those with high myopia.

If left untreated, a macular hole may continue to enlarge, leading to further deterioration in central vision, but a small macular hole may close spontaneously. The primary treatment is surgery with vitrectomy, replacing the vitreous with a gas bubble to help the macula heal. The success rate is about 95%, but the final outcome depends on the size and duration of the hole [25] (refer to College of Optometrists' CMGs for:—Vitreomacular traction and macular hole).

EPIRETINAL MEMBRANE (ERM)

An ERM, also known as macular pucker or cellophane maculopathy, is a thin, transparent layer of scar tissue that grows across the central (macular) area of the retina. It appears as a greyish semitranslucent avascular membrane over the internal limiting membrane (ILM) on the surface of the retina (Figure 3.23).

An ERM (Figure 3.23) can be caused by trauma, inflammation or other conditions but in most cases is due to age-related degeneration of the vitreous gel, which pulls away from the retina and releases cells to form a membrane. This progressively affects central vision and causes visual distortion known as metamorphopsia. OCT is used to assess the extent of the membrane and its impact [24].

Treatment for an ERM is considered if the condition is causing significant vision problems. In many cases, the symptoms are mild and do not affect daily

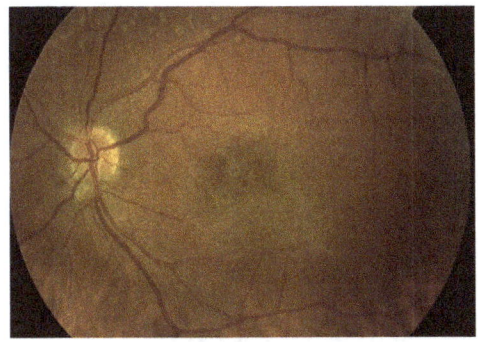

FIGURE 3.23 Epiretinal membrane (ERM) over the macula.

Source: (Courtesy of Dr. Fatima Mesa-Lugo, Hospital Universitario de Canarias, Spain)

activities, so treatment is not necessary. If vision is severely affected, the only treatment available is vitrectomy with removal of the vitreous gel and gentle peeling of the epiretinal membrane away from the retina. Surgery is performed under local anesthesia as an outpatient procedure.

Maculopathies

Patients rarely volunteer symptoms of distortion, so it is necessary to ask them to look at a straight line, such as a door frame (and comment if they see it distorted, bent or with a wavy line) or an Amsler chart as previously described. If so, it is likely that they have a macular problem.

Common maculopathies include diabetes, AMD, macular hole, epiretinal membrane and myopic maculopathy, managed with anti-VEGF to halt neovascularization. Yorston reviews maculopathies with a diagnostic flow diagram [26].

Neurodegenerative Conditions

The use of OCT for assessing changes in neuro-inflammatory and neurodegenerative diseases, identified as imaging biomarkers, across the retina and optic nerve has allowed much greater understanding of the pathological processes, as well as contributing to identifying early disease for better therapy [15]. In particular, it is possible to assess changes in the retinal nerve fibre layer, either of thinning due to loss of ganglion and amacrine cells in the macula or optic disc areas or an increase in the inner nuclear layer, reported as a sign of activation of Müller cells in patients with early diabetic retinopathy or multiple sclerosis.

Multiple Sclerosis (MS)

MS is a demyelinating disease of the central nervous system due to autoimmune-mediated inflammation. The course of MS is relapsing–remitting (RRMS) at onset in 85% of cases with episodes of neurological dysfunction followed by complete or incomplete recovery [27].

A common first presentation of RRMS is unilateral optic neuritis, characterised by the following:

- gradual onset monocular visual loss
- *pain when moving the eye*
- impaired colour vision

Visual loss rarely progresses beyond two weeks from onset, while some evidence of recovery is expected within one month; if recovery takes more than two weeks, it may not recover to baseline. If there is no recovery by one month, then the diagnosis needs to be revised.

On examination:

- Visual acuity is typically reduced.
- There may be a relative afferent pupillary defect—check with the *swinging flashlight test.*
- A central scotoma may be present—test with a red target on confrontation and Humphrey field tests.
- Colour vision may be impaired—test with Ishihara charts.
- Visual field test.

On fundoscopy, the optic disc may appear normal (retrobulbar neuritis) or swollen and may become pale and atrophic over time following the attack [27].

Routine ophthalmoscopy can detect the following:

- retinal periphlebitis
- optic disc swelling and atrophy
- localised notch in the retinal nerve fibre layer or a clear notch on the disc

The deterioration in the optic nerve is reflected in other myelinated pathways in the brain or spinal cord although on a patchy basis.

OCT is useful to show the following:

- The cup-to-disc ratio and related optic nerve head metrics.
- Thinning of the temporal nerve fibre layer.
- It can be suggestive of old optic nerve damage from previously undiagnosed optic neuritis.
- In patients with established MS, OCT may be used for follow-up.

The presence of OCT alterations consistent with acute optic neuritis or chronic optic neuropathy increases clinical suspicion for MS [28].

Alternatively, a recurring normal OCT decreases the likelihood of an underlying demyelinating disorder for patients with repeated or chronic visual symptoms.

For other neurodegenerative conditions, refer to T&F website Chapter S3.

For additional photographs and OCT images, including myelinated nerve fibres in the retina, optic disc head pit, choroidal naevus with drusen and age-related issues, refer to Supplementary Chapter S3.

REFERENCES

1. Vision Loss Expert Group of the Global Burden of Disease Study & the GBD 2019. Eye 2024. PMID: 38565601 (https://doi.org/10.1038/s41433-024-02995-5).
2. College of Optometrists. Clinical Management Guidelines. Glaucoma (Chronic Open Angle (COAG) 2025. Accessed 03/09/25).
3. Ruia S, Tripathy K. Statpearls [Internet]. PMID: NBK585112 (vision https://www.ncbi.nlm.nih.gov/books/NBK585112/).
4. Eyeguru. How to Interpret Visual Fields: 5 Most Common Patterns 2024. Accessed 18/08/25 (https://eyeguru.org/essentials/visual-fields/).
5. NICE. Glaucoma: Diagnosis and Management. NICE Guideline NG81 2022. Accessed 18/8/25 (https://www.nice.org.uk/guidance/ng81/).
6. Royal College of Ophthalmologists. Ophthalmic Services Guidance Designing Glaucoma Care Pathways Using GLAUC-STRAT-FAST 2022. Accessed 18/08/25 (https://www.rcophth.ac.uk/wp-content/uploads/2022/04/Designing-Glaucoma-Care-Pathways-using-GLAUC-STRAT-FAST.pdf).
7. European Glaucoma Society. Terminology and Guidelines for Glaucoma. 5th ed. 2020 Accessed 18/8/25 (https://www.eugs.org/).

8. College of Optometrists. Clinical Management Guidelines (Ocular hypertension (OHT)—College of Optometrists) 2025. Accessed 03/09/25.

9. College of Optometrists. Clinical Management Guidelines.Primary Angle Closure/Primary Angle Closure Glaucoma (PAC/PACG)—College of Optometrists 2025. Accessed 03/09/25.

10. Vision Loss Expert Group of the Global Burden of Disease Study & the GBD 2019. Eye 2024. PMID: 38965321 (https://doi.org/10.1038/s41433-024-03050-z).

11. Simo R et al. Diabetes Care 2014. PMID: 24652720 (https://doi.org/10.2337/dc13-2002).

12. Stewart M. Mayo Clin Proc 2012. Accessed 28/05/2025 (https://doi.org/10.1016/j.mayocp.2011.10.001).

13. Vision Loss Expert Group of the Global Burden of Disease Study & the GBD 2019. Eye 2024. PMID: 38937557 (https://doi.org/10.1038/s41433-024-03101-5).

14. Zachariah S et al. Comm Eye Health J [Internet] 2016. PMID: 38937557 (https://cehjournal.org/articles/475).

15. Vujosevic S et al. Eye 2023. PMID: 35428871 (https://doi.org/10.1038/s41433-022-02056-9).

16. Wong T et al. Brit Med Bull 2005. PMID: 16148191 (https://doi.org/10.1093/bmb/ldh050).

17. Henderson AD et al. Rev Neurol Dis 2011. PMID: 21769065 (https://pubmed.ncbi.nlm.nih.gov/21769065).

18. Scott CJ et al. Arch Ophthalmol 2010. PMID: 20547947 (https://doi.org/10.1001/archophthalmol.2010.94).

19. McGee S. Chapter 21: The Pupils. In: Evidence-Based Physical Diagnosis 2018, pp 161–180e3. ISBN: 978-0-323-39276-1 (https://doi.org/10.1016/B978-0-323-39276-1.00021-4).

20. Broadway D. Comm Eye Health J [Internet] 2005. PMID: 16148191. Accessed 28/05/2025 (https://pmc.ncbi.nlm.nih.gov/articles/PMC3588138/).

21. College of Optometrists. Clinical Management Guidelines. Retinal Vein Occlusion—College of Optometrists 2025. Accessed 03/09/25.

22. College of Optometrists. Clinical Management Guidelines. Retinal Vein Occlusion—College of Optometrists 2025. Accessed 03/09/25.

23. Hazlewood J et al. Eye 2025. PMID: 39856427 (https://www.nature.com/articles/s41433-025-03613-8).

24. Yorston D. Comm Eye Health J [Internet] 2025. PMID: 40151367. Accessed 28/05/2025 (https://cehjournal.org/articles/833/files/679a4f881037c.pdf).

25. College of Optometrists. Clinical Management Guidelines. Vitreomacular Traction and Macular Hole—College of Optometrists 2025. Accessed 03/09/25.

26. Yorston D. Comm Eye Health J [Internet] 2025. PMID: 40151368. Accessed 28/05/2025 (https://cehjournal.org/articles/825).

27. Cleveland Clinic. Optic Coherence Tomography (OCT) in the Diagnosis and Management of Multiple Sclerosis 2025. Accessed 18/08/25 (https://www.sciencedirect.com/science/article/pii/S147021182403519X?via%3Dihub).

28. Ford H. Clin Med 2020. PMID: 32675142 (https://my.clevelandclinic.org/departments/neurological/depts/multiple-sclerosis/ms-approaches/optic-coherence-tomography).

4: Dry Eye Disease (DED) and Inflammatory Conditions

CORE MESSAGES

Ocular surface disorders affecting the tear film include dry eye disease (DED), Sjögren's disease (syndrome), blepharitis and the scarring diseases.

a) DED is one of the most commonly presenting conditions in primary care and is associated with ocular discomfort of varying severity, quantitative and qualitative changes to the preocular tear film and inflammation and damage to the ocular surface.

b) Posterior blepharitis is associated with meibomian gland dysfunction and is a major cause of tear instability and evaporative dry eye. Refer to Chapter 6 for anterior blepharitis (infective/seborrheic). Often, elements of both anterior and posterior blepharitis are present together.

c) Sjögren's disease (syndrome) is an autoimmune disease affecting exocrine glands, leading to dry eyes and mouth.

d) Ocular rosacea has combined pathologies of DED, folliculitis caused by *St. aureus*, immune reaction and lipid keratopathy that can result in progressive keratitis.

e) Allergic eye disease can present in different ways, including seasonal allergic conjunctivitis (SAC), perennial allergic conjunctivitis (PAC), vernal keratoconjunctivitis (VKC) and atopic keratoconjunctivitis (AKC). Conjunctival scarring disorders are often progressive and destructive.

f) Inflammatory diseases of the ocular surface and adnexa include episcleritis and scleritis. Management of these entities involves non-pharmacological interventions, topical treatments and systemic therapy in some patients.

a) Dry Eye Disease (DED)

Dry eye disease (DED) is a common condition that presents a challenge for both affected patients and eye care practitioners. The complexity of its aetiology, heterogeneity in clinical presentation and association with other ocular and systemic conditions requires tailored management of the condition.

The pathogenesis of DED is complex and involves a mechanism that operates at the cellular, humoral, endocrine and neuronal levels. The main distinction is made between DED with increased evaporation of tears (evaporative dry eye) and reduced tear production (aqueous deficient dry eye). Although identifying the primary DED subtype (aqueous deficient or evaporative) remains important for classification, the current consensus is that these subtypes are part of a spectrum of disease, rather than being distinct pathophysiological entities [1].

48

DOI: 10.1201/9781003606789-5

Inflammation plays a key role in the development and progression of DED. This is expressed in the current definition of dry eye taken from the 2025 Tear Film and Ocular Surface Society Dry Eye Workshop III (TFOS-DEWS III): "Dry eye is a multifactorial, symptomatic disease characterized by a loss of homeostasis of the tear film and/or ocular surface, in which tear film instability and hyperosmolarity, ocular surface inflammation and damage, and neurosensory abnormalities are aetiological factors" [2].

In DED, the underlying mechanism appears to be an increase in tear osmolarity, which triggers a series of signaling events in ocular surface epithelial cells, leading to the release of inflammatory mediators and proteases. The result of this process is the characteristic superficial punctate epitheliopathy and tear film instability that characterises DED. The combination of epithelial injury and tear hyperosmolarity also stimulates corneal sensory nerve endings, causing ocular discomfort of variable severity. DED characterised by aqueous deficiency is associated with reduced lacrimal secretion caused by lymphocytic infiltration of the lacrimal gland, an age-related decline in lacrimal secretion, or obstruction of lacrimal gland ducts in the case of cicatricial disease. Symptoms of DED can be exacerbated by lifestyle and environmental factors. Triggering factors include contact lens wear, prolonged use of digital devices, air pollution, cigarette smoke, low humidity, air conditioning and wind [3].

Diagnostic Testing for Dry Eye Disease

Many conditions can mimic symptoms and/or signs of DED. There is no single gold standard test for diagnosing DED; instead, a variety of tests and techniques should be employed to assess loss of the homeostasis of the tear film and the integrity of the ocular surface [2].

Symptoms

Patients presenting with DED will often describe bilateral symptoms of grittiness and burning alongside a sensation of dryness. Symptoms vary in severity from mild to severe and may vary throughout the day. To evaluate symptoms, several validated questionnaires are available that allow (semi-)quantified assessment. However, in routine practice, it is important that the questionnaire is not burdensome for the patients and is easy to score (Chapter 8). TFOS-DEWS III have recently recommended the use of the six-item Ocular Surface Disease Index (OSDI-6), which is an adaptation of the original 12-item OSDI. OSDI-6 has subscales covering symptoms and visual disturbance, visual function/tasks and environment. OSDI-6 results can be indexed to severity, as normal (0–3 points), mild-to-moderate DED (4–8 points) and severe DED (> 8) [2].

Tear Film Breakup Time (TBUT)

Evaluation of the TBUT is a relatively simple and frequently performed test in the clinic. TBUT can be evaluated invasively at the slit lamp following the installation of fluorescein (to enhance the visibility of the tear film) and measuring the time interval/sec between a blink and the first break in the tear film. Alternatively, tear stability can be assessed non-invasively by projecting a grid or pattern onto the tear film and measuring the time until the pattern distorts. Non-invasive tear breakup time (NIBUT) eliminates the physical disturbance of the tear film and is recommended by the Dry Eye Workshop (DEWS III) [2]. A NIBUT of < 10 s is considered as a positive sign of tear stability. Where there is no access to a NIBUT device, fluorescein TBUT should be performed with a minimal volume of fluorescein applied and a diagnostic cut-off of < 5 s used as an indicator of instability.

Tear Meniscus Assessment and Schirmer Test

Tear meniscus height measured at the slit lamp provides a useful measure of aqueous component of the tears. The tear meniscus height should be measured directly below the pupil midline with the eye in the primary position. A cut-off value of ≤ 0.20 mm has been proposed as an indicator of aqueous deficiency.

The Schirmer test is most useful in the diagnosis of patients with severe aqueous deficiency, e.g. Sjögren's disease patients [4]. It is performed by placing a defined paper test strip in the lateral third of the lower eyelid. After five minutes, the length of the moistened portion of the strip is measured. The Schirmer test can be performed without anaesthesia (Schirmer I), measuring basic and reflex tearing. Schirmer II test is done following nasal stimulation and measures reflex tearing only. "Schirmer with anaesthesia" or the basic secretion test is also commonly performed and measures basal tear secretion. Basic secretion with less than 10 mm of wetting is considered diagnostic for aqueous deficiency. The Schirmer test is often criticized for its variability and poor reproducibility and is of limited value in mild cases.

Ocular Surface Integrity Assessment by Staining

Several vital dyes are used to semi-quantitatively evaluate the cell damage at the ocular surface, and the subsequent staining of the tissues is an important diagnostic sign in DED. Fluorescein is the most commonly used stain, and lissamine green has largely replaced rose bengal since it is less toxic to the ocular surface and is better tolerated. Lissamine green is particularly useful in detecting damage to conjunctival epithelial cells.

The degree of staining can be graded using various scales. The most common grading scale was introduced by van Bijsterveld [5]; the interpretation of staining is based on intensity and location. The nasal and temporal conjunctiva and the cornea are graded on a scale of 0–3 with a maximum possible score of 9. Similarly, the Oxford grading score rates the intensity of the punctate staining of the cornea and conjunctiva on a 0–5 scale depending on severity. Pictorial representation of staining intensity is used for the scoring [6].

Tear Osmolarity

Elevated osmolarity and increased variability of osmolarity of the tears are characteristics of DED. Osmolarity values typically increase with disease severity. Various cut-off values have been reported, with 308 mOsm/L used as a threshold to diagnose mild-to-moderate disease, whereas 316 mOsm/L has been used as a cut-off for more severe disease.

Tear osmolarity can be determined using the TearLab Osmolarity System [7] (TearLab, San Diego, CA—the I-PEN® Tear Osmolarity System) (https://imedpharma.com/product/i-pen/), which measures the osmolarity of a 50 nL tear sample. Normal values are considered to be 296±9.8 mOsm/L. Osmolarity greater than 308 mOsm/L or an interocular difference of > 8 nOsm/L are considered to indicate at least mild dry eye and has been demonstrated to serve as an early indicator of ocular surface instability. TFO testing needs to be evaluated in conjunction with other signs and symptoms of DED.

Evaluation of Lid Margin Health

The term "blepharitis" is most commonly used to describe anterior blepharitis, which represents a chronic inflammation of the lid margin anterior to the grey line. Anterior blepharitis is characterised by squamous debris around the base of the lashes and lid margin hyperaemia. Anterior blepharitis is more likely to have an infectious aetiology (see Chapter 6).

Posterior blepharitis, commonly referred to as meibomian gland dysfunction (MGD), is a major contributing factor to DED. MGD is associated with altered meibomian secretions, plugging of duct orifices and lid margin hyperaemia (Figures 4.1 and 4.2). Quantitative and qualitative changes in meibomian gland secretion leads to tear film instability, reduced TBUT and an evaporative dry eye. Meibomian gland function can be assessed by evaluating meibum quantity, quality and expressivity at the slit lamp. However, enhanced visualization is obtained using meibography based on infrared imaging systems [2].

There is a growing interest in an area of the lid margin known as the "lid wiper", where the lid margin contacts the ocular surface. Damage to the marginal conjunctival epithelium at the lid wiper zone (known as lid wiper epitheliopathy) has been proposed as an additional clinical sign in DED. Lid wiper epitheliopathy is most commonly graded using the Korb grading system [8], which uses the

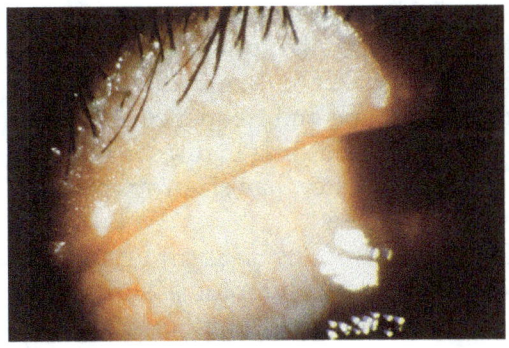

FIGURE 4.1 Abnormal secretions from the meibomian glands.

Source: (Seal D, Pleyer U. Ocular Infection, 2nd Edition 2007)

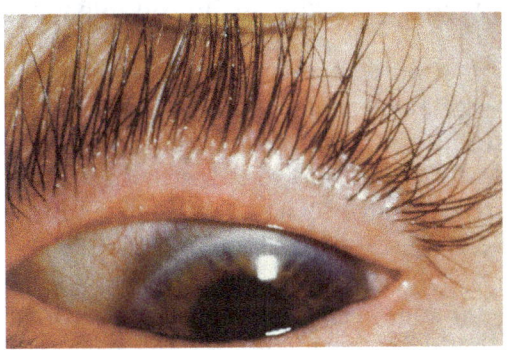

FIGURE 4.2 Thickened and hyperaemic lid margin in MGD.

Source: (Seal D, Pleyer U. Ocular Infection, 2nd Edition 2007)

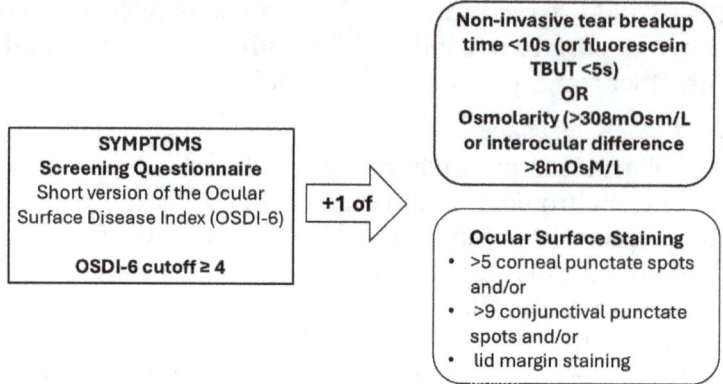

FIGURE 4.3 TFOS-DEWS III diagnostic algorithm.

combination of the horizontal length of staining in mm and the sagittal width of the staining.

Given the overlap in clinical presentation between DED and other ocular surface diseases, it is important to adopt a standardised diagnostic approach. The TFOS-DEWS III has provided a useful diagnostic algorithm that encompasses symptoms and key clinical signs of DED (Figure 4.3) [2].

Management and Therapy

Tear supplements and ocular lubricants, which enhance or stabilise the tear film, are the mainstay of treatment for DED. A large number of supplements are available (see Appendix 1), and these can generally be purchased over the counter in most countries without a prescription. There is no high quality evidence on which supplements are most effective in treating DED [9], and therefore, the selection of the most appropriate tear supplement type and frequency of administration is normally based on a stepwise approach according to disease severity. Patients requiring high frequency administration (greater than six drops per day) are likely to benefit from preservative-free formulations.

In patients with aqueous deficient DED, punctal occlusion is an established intervention when tear supplements do not improve symptoms sufficiently. Plugging of the puncta using semi-permanent silicone or temporary collagen punctal plugs aims to conserve naturally produced tears by totally or partially blocking the lacrimal drainage system. Although evidence from clinical trials suggest that punctal plugs can be effective, improvements in clinical outcomes are inconsistent [9].

In addition to tear replenishment, patients should be advised to avoid environmental and lifestyle factors that could precipitate symptoms of DED—e.g. avoid prolonged reading, take frequent breaks when using digital devices, make a conscious effort to blink more frequently and use humidifiers to enhance humidity.

Lid hygiene is the mainstay of clinical treatment for MGD, consisting of a combination of warm compresses or heat application, mechanical lid massage and the use of lid scrubs [10].

Oral tetracyclines—e.g. doxycycline (100 mg once daily for two to three months)—can be given to inhibit bacterial lipase production by *Staphylococcus epidermidis*, found on the lid margins. This action reduces the release of toxic fatty acids in excessive meibomian secretion that contribute to inflammation and symptoms of irritation.

b) Sjögren's Disease

In 1933, the Swedish ophthalmologist Henrik Samuel Conrad Sjögren described in his dissertation "On the Knowledge of Keratoconjunctivitis Sicca" a series of cases of 19 patients who had sicca symptoms, with inflammatory dry eyes and mouth as the main symptom. It was not until the translation into English (1943) that the term Sjögren's syndrome became established worldwide. In 2016, the EU-USA societies (ACR and EULAR) updated the classification criteria for Sjögren's syndrome (disease) with the help of a score [11]. These classification criteria are used for diagnostic orientation. In 2025 (11/06), *Nature Reviews Rheumatology* published the international consensus formalising the name change from Sjögren's syndrome to Sjögren's disease [12].

Definition and Terminology

Sjögren's disease is a chronic inflammatory autoimmune disease of unknown origin, which leads to the main symptoms of keratoconjunctivitis sicca and xerostomia due to the involvement of exocrine glands. The clinical picture can also include a wide range of manifestations, including extraglandular and systemic involvement of different organs. In addition, typical chronic fatigue determines the quality of life of patients.

The distinction between primary Sjögren's disease (syndrome) (pSS) and a secondary or associated form (sSS) is important therapeutically and prognostically; sSS occurs as a concomitant disease in the context of other autoimmune diseases (Table 4.1). Patients with pSS have a substantially increased risk (5%) of developing non-Hodgkin's lymphoma of the B-cell series. Anti-Ro (-SSA) and/or anti-La (-SSB) autoantiobodies are considered immunological hallmarks of the disease; they are found in 50 to 70% of patients and are associated with increased severity [13].

sSS is generally less severe, with prognosis and therapy based on the underlying disease. In addition, a differential diagnosis of "sicca" symptoms must be distinguished from other diseases without an autoimmune basis (Table 4.2), as well

TABLE 4.1 Consensus Criteria for the Classification of Primary Sjögren's Disease (Syndrome) (ACR/EULAR)

Unstimulated pathological total saliva test ≤ 0.1 ml/minute (1 point)

Schirmer test pathological (< 5 mm in five minutes) (1 point)

Pathological findings in the lissamine green or fluorescein stain
(≥ 5 in the ocular staining score or ≥ 4 in the Van Bijsterveld score) (1 point)

Autoantibody Detection: Anti-Ro/SS-A (3 points)

Histology—focal lymphocytic sialadenitis, Focus-Score ≥ 1 foci/4 mm²; 1 Focus = 50 lymphocyte/4 mm² (3 points)

Diagnosis is considered confirmed at ≥ 4 points, after application of the inclusion and exclusion criteria.

Inclusion criteria: Dry eyes and/or mouth for at least three months without any other explanation (e.g. medication, infection)

Exclusion criteria: Condition after irradiation of the head/neck region, "Human immunodeficiency virus (HIV)" infection/AIDS, sarcoidosis, active infection with hepatitis C virus, amyloidosis, graft-versus-host disease and IgG4-associated disease. The condition for classification as pSS is the absence of any other potentially associated disease.

Source: [11]

TABLE 4.2 Frequency of Associated Sjögren's Disease (Syndrome)

Disease	Frequency [%]
Systemic lupus erythematosus	15–36
Rheumatoid arthritis	22–32
Systemic sclerosis	11–24
Primary biliary cirrhosis	8–15
Polymyositis	9–18

as limited lacrimal gland function in old age due to glandular involution with hormonal changes in menopause.

c) Ocular Rosacea

Ocular rosacea is the ocular manifestation of rosacea, a chronic inflammatory skin disease affecting the centrofacial region (cheeks, chin, nose and central forehead), although ocular features can occur prior to skin involvement. Ocular rosacea affects adult males and females equally, is uncommon in children and usually starts after the age of 30 years.

Signs include bilateral hyperaemic thickened lid margins, telangiectasia of the lid margins (Figure 4.4) and tear film instability. This is primarily due to meibomian gland dysfunction. Corneal involvement occurs in up to 30% of patients ranging from punctate staining to corneal vascularization, infiltration and thinning (Figures 4.5 and 4.6). The diagnosis of ocular rosacea is largely based on clinical findings. The main symptoms include red, burning and itchy eyes, dryness, sensitivity to light and blurred vision.

The aetiology of ocular rosacea is considered multifactorial (Figure 4.7) with genetic predisposition, environmental impact, demodex and susceptibility to *St. aureus* colonisation of the lid margin with enhanced delayed-type hypersensitivity due to CMI (Chapter 10) [14, 15].

Treatment is summarised in Table 4.3. Ciclosporin (Chapter 10) has given a better response rate than doxycycline (tetracycline) for managing blepharitis associated with rosacea. In a comparative trial, ciclosporin was more effective in symptomatic relief and in treatment of eyelid signs ($P = 0.01$). In addition, there was a statistically significant increase in the mean Schirmer score with

TABLE 4.3 Treatment Options for Ocular Rosacea

Mild	Lid hygiene and unpreserved tear substitute (Appendix 1)
Moderate	Topical antibiotic and anti-inflammatory drops (Appendix 1)
	Fusidic acid (1% viscous eye drops) gave a 75% response rate of symptomatic relief for blepharitis and rosacea in a placebo-controlled trial compared to 50% for tetracycline, with no additional benefit for the combination [15]. Fusidic acid has good anti-staphylococcal properties as well as a ciclosporin-like activity (later) suppressing cell-mediated immunity (DTH). It is now available as a non-proprietary product.
Moderately severe	Oral antibiotics (doxycycline*, azithromycin**)
Severe, loss of vision	Amniotic membrane transplantation, corneal graft

* also has an anti-inflammatory effect modulating T-cell activation and production of pro-inflammatory cytokines [16].

** also has an anti-inflammatory effect inhibiting production of pro-inflammatory cytokines such as TNF, IL-1, IL-6 and IL-8 (Chapter 10).

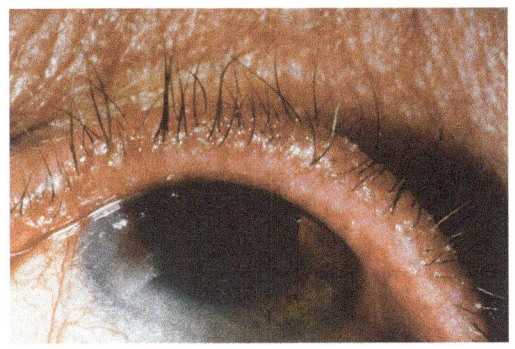

FIGURE 4.4 Rosacea blepharophyma with thickened lid edges, folliculitis due to *St. aureus*, lid margin telangiectasia and meibomian gland dysfunction (MGD).

Source: (Seal D, Pleyer U. Ocular Infection, 2nd Edition 2007)

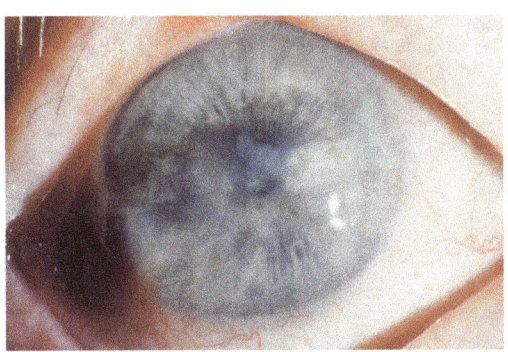

FIGURE 4.5 Rosacea with corneal neovascularization arising from the lateral limbus, forming a pannus with lipid keratopathy.

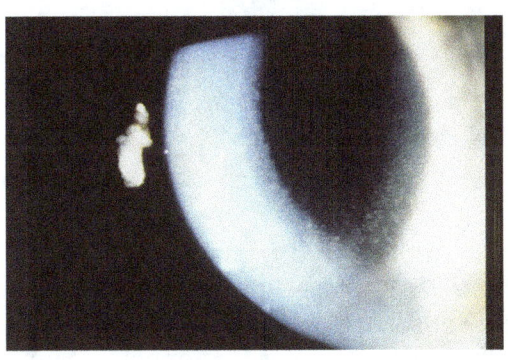

FIGURE 4.6 Slit lamp image showing lipid keratopathy in rosacea.

anaesthesia and TBUT scores in the ciclosporin treatment group compared to the doxycycline treatment group ($P < 0.05$) [17]. Although ciclosporin emulsion is used as an off-label treatment for ocular rosacea, the available preparations are expensive [18] (refer to College of Optometrists' CMGs for—Ocular rosacea).

For more photographs, refer to Supplementary Chapter S4.

d) Episcleritis and Scleritis

Episcleritis is an acute inflammation of the loose connective tissue between the conjunctiva and sclera. Episcleritis is idiopathic in 70% of cases. However, in up to a third of cases, it is associated with particular systemic diseases, such as rheumatoid arthritis, Crohn's disease, ulcerative colitis or other autoimmune conditions.

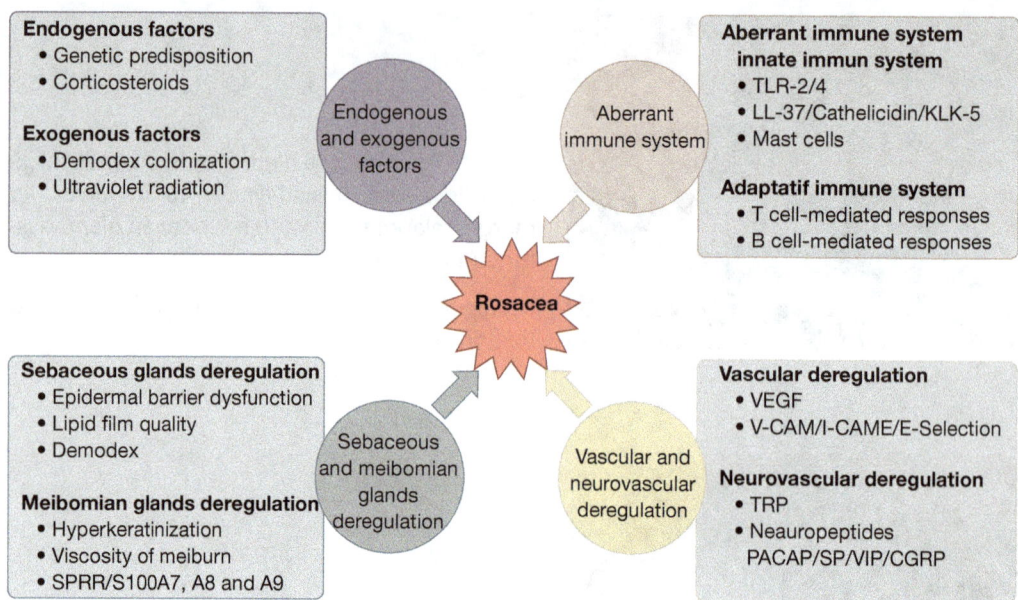

Endogenous factors
- Genetic predisposition
- Corticosteroids

Exogenous factors
- Demodex colonization
- Ultraviolet radiation

Endogenous and exogenous factors

Aberrant immune system

Aberrant immune system innate immun system
- TLR-2/4
- LL-37/Cathelicidin/KLK-5
- Mast cells

Adaptatif immune system
- T cell-mediated responses
- B cell-mediated responses

Rosacea

Sebaceous glands deregulation
- Epidermal barrier dysfunction
- Lipid film quality
- Demodex

Meibomian glands deregulation
- Hyperkeratinization
- Viscosity of meiburn
- SPRR/S100A7, A8 and A9

Sebaceous and meibomian glands deregulation

Vascular and neurovascular deregulation

Vascular deregulation
- VEGF
- V-CAM/I-CAME/E-Selection

Neurovascular deregulation
- TRP
- Neauropeptides PACAP/SP/VIP/CGRP

FIGURE 4.7 Pathophysiology factors in rosacea.

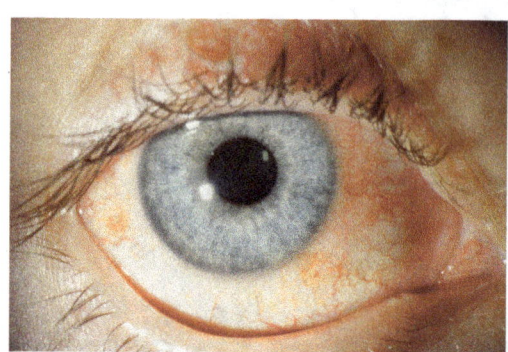

FIGURE 4.8 Episcleritis (mild).

Episcleritis is commonly found in young to middle-aged females and rarely in children [19] (refer to College of Optometrists' CMGs for—Episcleritis).

Symptoms in episcleritis include an acute onset, redness, mild ocular discomfort or pain and normal visual acuity without discharge or photophobia. Signs show hyperaemia from dilated episcleral vessels in one or more quadrants of one or both eyes (Figures 4.8). Nodular episcleritis, which occurs in around 20% of cases, is characterised by a discrete raised nodule of inflamed episclera. The differential diagnosis for nodular episcleritis is phlyctenular keratoconjunctivitis (Chapter 6).

In episcleritis, the patient may be asymptomatic and so requires no therapy; the condition is usually self-resolving in seven to ten days. If the episcleritis is symptomatic, it can be managed with artificial tears for one to two weeks and oral NSAIDs—e.g. flurbiprofen—as needed (Appendix 1). More severe cases, including the nodular type, may require a topical steroid (fluorometholone or loteprednol) for one to two weeks, with gradual tapering as the inflammation resolves.

The most important differential diagnosis in episcleritis is scleritis, which may be idiopathic, but in 30–40% of cases is associated with an autoimmune disease, most commonly rheumatoid arthritis. Anterior scleritis (Figure 4.9) is the most common form of scleritis (occurring in 90% of cases) and is characterised by inflammation of the sclera anterior to the rectus muscle insertions. Posterior scleritis is defined as the involvement of the sclera posterior to the insertion of the rectus muscles.

A patient with scleritis will generally have severe pain, which often radiates to the periorbital regions, photophobia, tearing and possibly reduced visual acuity. The majority of patients with scleritis present with diffuse oedema of episcleral and scleral tissues, with injection of both the superficial and deep episcleral vessels. Patients with nodular scleritis typically experience one or more firm, tender nodules on the sclera. Necrotising scleritis (Figure 4.10) is the most severe sight-threatening form of scleritis, which can lead to scleral thinning and perforation of the globe.

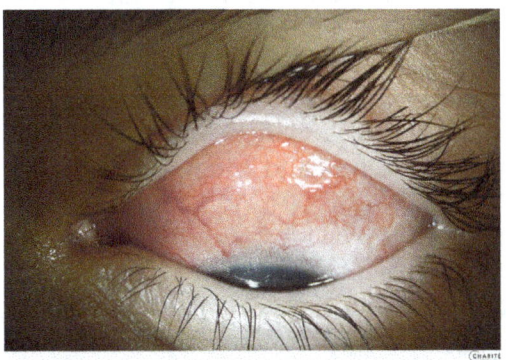

FIGURE 4.9 Diffuse scleritis (moderate).

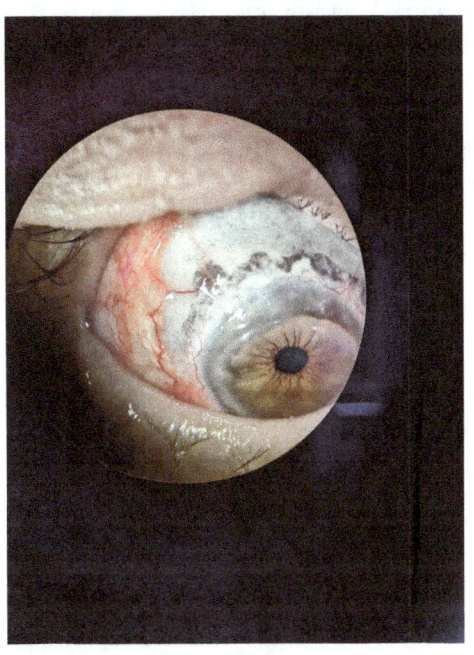

FIGURE 4.10 Necrotising scleritis with corneal involvement.

Pharmacological testing may be useful in differentiating between episcleritis and scleritis. This is achieved by instilling one drop of 2.5% phenylephrine to the affected eye and evaluating the episcleral vessels after 15 minutes. If the inflammation is localised to the episcleral tissue, then the vessels will blanch, and the eye will be relatively white and asymptomatic. Scleral vessels do not blanch with phenylephrine, and the eye continues to show significant hyperaemia.

Treatment for mild to moderate non-necrotising scleritis includes high-dose oral NSAIDs (e.g. flurbiprofen) or paracetamol if NSAIDs are contraindicated. For cases of necrotising anterior and posterior scleritis, emergency (same day) referral is required [20] (refer to College of Optometrists' CMGs for—Scleritis).

e) Allergic Eye Disease

Allergic eye disease is a common clinical presentation in primary eye care. Seasonal allergic conjunctivitis (SAC), the ocular manifestation of hay fever, is the most common form of allergic conjunctivitis that involves a type 1 (mast cell-mediated) hypersensitivity response of the conjunctiva to seasonal airborne allergens, particularly grass pollen. Perennial allergic conjunctivitis (PAC) persists throughout the year due to an allergic reaction to non-seasonal allergens, e.g. pet fur or house dust mite. The symptoms of SAC and PAC are similar and consist predominantly of itching and watering of the eyes. Signs include the following: mild to moderate lid oedema, conjunctival hyperaemia and chemosis and a diffuse papillary reaction (Figure 4.11).

Cool compresses and ocular lubricants can provide symptomatic relief. Patients should be advised against eye rubbing, which causes mechanical mast cell degranulation and exacerbates symptoms. In SAC, if nasal symptoms such as nasal discharge and sneezing are present, consider an oral antihistamine—e.g. cetirizine—as an alternative or alongside topical ocular treatment.

Topical treatments for SAC and PAC consist of antihistamines and mast cell stabilisers (Appendix 1). Mast cell stabilisers work best when started prior to the hay fever season and then used regularly; they can be effective in preventing recurrence of symptoms.

Antihistamine eye drops work immediately to treat symptoms. Several of the currently available formulations demonstrate dual-acting antihistamine and mast cell stabilising properties, e.g. olopatadine, and require only twice daily administration [21] (refer to College of Optometrists' CMGs for—Conjunctivitis (seasonal and perennial allergic).

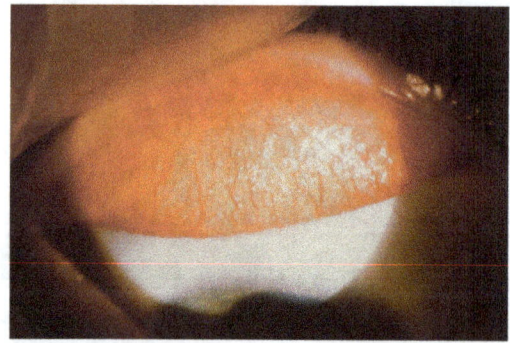

FIGURE 4.11 Fine papillary reaction of the tarsal conjunctiva.

Less common types of allergic conjunctivitis include vernal keratoconjunctivitis (VKC), in children, and atopic keratoconjunctivitis (AKC) in adults, which are severe and potentially sight-threatening diseases characterised by chronic inflammation of the ocular surface. VKC and AKC have complex immunopathology with features of a mixed type I and type IV (DTH) hypersensitivity response (Chapter 10) [22].

VKC is a rare and potentially sight-threatening allergic disorder of children. It usually presents in children under 10 years of age with a history of asthma and eczema. It is relatively rare in Western Europe but is more common in other parts of the world, e.g. Mediterranean region, parts of Africa, Indian subcontinent. Patients tend to be more symptomatic during the spring pollen season, with intense itching and stringy mucous discharge. Pain and photophobia may be present with corneal involvement. Signs of VKC include the following: conjunctival hyperaemia and chemosis, giant tarsal palpebral papillae (> 1 mm in diameter) (Figure 4.12), limbal inflammation (Figure 4.13) and corneal involvement, which can be sight-threatening. Chronic eye rubbing can lead to the development of keratoconus and other corneal ectasias [23] (refer to College of Optometrists' CMGs—Vernal keratoconjunctivitis (spring catarrh)).

AKC occurs most commonly in young adults, as an ocular complication of atopic dermatitis. Patients typically present with bilateral ocular itching, burning and watering. In more severe cases with corneal involvement, there may be blurred vision and photophobia. Signs of AKC include the following: thickened, crusted and fissured eyelids, chronic blepharitis, conjunctival hyperaemia and giant and limbal follicles (Trantas dots). Corneal involvement, which may be sight-threatening, ranges from punctate epitheliopathy to corneal erosions, progressive corneal subepithelial scarring (Figure 4.14), neovascularization/pannus formation

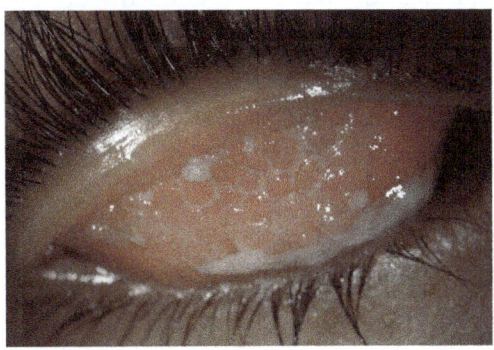

FIGURE 4.12 VKC tarsal type: showing giant papillary reaction ("cobblestones") with extensive mucus secretion.

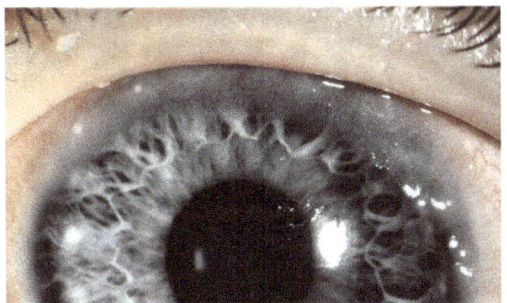

FIGURE 4.13 VKC limbal type: presenting with "Trantas dots" at the superior limbal region.

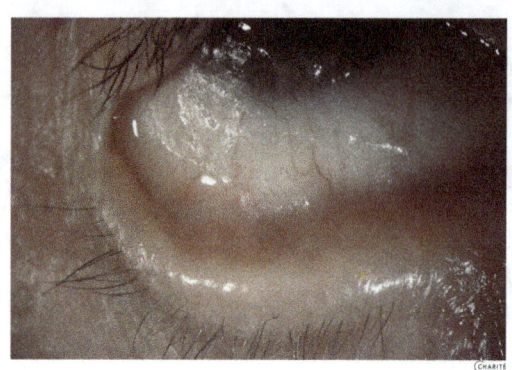

FIGURE 4.14 AKC presenting with conjunctival (symblepharon) and corneal involvement (neovascularization).

and thinning. Patients with AKC are prone to herpes simplex keratitis (which may be bilateral), corneal ectasia such as keratoconus and atopic cataracts [24] (refer to College of Optometrists' CMGs for—Atopic keratoconjunctivitis (AKC)).

Both VKC and AKC require prompt treatment to prevent sight-threatening complications. Treatment options include a combination of mast cell inhibitors, antihistamines, corticosteroids and calcineurin inhibitors.

f) Conjunctivitis Medicamentosa

Chemical irritation (toxicity) or delayed hypersensitivity response of ocular tissues caused by an applied topical drug, contact lens care product, cosmetic or environment substance can cause diffuse punctate staining of the cornea and conjunctiva. Patients will complain of a deterioration of condition despite being compliant with treatment advice (usually following an initial improvement in symptoms). Treatment includes evaluating the non-prescribed/prescribed medication for preservatives and referring back to the original prescriber. Caution should be applied; do not discontinue a medication when the consequences of interruption are more serious than conjunctivitis medicamentosa [25] (refer to College of Optometrists' CMGs for—Conjunctivitis medicamentosa (also known as dermatoconjunctivitis medicamentosa)).

g) Contact Lens–Associated Papillary/Giant Papillary Conjunctivitis

Refer to Chapter 9.

h) Conjunctival Scarring Disorders

For *ocular mucosal pemphigoid, Stevens–Johnson syndrome* and *graft-versus-host disease*, refer to Supplementary Chapter S4.

REFERENCES

1. Craig JP et al. TFOS DEWS II Definition and Classification Report. Ocul Surf 2017. PMID: 28736335 (https://doi.org/10.1016/j.jtos.2017.05.008).
2. Wolffsohn JS et al. TFOS DEWS III Diagnostic Methodology. Am J Ophthalmol 2025. PMID: 40451408 (https://doi.org/10.1016/j.ajo.2025.05.03) Online ahead of print.
3. Stapleton F et al. TFOS DEWS III Digest Report. Am J Ophthalmol 03/06/2025:S0002-9394(25)00276-4. PMID: 40472874 (https://doi.org/10.1016/j.ajo.2025.05.040) Online ahead of print.
4. Brott N et al. Schirmer Test. StatPearls [Internet]. PMID: 32644585. Accessed 28/05/2025 (https://www.ncbi.nlm.nih.gov/books/NBK559159/).

5. van Bijsterveld OP. Diagnostic tests in the Sicca syndrome. Arch Ophthalmol 1969 PMID: 4183019 (doi: 10.1001/archopht.1969.00990020012003).

6. Bron AJ et al. Grading of Corneal and Conjunctival Staining in the Context of Other Dry Eye Tests. Cornea 2003. PMID: 14508260 (https://doi.org/10.1097/00003226-200310000-00008).

7. I-MED PHARMA. The I-PEN® Tear Osmolarity System 2025. Accessed 18/08/25 (https://imedpharma.com/product/i-pen/).

8. Korb DR et al. Lid Wiper Epitheliopathy and Dry Eye Symptoms. Eye Cont Lens 2005. PMID: 15665665 (https://doi.org/10.1097/01.icl.0000140910.03095.fa).

9. Jones L et al. TFOS DEWS III Management and Therapy Report. Am J Ophthalmol 2025. PMID: 40467022 (https://doi.org/10.1016/j.ajo.2025.05.039) Online ahead of print.

10. Hofmann SC, Günther C, Böckle BC, Didona D, Ehrchen J, Gaskins M, Geerling G, Gläser R, Hadaschik E, Hampl M, Haßkamp P, Jackowski J, Kiritsi D, Nast A, Pleyer U, Reichel C, Roth M, Schumann M, Sticherling M, Worm M, Zillikens D, Goebeler M, Schmidt E. S2k Guideline for the Diagnosis and Treatment of Mucous Membrane Pemphigoid. J Dtsch Dermatol Ges 2022 Nov;20(11):1530–1550. Epub 2022 Nov 10. PMID: 36354061 (https://doi.org/10.1111/ddg.14905).

11. Franceschini F et al. BMC Med 2017. PMID: 28359271 (https://pubmed.ncbi.nlm.nih.gov/28359271/).

12. Ramos-Casals M et al. 2023 International Rome Consensus for the Nomenclature of Sjögren Disease. Nat Rev Rheumatol 2025. PMID: 40494962 (https://doi.org/10.1038/s41584-025-01268-z) Online ahead of print.

13. Bjordal O et al. Surv Ophthalmol 2020 [Internet]. Accessed 28/05/2025 (https://www.surveyophthalmol.com/article/S0039-6257(19)30283-8/fulltext).

14. Rodrigues-Braz D. Mol Vis 2021. PMID: 34035646 (http://www.molvis.org/molvis/v27/323).

15. Seal D et al. Brit J Ophthalmol 1995. PMID: 7880791 (http://doi.org/10.1136/bjo.79.1.42).

16. Krakauer T et al. Antimicrob Ag and Chemother 2003. PMID: 7880791 (https://doi.org/10.1128/aac.47.11.3630-3633.2003).

17. Arman A et al. Int J Ophthalmol 2015. PMID: 26086005 (https://www.ncbi.nlm.nih.gov/pmc/articles/PMC4458660/).

18. College of Optometrists. Clinical Management Guidelines. Ocular Rosacea 2025. Accessed 03/09/25.

19. College of Optometrists. Clinical Management Guidelines. Episcleritis 2025. Accessed 03/09/25.

20. College of Optometrists. Clinical Management Guidelines. Scleritis 2025. Accessed 03/09/25.

21. College of Optometrists. Clinical Management Guidelines. Conjunctivitis (Seasonal & Perennial Allergic) 2025. Accessed 18/08/25.

22. Royal College of Ophthalmologists. College-News-Focus. Chronic Allergic Eye Disease 2021. Accessed 18/08/25 (https://www.rcophth.ac.uk/wp-content/uploads/2021/01/College-News-FOCUS_July2018.pdf).

23. College of Optometrists. Clinical Management Guidelines. Vernal Conjunctivitis (Spring Catarrh) 2025. Accessed 03/09/25.

24. College of Optometrists. Clinical Management Guidelines. Atopic Keratoconjunctivitis (AKC) 2025. Accessed 03/09/25.

25. College of Optometrists. Clinical Management Guidelines.Conjunctivitis Medicamentosa (Also Known as Dermatoconjunctivitis Medicamentosa) 2025. Accessed 03/09/25.

5: Uveitis (Inflammatory, Autoimmune Disease or Infectious Causes)

CORE MESSAGES

Anterior uveitis is the most common form of intraocular inflammation, primarily affecting the iris and/or ciliary body. Patients typically present with gradual onset of moderate ocular pain, tearing and reduced vision.

Signs Include

Circumcorneal injection is characteristic due to congestion of perilimbal episcleral vessels.

Increased protein content in the aqueous humour may lead to secondary open-angle glaucoma.

Inflammatory cells circulating in the aqueous can deposit as keratic precipitates on the corneal endothelium, causing corneal haze due to stromal and epithelial oedema. These precipitates can be granulomatous or non-granulomatous, consisting of macrophage and lymphocyte aggregation or lymphocytes and neutrophils, respectively.

Pupillary miosis is often observed.

Management of anterior uveitis involves addressing the underlying cause, which may be infectious or autoimmune. Treatment typically includes corticosteroids to reduce inflammation and cycloplegic agents to relieve pain and prevent synechiae formation. Early diagnosis and appropriate treatment are crucial to prevent complications and preserve vision.

Intermediate uveitis is an inflammation centred on the vitreous specifically involving the pars plana, peripheral retina and vitreous body. Patients usually experience little pain but complain of floaters and blurred vision. It is associated with systemic diseases, such as multiple sclerosis or sarcoidosis, and infections, including Epstein–Barr virus and Lyme disease.

Posterior uveitis is the inflammation of the posterior part of the uveal tract, and managing patients with acute posterior uveitis remains a challenge. Vision may be acutely endangered. There are a great variety of aetiologies, and therapy is based mainly on systemic application—with all the risk that might be associated with it. In particular, the distinction between an infectious cause and a presumed autoimmune response is important since it will determine subsequent treatment. However, even an experienced clinician may be confused by certain manifestations such as syphilis ("The Great Mimicker") or intraocular lymphoma, as a masquerade syndrome. Because the clinical reaction to an inflammatory stimulus is limited, there is a common pattern that follows the general principles of inflammation:

Cellular infiltration of the vitreous
Retinochoroidal inflammation (infiltration)

DOI: 10.1201/9781003606789-6

Vasculitis

Exudative changes (either as circumscribed oedema—such as macular oedema, or papilloedema—or extensive, such as complete exudative retinal detachment)

Pan uveitis refers to inflammation that affects all parts of the uveal tract. Symptoms include a red painful eye, blurred vision, photophobia and floaters. Treatment depends on whether the cause is infectious or non-infectious.

INTRODUCTION

Uveitis is a relatively common inflammatory eye disease with an annual incidence between 17 and 52.4 per 100,000 person-years and prevalence between 38 and 370 per 100,000. It is the most common form of inflammatory eye diseases and an important cause of visual impairment and blindness. Given that uveitis predominantly affects the young adult population in their most productive years, the personal and socio-economic burden is significant.

The classification of intraocular inflammation is commonly described by the anatomical location of the primary site of inflammation. This relatively simple classification system has proven to be beneficial since it may provide clues on the association with an underlying aetiology.

1) Anterior uveitis
2) Intermediate uveitis
3) Posterior uveitis
4) Panuveitis

1) Anterior Uveitis

Anterior uveitis is the most frequent form of intraocular inflammation that involves the iris and ciliary body (Figures 5.1 and 5.2). Uveitis presents with a gradual onset of moderate ocular pain often localized to the distribution of the ophthalmic branch of the trigeminal nerve (V1), which is exacerbated on induced pupillary constriction (direct, near or consensual). Patients will also complain of photophobia, redness, tearing and reduced vision of variable degree [1] (refer to College of Optometrists' CMGs for—Uveitis (anterior)).

There is conjunctival injection and a characteristic limbal flush due to the congestion of perilimbal episcleral vessels.

The protein content of the aqueous humour is increased by a rise in vessel permeability and detected as an aqueous flare in the beam of the slit lamp. This may give rise to a secondary open-angle glaucoma. A fibrin coagulum may be present, particularly in HLA-B27+ individuals. Inflammatory cells circulating in the thermal currents of the aqueous may be deposited in acute cyclitis as keratic precipitates on the corneal endothelium with widespread opacities in the vitreous. These precipitates may damage the corneal endothelium and cause corneal haze due to stromal and epithelial oedema.

Precipitates have been described as granulomatous (mutton fat) or non-granulomatous (fine, stellate) and have been considered as a different type of cellular infiltrate. Granulomatous deposits may consist of macrophage and lymphocyte aggregation, whereas lymphocytes and neutrophils are considered non-granulomatous. Pupillary miosis is due to a sensory reflex and the release of

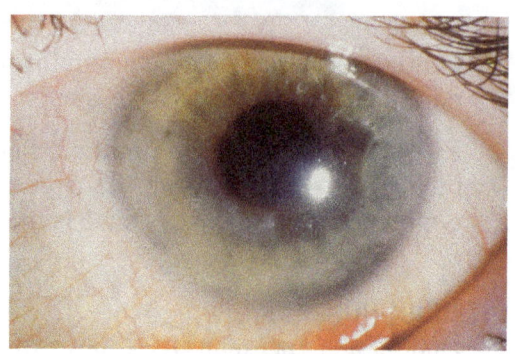

FIGURE 5.1 Acute uveitis with ciliary injection and fibrin exudation due to an autoimmune aetiology.

Source: (Seal D, Pleyer U. Ocular Infection, 2nd Edition 2007)

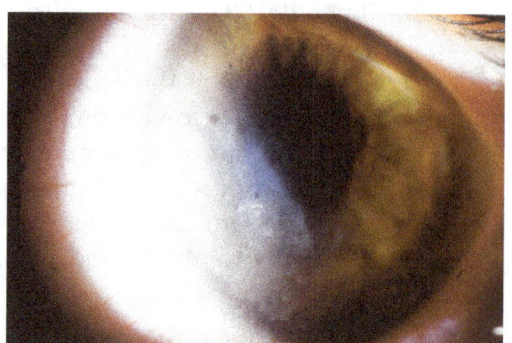

FIGURE 5.2 Acute uveitis (high magnification).

inflammatory mediators, but on dilatation, the pupil may become irregular at the site of posterior synechiae. A small, irregular pupil on presentation may remain following previous inflammation.

Aetiology

The cause of acute uveitis is often not established, but patients are investigated for both infectious and autoimmune aetiologies. Anterior uveitis may be part of a systemic illness, such as spondylo-arthropathy. It may also arise from an infection, such as *herpes simplex*; be part of an ocular syndrome, such as Fuchs' uveitis syndrome; be part of trauma, as in cataract surgery; or result from an idiopathic eye disease with a presumed immune pathogenesis.

The Standardisation of Uveitis Nomenclature (SUN) working group has developed an international standard for classifying uveitis (https://www.college-optometrists.org/clinical-guidance/clinical-management-guidelines):

Onset: sudden (acute) or insidious
Duration: limited ≤ 3 months or persistent > 3 months
Recurrent: repeated episodes separated by periods of inactivity without treatment ≥ 3 months
Chronic: persistent—characterized by relapse in < 3 months after stopping therapy

Non-Infectious Anterior Uveitis

In Europe and North America, up to 50% of patients with anterior uveitis are HLA-B27+. The clinical presentation of uveitis in patients associated with ankylosing spondylitis (AS) or reactive arthritis (ReA) is relatively consistent. Most patients present with acute onset of inflammation. The inflammation is active in one eye, but the attacks tend to recur, often in the contralateral eye. Intraocular pressure is often lower in the affected eye.

Infectious Anterior Uveitis

Several studies emphasize the role of herpes viruses in the aetiology of anterior (and posterior) uveitis. In fact, the number of patients affected by viral infection may be underestimated. In a prospective study of 110 patients analysing aqueous humour samples, viral infections were present in 15% with a predominance of HSV. In another investigation, intraocular antibody synthesis was positive for HSV in 23.5% of patients.

This high incidence may be biased by patient selection and referral pattern; however, it indicates that herpes viruses are an important cause of anterior uveitis *often in the absence* of keratitis.

Herpes viruses demonstrate some similar clinical patterns, such as unilateral non-granulomatous or granulomatous iritis or iridocyclitis, iris atrophy, increased intraocular pressure (IOP) and a high tendency to recur. They have been associated with other entities, such as Posner-Schlossman syndrome [12].

Herpes Simplex Virus (HSV)

The condition presents with recurrent non-granulomatous or granulomatous iritis or iridocyclitis in the absence of keratitis. Keratic precipitates and iris atrophy are frequently present. Often, increased IOP is seen caused by trabeculitis. Analysis of aqueous humour by polymerase chain reaction (PCR) or local antibody synthesis is helpful to differentiate the infectious cause from other diagnoses.

Varicella Zoster Virus (VZV)

Intraocular inflammation caused by VZV can present as zoster *sine herpete* (without cutaneous vesicles) or as reactivation in chickenpox or herpes zoster ophthalmicus.

Anterior uveitis caused by zoster *sine herpete* is infrequently reported and affects otherwise healthy, immunocompetent individuals. Clinical hints for the diagnosis include unilateral iritis or iridocyclitis, increased IOP, iridoplegia and sectorial iris atrophy. Hypopyon and hyphema may occur.

Histopathology demonstrates vasculitis, necrosis and lymphocyte infiltration in both iris and ciliary body. Intraocular inflammation may become recurrent and result in posterior synechia, cataract formation and secondary glaucoma. More frequently, uveitis can be observed in patients affected by herpes zoster ophthalmicus. It has been reported in approximately 50% of immunocompetent and immunocompromised patients.

The clinical presentation is similar to VZV uveitis *sine herpete* but is accompanied by cutaneous vesicles. Herpetic kerato-uveitis should be differentiated into either stromal or disciform types since it requires additional corticosteroids, whereas isolated anterior uveitis responds to (systemic) antiviral treatment. Often, the diagnosis can be based on clinical grounds, but in patients suspicious for "VZV uveitis *sine herpete*," aqueous or vitreous viral PCR (Appendix 5) or antibody analysis is helpful.

Cytomegalovirus (CMV)

CMV is typically associated with retinitis but recently has been shown associated with anterior uveitis. Clinical presentation and symptoms are similar to those associated with other viruses of the herpes family. In some patients, multiple fine stellate-shaped endothelial precipitates have been described as characteristic. A spillover from the posterior chamber in CMV retinitis is important to rule out. As in the previous infections, aqueous humour analysis for CMV is helpful to establish the diagnosis.

Bacterial Infections

Isolated cases of anterior uveitis due to bacteria are rare. Spontaneous, acute anterior uveitis is usually associated with systemic infection, such as syphilis, borreliosis, tuberculosis, cat scratch disease, Whipple's disease or others. In these patients, it is often not clear whether the infectious cause is directly related to intraocular inflammation or due to an associated immune response. The frequent association of anterior uveitis with gastrointestinal infection with Gram-negative bacteria—such as those of salmonella and shigella from a recent infection, such as diarrhoea, particularly in HLA-B27+ individuals—has raised the question whether it is directly linked or indirectly associated with a low-grade infection. Although intraocular antibodies have been detected in some patients, no direct evidence for intraocular infection can be provided in most cases, suggesting molecular mimicry (refer later).

Uveitis can also be due to an immune reaction to circulating microbial antigens, such as yersinia, or chlamydia, associated with urethritis. Occasionally, it presents following a sore throat caused by *Streptococcus pyogenes* in a patient of genetic predisposition, such as possessing the HLA-B27+ marker. Precise pathogenesis is not clear but may involve molecular mimicry by bacterial antigens cross-reacting with ocular and synovial tissue, also giving rise to arthropathies, with deposition of circulating cell wall antigens in tissue. Treatment in the latter case involves anti-inflammatory drugs rather than anti-infectives since the intact microbe is usually eradicated from the patient at the time of presentation.

Spirochetal Infection   Anterior and, more frequently, posterior uveitis can be caused by spirochetal infection including *Treponema pallidum* (syphilis) and *Borrelia burgdorferi* (Lyme's disease). Severe uveitis can be due to syphilis, diagnosed by a serology test for *T. pallidum*, when systemic treatment is given with penicillin for two weeks.

Mycobacterial Infection   Uveitis can also be associated with mycobacterial infection. Active tuberculosis may cause a tuberculous iritis due to *live* bacilli within a granulomatous reaction. In the early stages, there are minute, gray and translucent iris nodules and, at a later stage, a yellowish nodule surrounded by numerous satellite lesions. The presence of keratic precipitates indicates involvement of the ciliary body. Pseudohypopyon composed of caseating material may occur.

If the iritis is exudative rather than granular, then it may be due to an inflammatory response to circulating antigen similar to the phlyctena response (Chapter 6).

If a mycobacterial infection is suspected, patients require intensive investigation. Anterior uveitis also accompanies leprosy. Lepromatous leprosy causes more severe disease than the tuberculoid variety; systemic treatment is required.

Parasitic Infection In onchocerciasis, inflammation of part or all of the uvea occurs when microfilariae penetrate the sclera and can result in blindness from secondary glaucoma, optic nerve atrophy or phthisis bulbi (refer to Chapter 7). Toxoplasmosis is the most common cause of infectious posterior uveitis and, although rarely, it can also present as anterior uveitis.

Treatment
Initiate therapy of intense topical corticosteroids, using prednisolone 1% or dexamethasone 0.1% drops (Appendix 1) hourly, until the inflammation is controlled. Also give a topical cycloplegic after first checking for possibility of angle closure using cyclopentolate 1% tds for up to seven days.

Make a prompt review within three days and if the uveitis is responding well to treatment, then reduce the topical steroid to every two hours for five days and start tapering off over not less than six weeks. If no improvement occurs in one week, refer to an ophthalmologist. The IOP should be monitored due to the risk of steroid-induced ocular hypertension [2] (refer to College of Optometrists' CMGs for—see Steroid-related ocular hypertension and glaucoma).

2) Intermediate Uveitis (IU)
This involves the posterior ciliary body (pars plana) and the anterior choroid. IU primarily affects the vitreous and peripheral retina, often involving the ciliary body and the area just behind it. It is associated with systemic diseases, such as multiple sclerosis or sarcoidosis, and infections, including Epstein–Barr virus and Lyme disease. It is characterized by an inflammation in the vitreous causing dense floaters and blurred vision. It occurs most commonly in young adults and can affect both eyes simultaneously. IU may be chronic, persisting for more than three months, and can recur. Treatment methodologies may include corticosteroids and/or immunosuppressants.

3) Posterior Uveitis

Introduction
Symptoms in patients with posterior uveitis are relatively uniform but may depend on the morphological manifestations, including the following:

Floaters
Blurring of vision
Impaired vision
Metamorphopsia

Anatomy and Vascular Supply
The retina, which lines the choroid, has two layers of epithelium. The anterior epithelium of the iris is continuous with the outer epithelial layer of the ciliary body, and this is continued into the pigment epithelium of the retina, a single

layer of hexagonal cells lying immediately adjacent to Bruch's membrane next to the choroid.

The posterior epithelium of the iris, which is pigmented, passes into the inner non-pigmented layer of the ciliary body, which changes at the ora serrata into the neurosensory retina. This consists of three strata of cells:

(i) The visual cells lying externally (rods and cones).
(ii) A relay of bipolar cells (the outer plexiform layer), whose synapses form the inner and outer plexiform layers.
(iii) A layer of ganglion cells lying internally with, innermost, the nerve fibre layer composed of ganglion cell axons running centrally into the optic nerve. These neural cells are bound together by neuroglia with a supportive and nutritive function.

The arteries of the eye are derived from the ophthalmic artery, which is a branch of the internal carotid. Most of the venous return passes to the cavernous sinus, although there are lesser anastomoses within the orbit. The retina is supplied by the central retinal artery, which divides on the surface of the disc into the main retinal trunks. These are end arteries and have no anastomoses at the ora serrata. The uveal tract is supplied by the ciliary arteries.

Posterior uveitis refers to inflammation of the retina and/or choroid. When the inflammation originates in the choroid, it can spread to the adjacent retina, resulting in retinochoroiditis. It may be due to *bacteraemia, fungaemia, or larva migrans* and evolve into endophthalmitis. More commonly, *there is a non-purulent chronic granulomatous reaction*. The commonest causes of retinochoroiditis in Europe are due to *Toxoplasma gondii* infection and larva migrans from a *Toxocara canis* infection [3].

Parasitic Infections

Toxoplasma Retinochoroiditis

The intracellular protozoan parasite, *Toxoplasma gondii*, found in cats, pigs and most mammals is the commonest cause of posterior uveitis, accounting for approximately 10% of all cases [4]. It is excreted as oocysts by cats and ingested by humans from fecal contamination [5]. The cyst also resides in muscles of many animals and infects those eating raw or undercooked meat, especially pork. The infection can be congenital or acquired and is widespread in many parts of the world, with seroconversion rates up to 70%, although most of the human population remains asymptomatic.

Upon ingestion, sporozoites released from oocysts, or bradyzoites released from tissue cysts, infect human intestinal epithelial cells. These rapidly proliferate into tachyzoites, causing cell lysis and dissemination throughout host tissues, producing the acute phase of clinical disease. In response to host immunity, tachyzoites differentiate into slow-replicating bradyzoites within tissue cysts, establishing a chronic, latent infection. This stage is characterized by limited pathogenicity but lifelong persistence. Immunosuppression can trigger bradyzoite-to-tachyzoite conversion, resulting in reactivation of infection, cellular damage and clinical manifestations [4].

Acute infection is typically asymptomatic in immunocompetent individuals, but cervical lymphadenopathy or ocular disease, including anterior uveitis, can occur; it is followed by asymptomatic latent infection, during which the parasite encysts in various organs, including cardiac and skeletal muscles, brain parenchyma and retina. Latent infection can reactivate locally in the retina after many years, leading to significant loss of visual acuity (Figure 5.3). In pregnant women, acute infection acquired during or shortly before gestation can lead to congenital toxoplasmosis with fetal abnormalities, even though the mother remains asymptomatic.

Recurrent retinochoroiditis usually presents as a yellow inflammatory lesion, resulting in an overlying vitreous haze, at the margin of a pre-existing choroidal scar (Figure 5.4).

Another presentation is a juxtapapillary lesion at the margin of the optic disc, which causes a typical arcuate field defect. Small peripheral retinal lesions may be allowed to run their course, but lesions near the macula, optic disc or maculopapular nerve fibre bundle or those associated with severe vitritis should be treated.

Therapy is directed against both the dividing organism and the inflammatory host response. The problem is complicated by multiplication of the protozoan within "tissue cysts" within cells, which are impervious to drug penetration, so that recurrence can always be expected.

Toxoplasma infection is encountered in immunocompromised patients. The differential diagnosis of tuberculosis must always be considered. Atypical cases of toxoplasmosis are more frequently reported at a higher age and may mimic acute retinal necrosis.

The diagnosis is clinical, based on the characteristic fundus lesion and often marked by vitreous infiltration. Intraocular detection of toxoplasma is identified by PCR (Appendix 5) on a vitreous tap or retinal biopsy or by detecting specific local antibody, using a ratio between anterior chamber (aqueous) and serum levels. Direct evidence of *T. gondii* DNA in the intraocular fluids is more reliable because of the high seroconversion rate in many parts of the world.

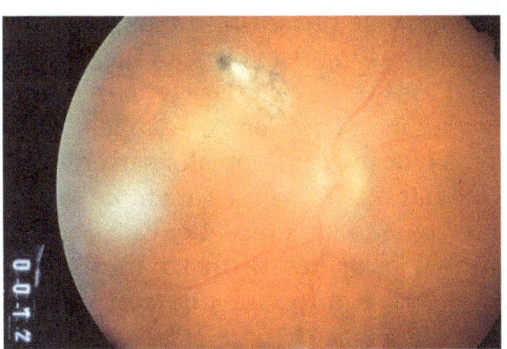

FIGURE 5.3 Acute chorioretinitis due to toxoplasma showing a new lesion and an old scarred lesion.

Source: (Seal D, Pleyer U. Ocular Infection, 2nd Edition 2007)

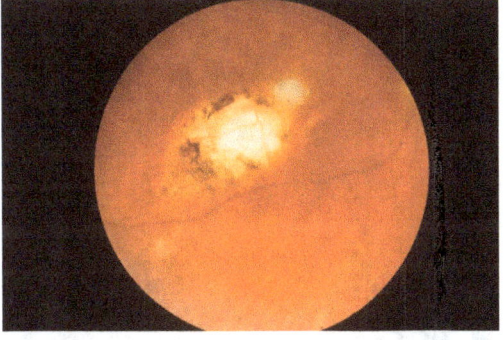

FIGURE 5.4 Active toxoplasmosis within a peripheral healed scar.

Source: (Seal D, Pleyer U. Ocular Infection, 2nd Edition 2007)

Treatment of systemic toxoplasmosis includes combinations of two antimicrobials, most often inhibitors of dihydrofolate reductase (DHFR) (pyrimethamine and trimethoprim) and dihydropteroate synthetase (sulfonamides, such as sulfadiazine, sulfamethoxazole and sulfadoxine), which block folic acid synthesis. Pyrimethamine, a key DHFR inhibitor, appears to be the most effective drug against *T. gondii* and is the basis for effective regimens. These include pyrimethamine-sulfadiazine, the gold standard against which other regimens are measured, and pyrimethamine combined with clindamycin, atovaquone, clarithromycin or azithromycin (refer to Appendix 6) [6].

Other regimens include trimethoprim in combination with sulfamethoxazole (co-trimoxazole) and atovaquone alone or in combination with sulfadiazine. Tetracycline is effective against the parasite, but it is often used in combination with other medications, viz. pyrimethamine and sulfonamides, for better efficacy, especially in immunocompromised patients. Secondary prophylaxis with trimethoprim-sulfamethoxazole, administered three times weekly for at least 12 months, can significantly reduce the risk of recurrence in ocular toxoplasmosis, especially in patients with central lesions or frequent relapses.

Unfortunately, all drugs used in clinical practice are only active against the tachyzoite stage of the parasite and have no activity against cysts containing bradyzoites, the latent stage of the parasite. No problem has occurred with drug resistance.

For toxocariasis, refer to Supplementary Chapter S5.
For ocular onchocerciasis, refer to Chapter 7.

Bacterial Infections
Brucellosis

Infection arises from unpasteurized milk, with *Brucella abortus* from the cow or *B. melitensis* from the goat. Initially, there is an acute phase of generalized fever and systemic disease with leukopenia, a relative lymphocytosis and a slightly enlarged liver and/or spleen. This is followed by a subacute phase with intermittent bouts of low-grade fever when the ocular manifestations can appear with reduced visual acuity from a chorioretinitis. A chronic granulomatous uveitis can also be present with secondary glaucoma. Ocular manifestations are more severe after a *B. melitensis* infection than after *B. abortus*, although the latter causes more severe systemic symptoms. Typically, the retinal lesion has distinct margins with a hemorrhage around it; it contains live bacilli that require antibiotic treatment by the systemic route (Figure 5.5).

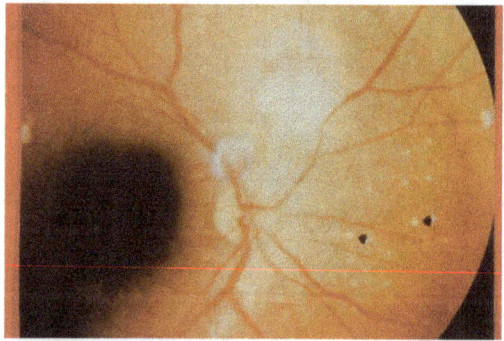

FIGURE 5.5 Acute chorioretinitis caused by *Brucella melitensis*—pale-yellow dots (black arrows)—is similar to that seen in tuberculosis, being foci of inflammation around live bacteria.

Source: (Seal D, Pleyer U. Ocular Infection, 2nd Edition 2007)

However, uveitis is the most common form of eye involvement. Patients living in endemic areas, such as Iran, who develop uveitis should be investigated for brucellosis [7]. Retinal biopsy and a PCR test gives definitive results.

Standard treatment is given with rifampin 600–900 mg/day and doxycycline 100 mg twice daily and, in case of eye involvement, with local and systemic corticosteroids for 2–4 weeks [7]. However, later appearance of retinochoroiditis can be treated with ofloxacin 800 mg and rifampicin 900 mg orally daily. During treatment, serial fundus examinations should be performed weekly, and progressive improvement should occur over six weeks when the choroidal lesion leaves a scar and the retinal lesion disappears (Figure 5.6). Occasionally, papillitis and retrobulbar neuritis can be present.

Tuberculosis—caused by Mycobacterium tuberculosis (also known as Koch's bacillus)

Ocular tuberculosis (OTB) is a rare manifestation of tuberculosis (TB) that can affect any part of the eye, including the conjunctiva, cornea, sclera and uveal tract. It is often associated with hematogenous spread from a primary focus but can also occur as a primary infection following an epithelial injury. The incidence of OTB has been increasing over the years, with a significant rise observed between 2010 and 2019. Despite the overall decrease in TB cases, the proportion of OTB among extrapulmonary TB cases has grown. OTB is more likely to be diagnosed in older individuals and those with diabetes. It is less likely to be laboratory confirmed compared to other forms of extrapulmonary TB, but patients are more likely to be tested by interferon gamma release assay (IGRA) and to be IGRA positive (Appendix 5).

Tuberculosis can affect any part of the uveal tract. Tuberculous choroiditis occurs in miliary and chronic disease. Miliary tubercles can be seen especially in tuberculous meningitis and used to be common at a late stage in children. The choroiditis appears as round, pale-yellow spots and vary in number from 3 to 70. They consist of giant cells around live bacilli. Before chemotherapy, their presence was a prelude to death, but recovery is now common with triple antituberculous therapy for a minimum of six months. A recent comparative study on OTB could not find an overall different clinical outcome in patients from endemic or non-endemic areas (Indonesia versus Netherlands) with the overall treatment outcomes comparable [8]. Choroidal tubercles (pale-yellow spots) can be an early sign of miliary tuberculosis, appearing before other systemic symptoms become apparent. They are visible during a fundus examination and can help to make an earlier diagnosis of miliary disease.

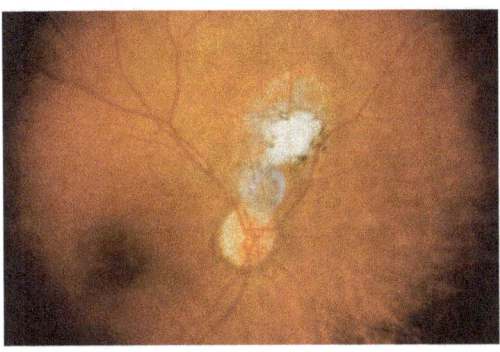

FIGURE 5.6 *Brucella melitensis* after successful treatment showing scarring.

Source: (Seal D, Pleyer U. Ocular Infection, 2nd Edition 2007)

OTB presents as raised lesions in active tuberculous chorioretinitis (Figure 5.7) or as a diffuse flat lesion if undergoing anti-tuberculous chemotherapy (Figure 5.8).

The healed lesion closely resembles that caused by toxoplasmosis (Figure 5.9). Disseminated choroiditis can occur with extensive development of granulomatous tissue, and (rarely) it can appear as a solitary mass resembling a neoplasm, such as a retinoblastoma or pseudoglioma.

A particular subtype of OTB may present as serpiginous-like choroiditis (Figure 5.10), a progressive type of posterior uveitis often leading to significant visual impairment [9].

This condition is characterized by the presence of serpentine-like lesions that spread from the optic disc towards the periphery of the retina. Active tuberculosis can exacerbate the inflammation, causing more extensive damage to the retinal and choroidal tissues. The diagnosis is based on clinical examination, imaging studies

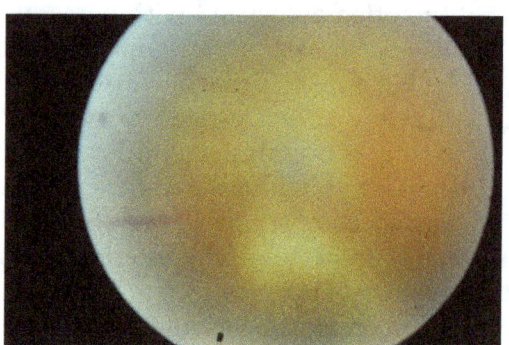

FIGURE 5.7 Active tuberculous chorioretinitis with raised pale-yellow lesions.

Source: (Seal D, Pleyer U. Ocular Infection, 2nd Edition 2007)

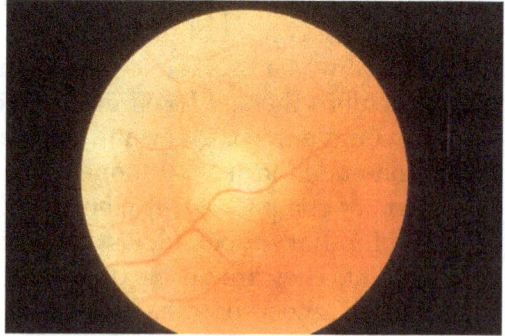

FIGURE 5.8 Choroidal tubercle healing on chemotherapy showing a flat lesion and loss of vessels.

Source: (Seal D, Pleyer U. Ocular Infection, 2nd Edition 2007)

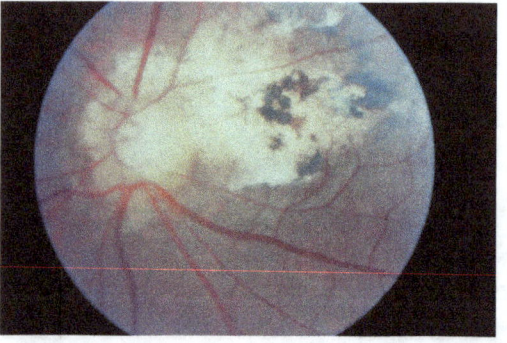

FIGURE 5.9 Extensive chorioretinal scar of healed tuberculosis.

Source: (Seal D, Pleyer U. Ocular Infection, 2nd Edition 2007)

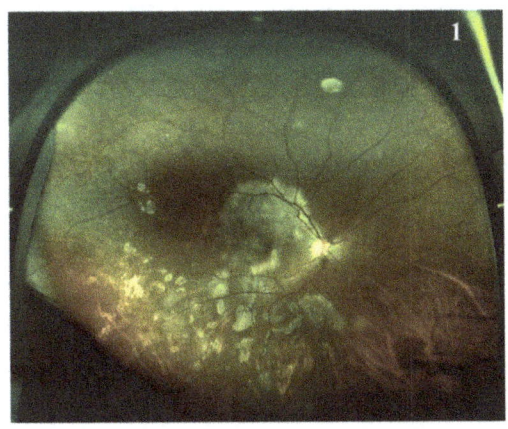

FIGURE 5.10 Serpiginous-like choroiditis due to *Mycobacterium tuberculosis*.

Source: (Courtesy of Drs. R. Bansal and V. Gupta)

and laboratory tests to exclude/confirm the presence of *Mycobacterium tuberculosis* (MTb). The exact mechanism is not clear but is due to a direct or indirect infectious trigger by MTb-causing choroiditis as an immuno-inflammatory reaction. The link of immune mechanisms with ocular inflammation caused by MTb is emerging and has been supported by both experimental and human data [9].

Treatment includes anti-tubercular therapy to address the underlying infection and corticosteroids to manage the inflammation. Early detection and prompt treatment are crucial to prevent severe visual loss and complications. Therapy is given with three anti-tuberculous drugs in association with specialist advice.

Syphilis (caused by the spirochaete *Treponema pallidum*)

Syphilis has regained importance because of reduced testing during the COVID-19 pandemic, a shift in sexual behaviours and a shortage of Penicillin G benzathine. Since late stages of the infection have a major impact on life quality and specific treatment is available, early detection is important. Both syphilis and borreliosis are caused by spirochetes that share some similarities with their presentation. Both may cause interstitial keratitis and anterior and posterior uveitis and are often accompanied by neural involvement of the peripheral or central nervous system [10].

For syphilis and borreliosis (Lyme disease), refer to Supplementary Chapter S5.

Viral Infections

Acute Retinal Necrosis (ARN) Syndrome

Acute necrotizing retinitis is a disorder caused by viruses of the herpes family (VZV, HSV, CMV). A set of criteria for diagnosis has been established that include the typical retinal necrosis features with a characteristic demarcation line. ARN has been described in both immunocompetent and immunosuppressed individuals. The clinical features differ according to immune status. Herpes zoster and H. simplex have been implicated more frequently in immunocompetent patients. HSV-associated ARN occurs in an earlier age group and is more frequently associated with the HSV-2 type. ARN tends to follow shingles in older patients.

ARN is characterized by a *rapid onset of painless loss of vision with areas of necrotizing retinitis*, often peripheral, which enlarge and coalesce.

There is marked vasculitis, macular oedema and acute optic neuritis. A prodromal phase with flu-like symptoms is common. The anterior segment is usually involved and may even mislead the diagnosis if pupil dilation is not performed and *the peripheral lesion overlooked. Mutton fat keratic precipitates, cells in the anterior chamber and elevated intraocular pressure are common.*

Prompt treatment with famciclovir (500 mg orally every eight hours) tapered slowly over 3–4 months as first-line therapy, or intravenous aciclovir at 500–800 mg/m2 eight-hourly for seven days (followed by 800 mg five times daily orally for 3–4 months) as second-line therapy, is effective in halting the progression of the infection and may prevent involvement of the other eye. Famciclovir has good bioavailability and is effective against aciclovir-resistant H. simplex.

Antiviral drugs, ganciclovir (200–2,000 ug per 0.1 mL) or foscarnet (1.2–2.4 mg per 0.1 mL), administered intravitreally can provide beneficial adjunctive therapy, especially if retinitis is threatening the macula or optic disc.

Corticosteroid (prednisone [0.5–2.0 mg/kg/day orally for up to six to eight weeks]) may have a beneficial therapeutic effect if initiated 24–48 hours after the start of antiviral therapy or once regression of retinal necrosis has been demonstrated.

Aspirin may minimize vascular thrombosis and propagation of further retinal ischaemia and necrosis. Topical corticosteroid drops and cycloplegics have been shown beneficial if there is anterior segment inflammation.

The outcome, however, may be poor. Occlusive vasculitis with optic neuropathy, macular oedema and retinal detachment are frequent and severely limit the outcome.

Acquired Immunodeficiency Syndrome (AIDS)

AIDS is treated nowadays with highly active antiretroviral therapy [11]. Human immunodeficiency virus (HIV), which causes AIDS, has been identified in tear fluid, conjunctival and corneal epithelium and the retina, but the principal ophthalmic manifestations of AIDS relate to the occurrence of florid opportunistic infections and to conjunctival and orbital involvement with Kaposi's sarcoma (Figure 5.11) and other neoplasms. Therapy is directed against the relevant organism and is prolonged compared to immunocompetent patients.

HIV, in the absence of other organisms, can cause a characteristic retinitis due to microvasculopathy of cotton wool spots, hemorrhages ("flame-shaped" in the nerve fibre layer or "dot-shaped" deeper in the retina) and microaneurysms (Figure 5.12). Macular exudates and oedema with optic neuropathy can occur. These forms of HIV retinopathy do not generally interfere with vision.

Cytomegalovirus is the commonest opportunistic ocular infection and produces a haemorrhagic necrotizing retinitis (Figure 5.13).

CMV retinitis is found in about 20% of terminal AIDS patients and is bilateral in about 17%, when the delay from presentation with HIV infection is shorter.

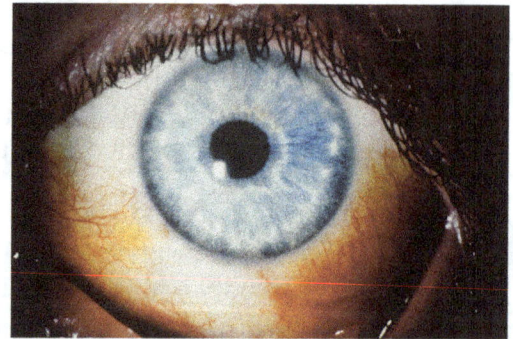

FIGURE 5.11 Kaposi's sarcoma in the conjunctiva in an HIV-positive patient.

Source: (Seal D, Pleyer U. Ocular Infection, 2nd Edition 2007)

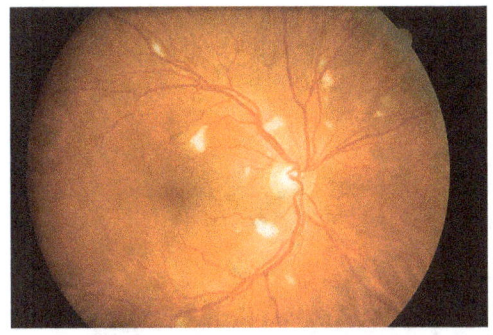

FIGURE 5.12 HIV microvasculopathy with white "cotton wool" spots and flame-shaped haemorrhages.

Source: (Seal D, Pleyer U. Ocular Infection, 2nd Edition 2007)

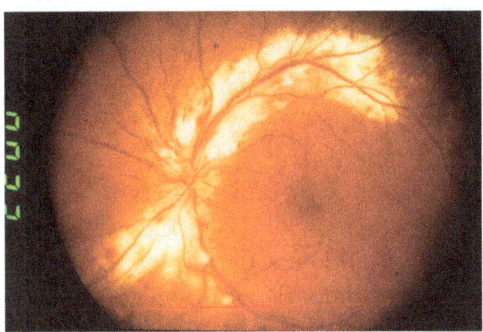

FIGURE 5.13 "Pizza pie" retinitis of severe CMV infection above and below the optic disc in an AIDS patient.

Source: (Seal D, Pleyer U. Ocular Infection, 2nd Edition 2007)

Occasionally, H. simplex virus, Epstein–Barr virus and toxoplasma cause clinically similar retinitis. CMV retinitis may also present in HIV disease in the absence of a severe depletion in the CD4 lymphocyte count.

Patients with CMV retinitis complain of visual field defects, flashing lights and symptoms of "floaters." If the central retina or optic nerve is involved, they complain of a reduction in visual acuity. CMV causes diffuse, full thickness retinitis that is sharply demarcated from the adjacent normal retina. It can present as a fulminant retinitis with yellow-white areas of necrosis surrounded by hemorrhages ("pizza pie" retinitis – Figure 5.13) or as a "granular" retinitis, in which hemorrhages are not a feature and may be absent. Both types follow a similar clinical course and may coexist together in the same eye.

Progression of CMV retinitis may be delayed in the short term by intravenous therapy with either ganciclovir or foscarnet, or the combination. Repeated intravitreal therapy is more effective and particularly valuable when there are no signs of disseminated CMV disease. The development of slow-release, intraocular implant systems for ganciclovir had provided further improvements in management but are no longer available. The prophylactic use of oral ganciclovir in persons with advanced AIDS has significantly reduced the risk of CMV, but active retinitis can still occur.

Fungal infections—refer to Chapter 7.
Non-infectious causes of posterior uveitis—refer to Supplementary Chapter S5
Acute posterior multifocal placoid pigment epitheliopathy (APMPPE) due to M. tuberculosis
Leber's idiopathic stellate neuroretinitis
Multiple evanescent white dot syndrome

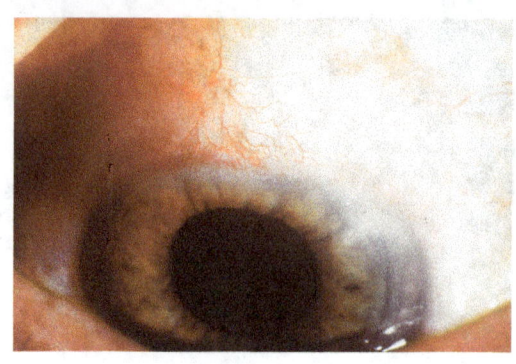

FIGURE 5.14 Panuveitis.

4) Panuveitis

The International Uveitis Study Group (IUSG) defines panuveitis as generalized inflammation of all three parts of the uvea (iris, ciliary body and choroid); in addition, the retina, vitreous, optic nerve or lens may be involved.

The cause is often unknown but includes exogenous or endogenous infection, injury with a perforating wound or an autoimmune disease. Possible endogenous infections include syphilis, tuberculosis, mumps and influenza. Other causes include immune-mediated conditions, such as Behcet syndrome. Secondary infection or trauma from cataract, glaucoma or vitreoretinal surgery can also cause panuveitis.

Symptoms include pain, light sensitivity, discharge, blurred vision, flashes and floaters. All parts of the uveal tract will be inflamed, yielding the diagnosis with evidence of anterior uveitis (iridocyclitis) and choroiditis (Figure 5.14). Slit lamp examination shows vitreous and aqueous cells, flare and keratic precipitates.

If there is an underlying cause, specific treatment should be given. Non-specific treatment includes cycloplegics, corticosteroids and immunosuppressive drugs. Biologic drugs currently used include anti-tumour necrosis factor, cytokine receptor antibodies and interferon-α.

REFERENCES

1. College of Optometrists. Clinical Management Guidelines. Uveitis (Anterior)—College of Optometrists 2025. Accessed 03/09/25.
2. College of Optometrists. Clinical Management Guidelines. Steroid-Related Ocular Hypertension and Glaucoma 2025. Accessed 03/09/25.
3. Gupta A et al. Ocular Toxocariasis. Statpearls [Internet]. PMID: 35015409. Last update 25/08/2023. Accessed 28/05/2025 (https://www.ncbi.nlm.nih.gov/books/NBK576384/).
4. Miyagaki M et al. Pathogens 2024. PMID: 39452769 (https://pmc.ncbi.nlm.nih.gov/articles/PMC11509995/).
5. Attias M et al. Parasit Vectors 2020. PMID: 33228743 (http://doi.org/10.1186/s13071-020-04445-z).
6. Yogeswaran K, Furtado JM, Bodaghi B, Matthews JM; International Ocular Toxoplasmosis Study Group; Smith JR. Current Practice in the Management of Ocular Toxoplasmosis. Br J Ophthalmol 2023 Jul;107(7): 973–979. Epub 2022 Feb 23. PMID: 35197262 (http://doi.org/10.1136/bjophthalmol-2022-321091).
7. Ghasemi Barghi R et al. Iran Red Crescent Med J 2011. PMID: 22737494 (https://pmc.ncbi.nlm.nih.gov/articles/PMC3371975/).
8. Alli H et al. Surv Ophthalmol 2022. PMID: 34626620 (https://doi.org/10.1016/j.survophthal.2021.10.001).
9. Bansal R et al. J Ophthalmic Inflamm Inf 2022. PMID: 36352169 (https://joii-journal.springeropen.com/articles/10.1186/s12348-022-00312-3).
10. Piergiorgio N et al. J Ophth Inflamm and Inf 2022. PMID: 35192047 (https://https://doi.org/10.1186/s12348-022-00286-2).
11. Kemnic T et al. HIV Antiretroviral Therapy. StatPearls [Internet] 2022. PMID: 30020680. Accessed 25/05/2025.
12. Lenglinger M, Schick T, Pohlmann D, Pleyer U. Cytomegalovirus-Positive Posner-Schlossman Syndrome: Impact on Corneal Endothelial Cell Loss and Retinal Nerve Fiber Layer Thinning. Am J Ophthalmol. 2022 May;237:290-298. doi: 10.1016/j.ajo.2021.12.015. Epub 2022 Jan 5. PMID: 34998717.

6: Diagnosis and Treatment of Ocular Infection

For the drugs formulary, refer to Appendix 1, and for further guidance, consult the Clinical Management Guidelines (College of Optometrists) and Appendix 6 for specialist use.

CORE MESSAGES

This chapter describes the common ocular infections found in practice, for both the adnexa and globe, including bacteria, chlamydia, viruses and protozoa (*Acanthamoeba*) in adults and children; fungi are covered in Chapter 7.

While some infections are mild and self-limiting, viz. viral conjunctivitis, others cause extreme pain and suffering, viz. *Acanthamoeba. The latter is a good example of the need for early recognition to gain therapeutic success within one month rather than six to twelve months for a late diagnosis with various complications.* Images are included to enable early identification, both within the text and Supplementary Chapter S6.

Orbital Cellulitis

Infections affecting the periorbital and orbital tissues can vary in severity, ranging from mild, self-limiting conditions to serious, potentially life-threatening emergencies [1] (refer to College of Optometrists' CMGs for—Cellulitis, preseptal and orbital).

Orbital Cellulitis—Postseptal

Orbital cellulitis is a postseptal infection of the extraocular orbital contents presenting with sudden onset of unilateral pain on ocular movement, lid oedema (warm and tender), eyelid redness, ptosis, proptosis, fever, severe malaise and *diplopia due to impaired extraocular muscle function.* The condition commonly affects children, where spread to the orbit occurs across the thin orbital plate of the ethmoid bone. A few cases follow penetrating injury, or are secondary to panophthalmitis, but the majority occur in association with sinusitis.

Postseptal infection is an ophthalmic emergency and requires multidisciplinary management in hospital with appropriate cultures because of the risk of extension to the eye or cranial cavity. Subperiosteal abscess with displacement of the globe, or cavernous sinus thrombosis with headache and neck stiffness, can develop. Loculated pus must be drained. Delayed or inadequate treatment may lead to blindness or death. CT X-ray scan and magnetic resonance imaging (MRI) identify the extension of the infection into the soft tissues and orbit (but children may require anaesthesia) [2].

Pathogens from the sinuses include *Streptococcus pyogenes, Staphylococcus aureus, Haemophilus influenzae* and anaerobic bacteria if there is a chronic

DOI: 10.1201/9781003606789-7

sinusitis. Phycomycetes (fungi) may be involved in diabetic patients. Post-traumatic orbital cellulitis is often polymicrobial, including anaerobic bacteria, viz. *Clostridia sp.*

Systemic antibiotic therapy is required in large doses with co-amoxiclav combined with a quinolone (moxifloxacin or ciprofloxacin) or a combination of a cephalosporin and metronidazole. If extension occurs into the meninges, then antibiotics that penetrate into the central nervous system are required, such as cefotaxime, levofloxacin, chloramphenicol or rifampicin in high dosage.

Cellulitis—Periorbital (Preseptal)

Periorbital (preseptal) cellulitis may resemble postseptal cellulitis—an acute onset of swelling, redness and tenderness of the lids with fever (Figures 6.1 and 6.2). However, although intense lid swelling is present, the *presence of normal ocular movements and the absence of globe inflammation* distinguishes it from orbital cellulitis. The infection lies anteriorly to the orbital septum, but delay in therapy can allow extension to the orbit (orbital cellulitis). The differential diagnosis can be resolved by MRI. Preseptal cellulitis is associated with sinusitis, conjunctivitis, dacryocystitis and an infected injury.

Parenteral therapy is designed to cover the common causative organisms:

In adults: *St. aureus, Streptococcus pneumoniae, Streptococcus pyogenes* and *H. influenzae*. In children: *H. influenzae* is the commonest cause.

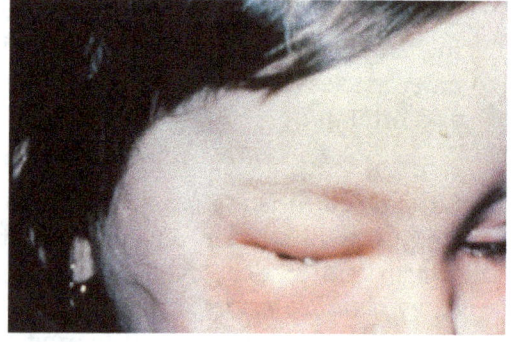

FIGURE 6.1 Periorbital (preseptal) cellulitis due to *Haemophilus influenzae*.

Source: (Seal D, Pleyer U. Ocular Infection, 2nd Edition 2007)

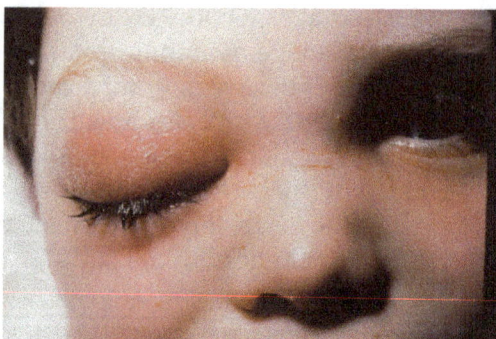

FIGURE 6.2 Periorbital (preseptal) cellulitis due to *Staphylococcus aureus*.

Co-amoxiclav or cefuroxime (for penicillin allergy) are drugs of choice to cover pathogens listed earlier, given in large dosage. In view of the emergence of multiple-resistant strains of *H. influenzae,* consideration should be given to the use of a 'third generation' cephalosporin, such as cefotaxime, particularly when the clinical response is poor or resistant organisms are isolated from nasal swabs.

In adults, therapy is directed against streptococci and *St. aureus* with high-dose intravenous benzylpenicillin alternating with flucloxacillin or, in advanced cases, clindamycin or vancomycin. Anaerobic cellulitis occurs following trauma, particularly with human or animal bites, and the latter can include infection by *Pasteurella sp.* or group G beta-hemolytic streptococci for which co-amoxiclav is used.

Necrotising Fasciitis of the Lid

This is due to infection by *Streptococcus pyogenes* above the fascial layer. It is serious and causes a spreading thrombosis of the overlying skin and subcutaneous tissue (Figure 6.3).

A CT scan (Figure 6.4) shows the inflammation and swelling exterior to the orbital contents.

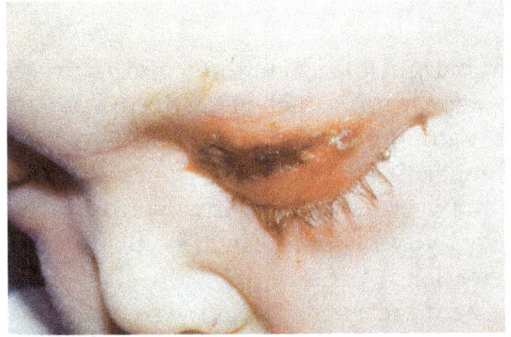

FIGURE 6.3 Necrotising fasciitis of the lid.

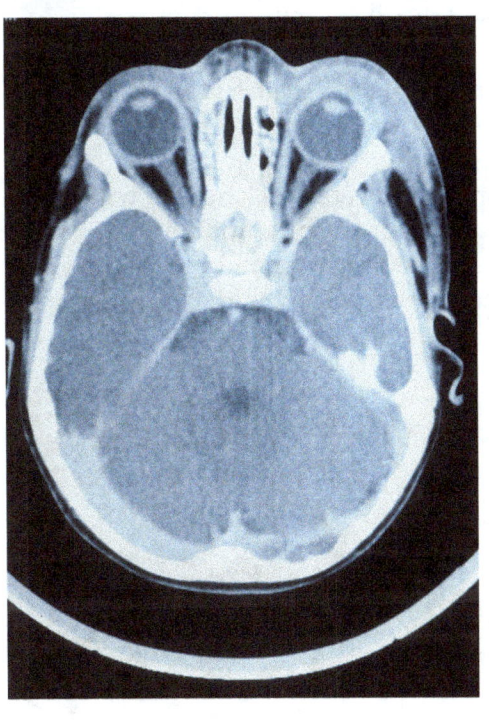

FIGURE 6.4 CT scan showing normal globe contents with inflammation exterior only.

Therapy includes large doses of penicillin and cloxacillin with drainage of the infection as required.

Blepharitis (Anterior)

Blepharitis is an inflammation of the lid margin, which may be anterior or posterior or mixed. Anterior blepharitis involves the lash line, while posterior blepharitis involves dysfunction of the meibomian glands. Both are associated with skin disease, including seborrhoea, atopy (allergy) and rosacea.

The term 'staphylococcal' blepharitis was coined by Thygeson 80 years ago to describe an anterior blepharitis with lash collarettes and crusting, lid ulceration and folliculitis (inflammation of eyelash follicles), associated with a positive culture for *St. aureus.* This syndrome does NOT include the isolation of coagulase-negative staphylococci (CNS), which are common skin commensals.

Symptoms include ocular discomfort, soreness, tearing, burning and itching. Blepharitis is diagnosed by clinical examination. The lid margin is examined with the slit lamp for evidence of folliculitis and collarettes. In the acute condition, there will be beads of pus and an ulcerated margin (Figure 6.5). When chronicity ensues, there is a loss or misdirection of lashes.

Blepharitis Due to *St. aureus*

Since *St. aureus* may colonise the normal lid margin (6–15%) without giving rise to blepharitis, it follows that positive culture alone is not sufficient for the diagnosis. 76% of patients with blepharitis associated with atopic dermatitis have a positive lid culture for *St. aureus*, and ulcerative blepharitis is almost entirely confined to patients in this group. The blepharitis of atopy presents in relative youth (19–31 years) and may wax and wane with the activity of the dermatitis. Blepharitis accompanying seborrhoeic dermatitis (refer later) preferentially affects young men in their second and third decades. Rosacea presents later, in the seventh and eighth decades, with a greater frequency in women.

St. aureus marginal ulcer presents with peripheral curvilinear infiltrates in the peripheral cornea, often where the lids cross the cornea, associated with loss of corneal epithelium; ulceration in the marginal zone *is separated from the limbus* by a clear corneal zone (Figure 6.6). It is an immuno-inflammatory reaction and not due to infection *per se.*

Autoimmune diseases can cause peripheral ulcerative keratitis with crescentic lesions, epithelial defect, thinning and stromal infiltration at the limbus with extension into the sclera. Mooren's ulcer is an autoimmune condition that presents with severe pain, photophobia and blurred vision, with circumferential

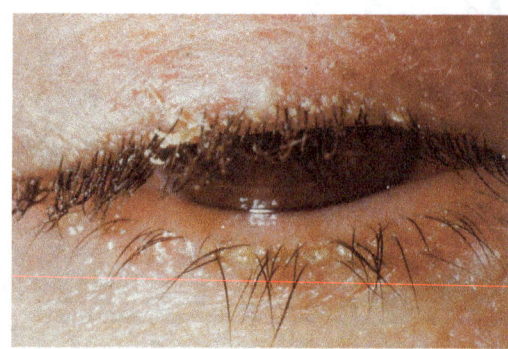

FIGURE 6.5 Severe folliculitis due to *St. aureus.*

Source: (Seal D, Pleyer U. Ocular Infection, 2nd Edition 2007)

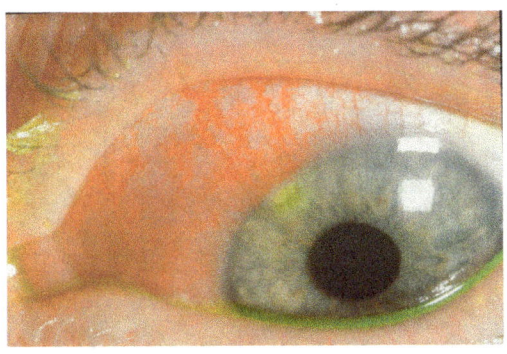

FIGURE 6.6 Inflammatory conjunctivitis, limbitis and marginal ulcer associated with *St. aureus* blepharitis.

peripheral stromal ulceration and progressive circumferential and central stromal thinning [3]. At early stages, both can be a differential diagnosis.

Several groups have suggested ways by which lid bacteria might contribute to both anterior and posterior blepharitis, either directly by infection and the release of exotoxins or indirectly through their action on lipids. Bacterial species in addition to *St. aureus* produce esterases and lipases capable of splitting cholesterol esters into cholesterol and fatty acids. Such fatty acids are conceived as potentially irritant to the eye, perhaps by the formation of soaps. *In vitro* cholesterol stimulates the growth of some *St. aureus* strains. Individuals whose meibomian secretions are rich in cholesterol show twice as many staphylococcal strains (*St. aureus* and CNS) on their lid margins. This mechanism could, therefore, increase the risk of colonisation, infection and immunisation.

Ficker et al. [3] found enhanced DTH (cell-mediated immunity) to protein A of *St. aureus* that exceeded the percentage of those who were culture positive. This suggests that CMI may provide the mechanism for inflammatory lid disease during episodes of recolonisation. In this view, eradication of *St. aureus* from the lids by antimicrobial therapy will reduce the opportunity of stimulating CMI-induced reactions [4] and the propensity for causing marginal ulceration.

Culture of the lid margin requires 'scrubbing' with a swab soaked in sterile broth and plating out directly on blood agar and a selective medium for *St. aureus*. Coagulase-negative staphylococci (CNS) may be cultured but should not be considered as pathogenic. CNS colonise over 80% of normal and blepharitic lid margins and are part of the normal lid flora; the presence of CNS alone is not an indication for treatment.

In chronic anterior blepharitis, lid hygiene should be attended to regularly, using lid scrubs with dilute baby shampoo or commercially available lid-cleansing products, and misdirected lashes must be removed.

If *St. aureus* is suspected (or culture-proven), treatment should commence with topical chloramphenicol; an alternative is fusidic acid but is more expensive. If laboratory cultures demonstrate resistance, tetracycline ointment can be used instead if the isolate is sensitive. In acute blepharitis, flucloxacillin or azithromycin can also be given by mouth (250 mg qds for four days). Avoid corticosteroid drops until the acute infectious episode is under control, and use with caution afterwards [5].

Seborrhoeic Blepharitis

Symptoms include irritation, itching and a 'burning' sensation in the eye. Signs include inflammation and thickening of the lid margin with flakey or scaly

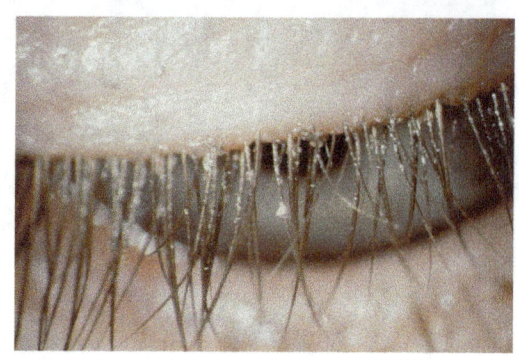

FIGURE 6.7 Scaly deposits on lid margin and lashes with normal conjunctiva and cornea.

crusting around the lashes (Figure 6.7). It is associated with seborrhoeic dermatitis (an itchy rash on the skin and scalp) and can be exacerbated by rosacea. There may also be early signs of a dry eye.

Management with lid cleansing, using wet warm compresses, to wipe away deposits from lid margins helps to improve symptoms in many patients. Treatment of associated 'dandruff' will also help. If associated with 'dry' eyes (refer later), lubricating drops may help.

Seborrhoeic Blepharitis Associated with *Demodex folliculorum*

D. folliculorum survives in hair follicles, especially in eyelashes, and ingests shed epidermal cells. It colonises most people without causing problems but gives symptoms when it multiplies in large numbers associated with immunosuppressants, chemotherapy, rosacea and use of facial hydrocortisone cream.

Symptoms include a burning sensation, *itchiness,* pustules and scales resembling eczema (Figure 6.8). There may be loss of lashes and thickened scaly lids. The mite can be recognised on microscopy of a skin scraping (Figure 6.9).

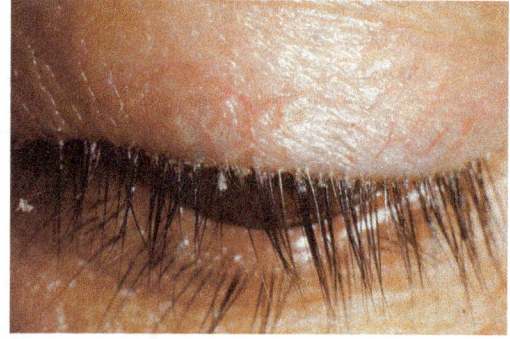

FIGURE 6.8 Cuffing of lashes with excessive *Demodex folliculorum.*

Source: (Seal D, Pleyer U. Ocular Infection, 2nd Edition 2007)

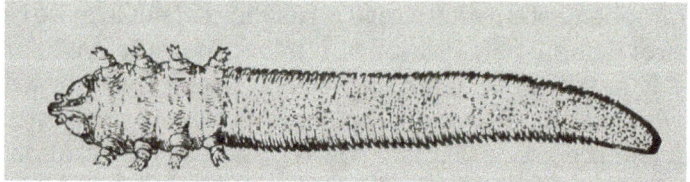

FIGURE 6.9 *Demodex folliculorum* (0.15–0.40 mm).

Source: (Seal D, Pleyer U. Ocular Infection, 2nd Edition 2007)

Treatment includes a combination of daily lid scrubs for six weeks in combination with lid wipes containing Terpinen-4-ol, a purified active extract from tea tree oil, mechanical debridement with lid hygiene and, if needed, topical permethrin cream (an insecticide that also kills scabies and lice) applied to the eyelashes and surrounding areas for a period up to six months; if needed, oral therapy is given with two doses of ivermectin, taken two weeks apart, or metronidazole for ten days together with topical permethrin.

Conjunctivitis

Conjunctivitis can be due to bacteria (*St. aureus*, streptococci, *Haemophilus influenzae*, *Neisseria* and *Gram* –ve rods), viruses, fungi, helminths and protozoa. Non-infective forms are frequently caused by allergy (refer later), dry eye (Chapter 4) or toxicity due to preservatives associated with eye drops or contact lens wear. Rarely, it may be due to systemic medication (Stevens–Johnson syndrome).

Bacterial conjunctivitis commonly has an acute or subacute manifestation with redness, discharge, swelling, tearing and irritation (Figure 6.10) [6] (refer to College of Optometrists' CMGs for—Conjunctivitis (bacterial)). The vision is not normally affected. Pain is an uncommon finding and may direct to differential diagnoses, such as (epi-)scleritis (Chapter 4). The discharge is mucopurulent or just purulent, consisting of cellular (leukocytes, bacteria, epithelial cells) and non-cellular (fibrin, protein, mucus) material. There is no strict association of the type of discharge and the aetiology of conjunctivitis; a mucopurulent exudate is most commonly seen in bacterial conjunctivitis. Formation of pseudo-membranes can occur with severe bacterial conjunctivitis, especially due to *Streptococcus pneumoniae* and *Corynebacterium diphtheriae*, not seen with diphtheria immunisation.

Neisseria gonorrhoeae or *N. meningitidis* may present hyper-acutely, with massive lid swelling and a characteristic, profuse yellow-green discharge (Figure 6.11).

Bacterial conjunctivitis is essentially a clinical diagnosis but may be supported by identification of the causative organism with a smear and/or culture. Laboratory investigations are necessary when the conjunctivitis is chronic (> 2 weeks), does not improve with antimicrobial medication and in young children.

Bacterial conjunctivitis often resolves in five to seven days. Topical antibiotics may modestly improve the condition and mean the patient is less infectious to others. Treatment options include chloramphenicol, 0.5% drops or 1% ointment, but it is *not* effective against *Pseudomonas aeruginosa*. Topical moxifloxacin 0.5% drops,

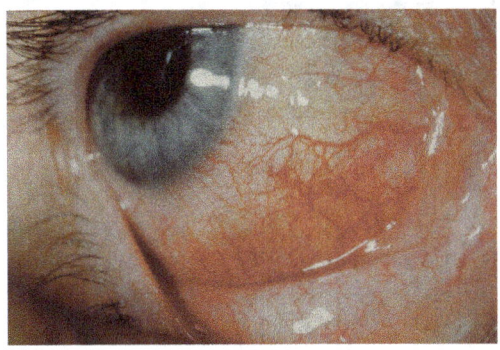

FIGURE 6.10 Bacterial conjunctivitis in an adult.

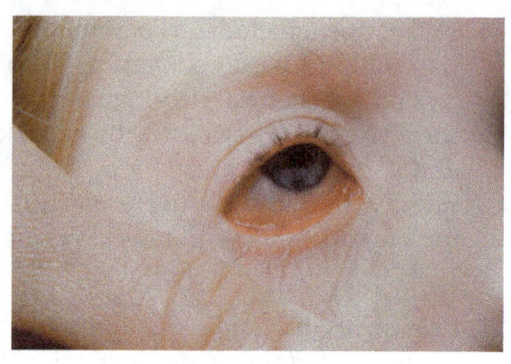

FIGURE 6.11 Conjunctivitis in adult due to *Neisseria gonorrhoeae*.

if the organism is not known, have enhanced broad-spectrum activity against *St. aureus*, streptococci, *Neisseria* and Gram –ve rods, including *Pseudomonas aeruginosa*.

Chlamydial inclusion conjunctivitis is an acute eye infection caused by *Chlamydia trachomatis* serotypes D-K, known as trachoma and inclusion conjunctivitis (TRIC), primarily associated with sexually transmitted infections (STIs).

- Occurs most commonly in sexually active young adults.
- Women are more susceptible than men.
- Most have concurrent genital tract infection.
- Transmitted by direct contact with infected genital secretion (hand-to-eye spread).

Clinical Features

Conjunctivitis is often unilateral but can involve both eyes, with acute muco-purulent conjunctivitis and discharge. It is associated with marginal ulcers and pannus (Figure 6.12). The follicular reaction on the upper tarsal plate is a key feature. No corneal scarring or blindness occurs (very different to trachoma).

Following urgent referral (within one week) to an ophthalmologist or general practitioner, patients are treated systemically with azithromycin (1 gm oral) as a single dose, doxycycline 100 mg bd for seven to ten days, tetracycline 100 mg qds for seven to ten days or erythromycin 500 mg qds for seven days [7] (refer to College of Optometrists' CMGs for—Conjunctivitis, chlamydial).

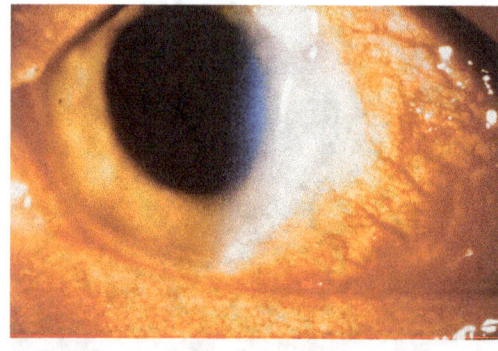

FIGURE 6.12 Conjunctivitis with a marginal limbal infiltrate (ulcer) due to chlamydia (trachoma and inclusion conjunctivitis—TRIC).

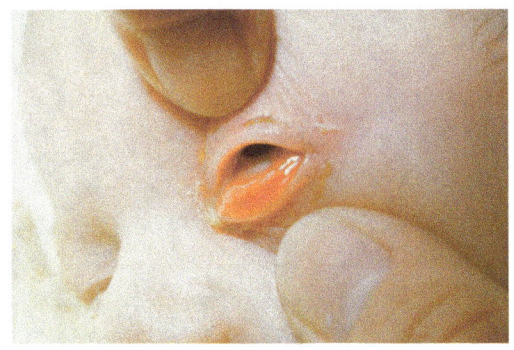

FIGURE 6.13 *N. meningitidis—eversion of lids* to reveal green-yellow pus.

Source: (Seal D, Pleyer U. Ocular Infection, 2nd Edition 2007)

Ophthalmia Neonatorum

Ophthalmia neonatorum is defined as any purulent discharge from the eyes during the first 28 days of life. Ophthalmia neonatorum occurs in developed countries in approximately 10% of live births, with gonococcal infection now rare. Elsewhere, the incidence of gonococcal conjunctivitis varies from 0.04% of live births in the Western countries to 1.0% in parts of Africa. The incidence of neonatal *chlamydial ophthalmia* in London has been estimated at less than 1%. Typical bacteria isolated include the following: *Haemophilus influenzae* (17%), *Staphylococcus aureus* (17%), *Streptococcus pneumoniae* (11%) and *Enterococcus* (8%).

Bacterial conjunctivitis in babies can be unilateral, viz. *Neisseria meningitidis*, presenting with a purulent conjunctivitis as early as three days (Figure 6.13). In the neonate, this infection can progress rapidly to keratitis and perforation, leading to blindness; urgent antibiotic therapy is needed [8] (refer to College of Optometrists' CMGs for—Ophthalmia neonatorum).

Treatment of Neonate with Conjunctivitis Due to *N. meningitidis* or *N. gonorrhoeae*

0.5% erythromycin ophthalmic ointment is used for neonatal prophylaxis against gonococcal infection in North America. Systemic treatment is essential for gonococcal keratoconjunctivitis (topical therapy alone is not adequate) with ceftriaxone (or cefotaxime, ciprofloxacin or benzyl penicillin). It is administered in a single dose of 25 to 50 mg/kg, up to a maximum of 125 mg, intramuscularly or intravenously. Additionally, newborns should be treated for seven days with ceftriaxone 25–40 mg/kg intravenously every 12 hours for three days or for benzylpenicillin in two daily doses for seven days, combined with topical saline lavage and antibiotic ointment (gentamicin, ofloxacin or levofloxacin). Single-dose intramuscular therapy may be appropriate when there is no corneal involvement [9].

Treatment of Neonate with Symptoms of Conjunctivitis (Cause Unknown)

Use ceftriaxone (50–100 mg/kg/day IM) as a single dose plus azithromycin (1 gm oral, single dose), which is added due to the frequent co-infection with *Chlamydia trachomatis*.

Neonatal chlamydial conjunctivitis is an eye infection caused by *Chlamydia trachomatis* serotypes D-K (Figure 6.14).

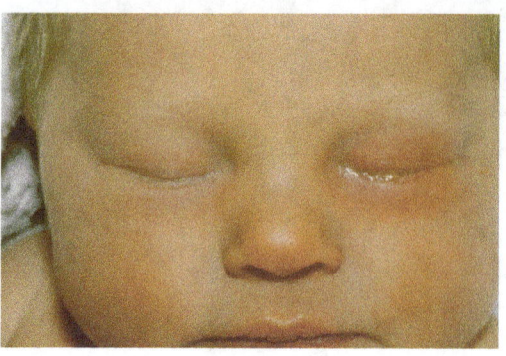

FIGURE 6.14 Bilateral conjunctivitis due to *Chlamydia* (TRIC).

Source: (Seal D, Pleyer U. Ocular Infection, 2nd Edition 2007)

- Transmitted from active, untreated *Chlamydia trachomatis* genital infection at delivery (passage through birth canal)
- Can also occur in babies delivered by Caesarean section
- Incubation period: 5–14 days after birth (< 5 days for gonococcal, 5–14 days for chlamydial and less severe)
- Clinical features: moderate conjunctival redness and watery mucoid secretions
  - Red eyes ('conjunctival injection'), swollen eyelids, affects both eyes
  - Acute watery, then mucopurulent discharge
  - Can lead to slow-onset pneumonia, if untreated (infant pneumonia syndrome)
  - Treat with oral azithromycin (and oral doxycycline if associated with a sexually transmitted disease)
  - No topical treatment

Viral Conjunctivitis

Adenovirus infection, like chlamydial conjunctivitis to a lesser degree, may present with a follicular conjunctivitis, usually absent from bacterial infections (Figure 6.15). This may be seen alone or part of pharyngoconjunctival fever (PCF) (both more common in children) or as acute hemorrhagic conjunctivitis (Figures 6.16 and 6.17) or epidemic keratoconjunctivitis (EKC). Adenovirus EKC is associated with epidemics from shipyards, close living quarters and eye clinics (via tonometers and staff handling of patients). Early diagnosis is required to bring outbreaks to a quick halt aided by rapid confirmation in the laboratory with PCR or other tests [10] (refer to College of Optometrists' CMGs for—Conjunctivitis (viral, non-herpetic)).

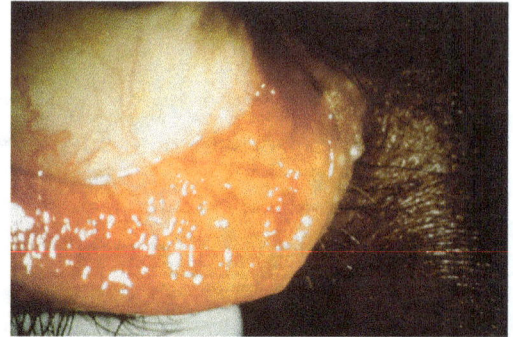

FIGURE 6.15 Acute follicular 'cobblestone' conjunctivitis due to a viral infection.

Source: (Seal D, Pleyer U. Ocular Infection, 2nd Edition 2007)

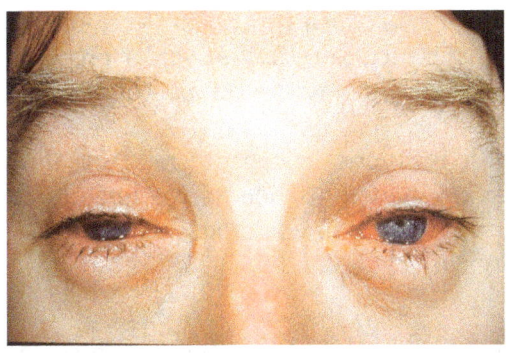

FIGURE 6.16 Acute haemorrhagic conjunctivitis (AHC) due to adenovirus serovar 11.

Source: (Seal D, Pleyer U. Ocular Infection, 2nd Edition 2007)

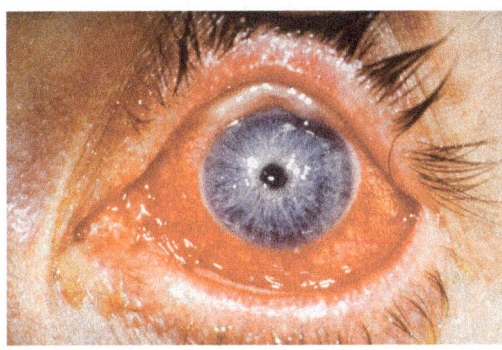

FIGURE 6.17 AHC—the cornea has fine punctate epithelial keratitis.

Source: (Seal D, Pleyer U. Ocular Infection, 2nd Edition 2007)

Acute follicular conjunctivitis is a self-limiting condition without sequelae, usually caused by adenovirus serotypes 1, 2, 4–6 and 19. Conjunctivitis begins unilaterally but commonly becomes bilateral. It lasts up to 21 days in its acute form.

Acute Hemorrhagic Conjunctivitis (AHC)

Enterovirus 70, associated with occasional paralysis, and coxsackie A24 variant virus have caused epidemics of AHC, especially in Southeast Asia (Hong Kong and Singapore) and India. Adenovirus 11 may also give rise to a form of AHC.

The infection involves an incubation period of 18 to 36 hours, with the sudden onset in one eye, followed by the other the same day. There is lid swelling, mild photophobia, irritation and a seromucous discharge, becoming watery on the second day. Preauricular lymphadenopathy develops in 65% of patients. The tarsal conjunctiva is hyperemic with small petechiae and is oedematous in the lower fornix. Small follicles develop on the second day in the lower, temporal conjunctiva and last up to ten days. The bulbar conjunctiva is edematous and shows subconjunctival hemorrhage. Bleeding can vary in size from a pinpoint to the whole of the bulbar conjunctiva and is exacerbated by clinical manipulation on examination. Bleeding decreases after the second day and absorbs gradually over one week. The cornea shows fine punctate epithelial keratitis, without nummular opacities, and no sequelae occur.

The infection is highly contagious, with rapid spread among people in homes and workplaces, including hospitals and clinics (refer to Appendix 2 for prevention control). Spread is mainly person-to-person, but during the acute infection, the virus can be detected in throat washings and stool specimens. Diagnosis is usually clinical. Virus culture (or PCR) should be performed if possible. Treatment is symptomatic and resolves within two weeks.

Conjunctivitis in measles, mumps, dengue, glandular fever (EBV infection) and hepatitis A are associated with systemic virus infection. *Herpes simplex* presents as primary blepharo-conjunctivitis and *Herpes zoster* with shingles of the Vth nerve (refer later).

The use of corticosteroids combined with antibiotics is controversial, *but their use is contraindicated for fungal (Chapter 7) or viral keratitis*, when they contribute to the progression of the infection by inhibiting the immune response. Herpes conjunctivitis should be treated with topical aciclovir.

Phlyctenular Keratoconjunctivitis

This is an inflammatory condition caused by a type IV delayed-type hypersensitivity (CMI) reaction to one or more antigens. The triggering antigen is usually a bacterial protein, in the past from systemic *Mycobacterium tuberculosis* but today more frequently from localised *Staphylococcus aureus*, or *Chlamydia trachomatis* in endemic areas, but may also be a virus, fungus (*Candida albicans*) or a nematode such as pin worms. Different presentations are shown in Figures 6.18 and 6.19.

Phlyctena are small raised nodules, pinkish-white or yellow in colour, that may ulcerate and are often surrounded by dilated blood vessels. The lesions are often triangular in shape, with the base at the limbus and the apex pointing towards the centre of the cornea.

A search should be made for the appropriate systemic or localised antigen, but it often cannot be identified. Corticosteroid suppresses the immune response, reducing inflammation and improving most symptoms; prednisolone or loteprednol drops are used, the latter preferred due to its lower risk of elevating intraocular pressure (Appendix 1).

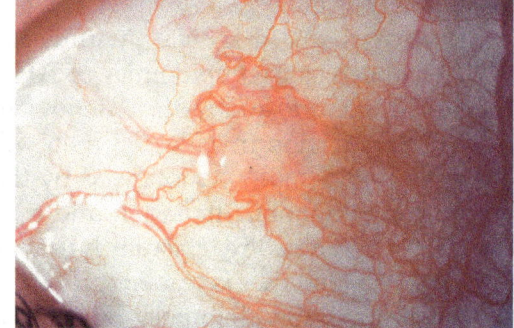

FIGURE 6.18 Conjunctival phlycten—causative antigen not known.

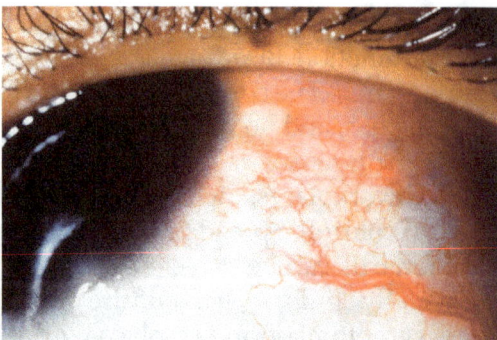

FIGURE 6.19 Multiple phlyctena at the limbus—causative antigen not known.

Source: (Seal D, Pleyer U. Ocular Infection, 2nd Edition 2007)

Dacryocystitis

Blockage of the naso-lacrimal duct, with excessive tearing, can occur due to chronic infection with *Arachnia (Actinomyces) propionica* that is often mixed with other bacteria. Pus, massaged along the canaliculus to the punctum, can be Gram stained to show typical, branching Gram +ve bacilli (Figures 6.20 and 6.21) and sulphur granules (Appendix 5). Prolonged anaerobic culture on blood agar plates is necessary to demonstrate actinomycetes. Thioglycolate broth should also be inoculated, since oxygen tension decreases with depth, so that the actinomycete ('breadcrumb') colonies grow and float at the appropriate level (Appendix 5). Sensitivity tests should be performed.

For acute dacryocystitis, treatment includes oral antibiotics that cover both Gram +ve and Gram −ve organisms, viz. amoxycillin (for *A. propionica*) and moxifloxacin; hot compresses relieve pain. In addition, initial treatment involves irrigating the canaliculus with penicillin.

If the condition does not respond, incision and drainage with direct antibiotic application to the lacrimal sac and duct, along with povidone-iodine, provide immediate pain relief and rapid control of the infection; the endoscopic, endonasal DCR approach is best, as it preserves the orbicularis oculi and its pumping mechanism and avoids facial scarring. The postoperative infection rate in patients undergoing DCR is reduced by intra-operative IV cefuroxime (750 mg) or a five-day course of oral cefalexin 250 mg four times daily. Occasionally, repeat surgery and further povidone-iodine and penicillin are required to effect a cure.

Keratitis

Details on how to take a corneal scrape and staining methods are given in Appendix 5.

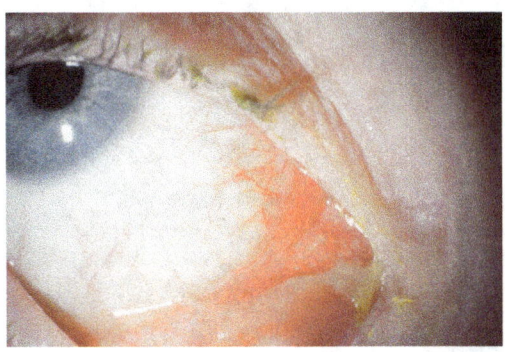

FIGURE 6.20 Pus exuding out of puncta (blocked naso-lacrimal) duct in a wet eye.

Source: (Seal D, Pleyer U. Ocular Infection, 2nd Edition 2007)

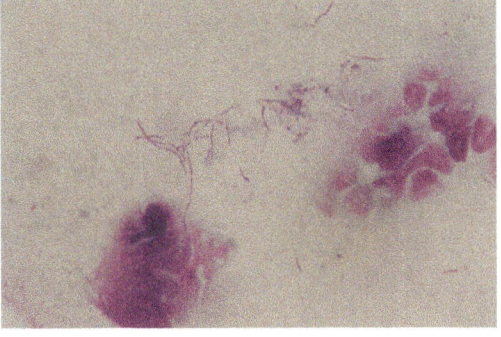

FIGURE 6.21 Gram stain of actinomycetes (long, branching Gram-positive rods) and neutrophils (pus) cells.

Source: (Seal D, Pleyer U. Ocular Infection, 2nd Edition 2007)

Bacterial Keratitis
Clinical Presentation

Suppurative bacterial keratitis presents clinically as a corneal stromal infiltrate or abscess with an overlying epithelial defect (Figures 6.22–6.24). Patients usually complain of unilateral pain (moderate to severe with usually an acute onset and rapid progression), lid swelling, redness, discharge (mucopurulent or purulent), photophobia (may be severe) and blurred vision. Bacterial invasion of the cornea causes inflammation and corneal ulceration, which may be followed by neovascularization. When the activity of proteinases, derived from bacteria or host neutrophils, leads to stromal melting, formation of a descmetocele may occur with risk of corneal perforation.

Some bacteria, particularly *Streptococcus pneumoniae* and other alpha-hemolytic streptococci, may induce focal infection with only minimal inflammation under an intact epithelium. These bacteria proliferate and multiply between the stromal

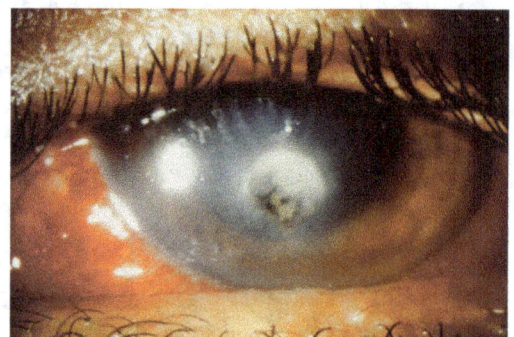

FIGURE 6.22 Infected corneal foreign body requiring removal (needle or blade).

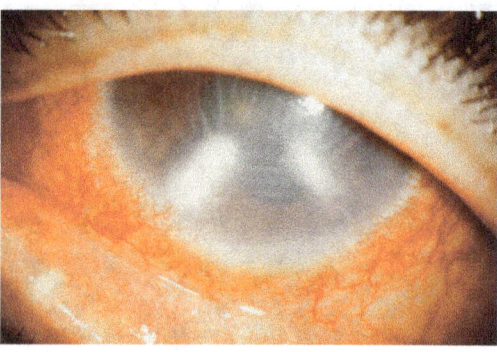

FIGURE 6.23 *Staphylococcus aureus* Gram positive cocci (GPC) infection of radial keratotomy incisions.

Source: (Seal D, Pleyer U. Ocular Infection, 2nd Edition 2007)

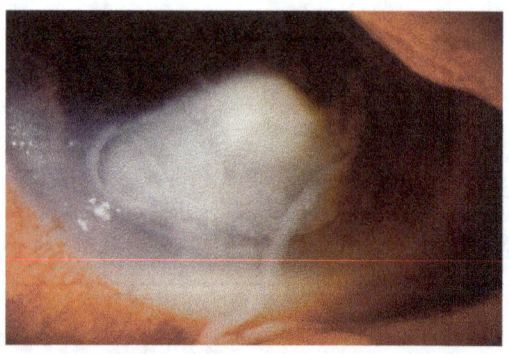

FIGURE 6.24 Corneal ulcer due to exposure infected with *Streptococcus pneumoniae* (GPC).

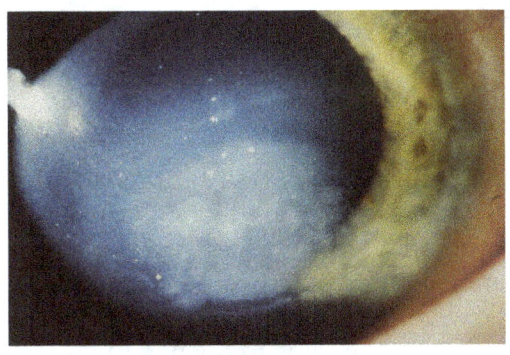

FIGURE 6.25 *Acanthamoeba* infection with secondary microaerophilic streptococcal infection causing a 'crystalline' keratopathy (also showing radial keratoneuritis).

lamellae, resulting in a needle-like or fern-like network opacity called crystalline keratopathy (Figure 6.25). It can also occur in large ulcers due to other causes, such as *Acanthamoeba*.

Injury is the commonest cause of keratitis in the tropics (Chapter 7), especially in agricultural workers with mixed bacterial and fungal infections, but in temperate climates, widespread use of soft contact lenses is the most important risk factor. Bacteria account for over 80% of ulcerative keratitis occurring in northern climates and 60% in southern climates, where fungal keratitis is more common. In temperate climates, Gram +ve bacteria predominate; *Candida sp.* is an occasional pathogen, and *Acanthamoeba* is associated with contact lens wear. This compares with *Pseudomonas aeruginosa* and filamentous mycelial fungi, which predominate in tropical and semi-tropical areas (Chapter 7).

Suppurative bacterial keratitis is usually central but may be peripheral. Because corneal thickness is only about 0.5 mm, such an ulcer may rapidly progress to perforation within 24 hours of onset. In the aphakic or pseudophakic eye with a capsulotomy, access to the vitreous space is facilitated and a secondary endophthalmitis may supervene. Bacterial keratitis needs urgent treatment with high doses of an effective antibiotic. Supplementary corneal transplantation, or other reconstructive surgery, may be required at a later stage in the management of corneal scarring or perforation. The presentation in children is similar to that in adults [11] (refer to College of Optometrists' CMGs for—Microbial keratitis (bacterial, fungal)).

Cultures and smears are not essential in every case of suspected infectious keratitis. In patients with only a small (< 2 mm), peripheral and non–sight-threatening lesion, laboratory workup may not be required. However, when the infiltrate is central, large, progressive and sight-threatening, cultures and smears are essential; an ulcer that is > 4 mm^2 in area is more likely to be infected. When performing the scrape, a sample for Gram stain should be obtained first and then another for culture (Appendix 5). In contact lens wearers, the lens, storage case and care solutions should also be cultured, including for *Acanthamoeba sp.. Acanthamoeba* and filamentous fungi, such as *Fusarium sp.*, can be detected in the cornea in vivo by confocal microscopy (if available).

Treatment

Emergency (same day) referral is indicated if:

- The infiltrate is > 1 mm
- There are two or more adjacent lesions

- The location is 3 mm or less from the centre of the cornea
- There is an anterior chamber reaction
- There are signs that may indicate fungal or *Acanthamoeba* keratitis
- Poor compliance with therapy

Therapy of infectious keratitis is ideally based on the results of smears and culture and subsequent in vitro sensitivity testing prior to initiating therapy. However, before culture results are available, treatment is started empirically, based on the clinical appearance, with commercial quinolone preparations, e.g. moxifloxacin 0.5% (Appendix 1); alternatives are levofloxacin 0.5% (5 mg/mL), ciprofloxacin 0.3% (3 mg/mL) (25) or ofloxacin 0.3% (3 mg/mL) at the same frequency. Ofloxacin treatment causes less irritation. Topical ciprofloxacin may leave microcrystalline deposits on the corneal surface, which take up to six months to dissolve, but has greater activity (two times to four times) against *Pseudomonas aeruginosa* (Appendix 6).

Drops should be given hourly day and night for the first three days, then two-hourly by day. Successful eradication of bacterial infection is reported in about 90% of patients treated in this way. Topical administration of levofloxacin (0.5% solution) gives greater penetration (two times to three times) into human corneal stroma and aqueous humour tissues than ofloxacin (0.3%) or ciprofloxacin (0.3%). However, the mean intracorneal concentrations of all three drugs following two drops exceeds the MIC90 for the majority of pathogens causing bacterial keratitis. Moxifloxacin offers an expanded anti-infective spectrum. In particular, moxifloxacin is effective against methicillin-resistant *Staphylococcus aureus*, and both are more effective against Gram –ve bacteria. Moxifloxacin is more effective than other quinolones against streptococci. For managing microbial keratitis in resource-limited settings, refer to [12] and Chapter 7.

Subconjunctival injections are not necessary, provided an intensive fortified drop regimen is used, as the latter will produce therapeutic levels in the cornea that are sustained and without large fluctuation. If frequent topical applications are not possible, as in a child or a disturbed individual, then subconjunctival injections of gentamicin 40 mg and cephazolin 100 mg can be used as an alternative, delivered under a general anesthetic. Inclusion of adrenaline 0.3 mL (of 1:1000) in 1 mL of solution prolongs the effective concentration of antibiotic in the cornea and aqueous from about six hours to over 24 hours.

Antibiotic ointment may be given at night in the later stages of therapy once infection is under control, but in the acute stages, it may interfere with absorption from drop therapy (Chapter S11). Systemic antibiotics have no place in the management of bacterial keratitis in the absence of limbal involvement or perforation. Antibiotics are modified according to the results of cultures and evaluation of the clinical response to initial therapy. If there is a clear clinical response, the same regime should be continued. Antibiotic sensitivities may be misleading because they are performed on lower tissue antibiotic levels than those achieved in the cornea during topical therapy. Therapy should be reduced by *increasing the interval* between drops every three to four days and not by reducing their concentration. The decision to terminate therapy is based on clinical response and the virulence of the causative organism.

If there is no response, all topical therapy should be stopped to allow the various drugs and preservatives to leach from the tissues. After 24 or 48 hours, the

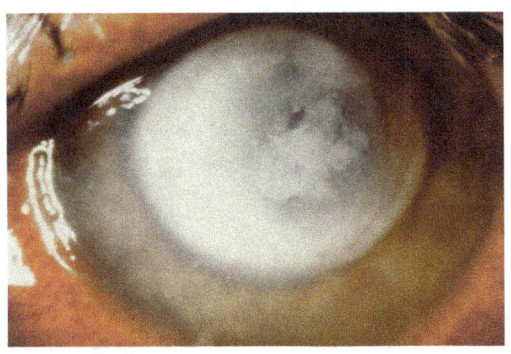

FIGURE 6.26 Severe keratitis with hypopyon due to *Pseudomonas aeruginosa* Gram negative rods (GNR) in a CLW.

clinical condition is reappraised, and the cornea is scraped again. On this occasion, a full search must be made for more exotic or fastidious organisms that may be unusual or have special cultural requirements, such as *Nocardia, Mycobacteria* (Chapter S6) and microaerophilic or anaerobic bacteria. A corneal biopsy may be required to identify the organism in the deeper stroma and has been successfully used for microaerophilic streptococci, *Fusarium sp.* and *Acanthamoeba*.

Contact lens wear (CLW) related microbial keratitis (refer also to Chapter 9).

In general, the risk of microbial keratitis is five times greater for soft than hard lens wearers and is greater with extended wear than daily wear. Silicone hydrogel (SH) contact lenses increase the oxygen diffusion to the cornea and reduce corneal oedema that occurs with overnight wear of hydrogels, which is a predisposing factor for microbial keratitis. The incidence is approximately 1 in 500 with extended wear (overnight) of hydrogel lenses and 1 in 2,500 with daily wear. Bacteria responsible include those associated with suppurative keratitis, but Gram −ve bacteria are more commonly encountered than Gram +ve, and *P. aeruginosa* is more frequent than other Gram −ve bacteria (Figure 6.26).

Contamination of contact lens storage solutions is an important source of bacterial keratitis. Use of tap water is a major risk factor for *Acanthamoeba* infection (refer later). Poor storage case hygiene is an important factor for all types of microbes (Chapter 9).

For further information, refer to Chapter 9 and [13].

Protozoal

For protozoan and filarial infections causing keratitis, refer to Chapter 7.

Keratitis due to the genus *Acanthamoeba* and other free-living unicellular protozoa, viz. *Vahlkampfia*, is usually, but not always, associated with contact lens wear (Chapters 7 and 9). As a eukaryotic organism, *Acanthamoeba* is organised into complex structures enclosed within a cell membrane. The nucleus is enclosed within a double-layered membrane similar to that of higher eukaryotes. Other membrane-bound organelles include mitochondria, vacuoles and lysosomes. They exist as motile trophozoites, moving by pseudopodia (Figure 6.27), and as resistant cysts (non-invasive phase) with ostioles (Figure 6.28) (https://www.microscopemaster.com/acanthamoeba.html).

Trophozoites ingest bacteria and fungal cells as a food source and are hence often present as a mixed infection. Pathogenic strains belong to group 2 (genotype 4) or group 3 [14].

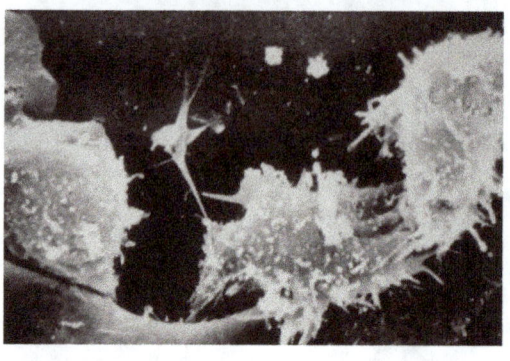

FIGURE 6.27 Scanning electron micrograph of trophozoites of *Acanthamoeba*.

Source: (Seal D, Pleyer U. Ocular Infection, 2nd Edition 2007)

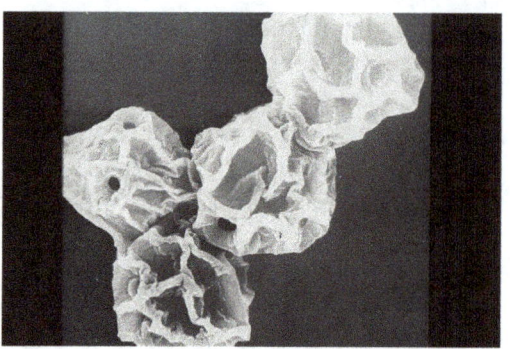

FIGURE 6.28 Scanning electron micrograph of cysts of Acanthamoeba showing ostioles.

Source: (Seal D, Pleyer U. Ocular Infection, 2nd Edition 2007)

Acanthamoeba is present in soil, pond water, swimming pools, hot tubs and domestic water supplies, often associated with scale and biofilm. *Acanthamoeba* is found in 18% of UK household bathrooms (tap, tap water, drain), while 64% of bathroom taps were colonised with Gram –ve bacteria [15].

If contact lenses are stored in tap water, instead of disinfecting solutions, then the amoeba attaches to the lens, often within a bacterial biofilm, and is carried by it to the corneal surface; here, the amoeba adheres to the corneal epithelium when the trophozoite releases proteases to initiate the invasive process. Unfortunately, some daily-wear contact lens wearers extend the economic life of their lenses by soaking them overnight in tap water and wearing them again instead of using them as daily disposables. Cosmetic users of nonprescription contact lenses, often young women, were the majority of patients in a recent study, when they received no hygiene instruction or optometric care [16].

It is vital to recognise early presentation of Acanthamoeba infection, which can be diagnosed within 14 days of symptoms beginning, to avoid a long, painful and complicated outcome that can be devastating. The patient complains of pain (which may be severe and is often out of proportion to the degree of inflammation, or conversely, it may be painless in the early stages), often intense redness and blurred vision in association with photophobia and wears contact lenses in most cases. Patients present to primary care or hospital emergency departments. Both the diagnosis and differential diagnosis should be considered; adenovirus (EKC) is described later, but signs of keratopathy appear later, after nine days. A corneal scraping is required for microscopy and culture, both for amoebae and for bacteria and fungi in case of a mixed infection (Appendix 5); if this is not possible on site, then the patient must be referred urgently (same day).

Early diagnosis (refer to figures later), therapeutic epithelial debridement (especially when the infection is still intraepithelial) and treatment with anti-amoebic drugs gives a good visual outcome within one month. Late diagnosis requires six months or more of anti-amoebic therapy with various complications, including excessive pain, limited vision and development of cataract and secondary glaucoma; if the infection is eventually controlled, the severe corneal scarring requires graft surgery, but this can succumb to reactivation of amoebae from the corneal rim. If uncontrolled, scleritis, iris atrophy, anterior synechiae and chorioretinitis develop to give a blind eye.

Clinical signs of *Acanthamoeba* infection are summarised later [17] (refer to College of Optometrists' CMGs for Microbial keratitis (*acanthamoeba sp.*)). Toxic epitheliopathy caused by contact lenses (Chapter 9) is a differential diagnosis in early disease.

A) The earliest evidence is swollen lids (Figure 6.29) with a diffuse, irregular oedema within the corneal epithelium, giving it a grey-dirty appearance (Figure 6.30) that may result in a dendritiform ulcer. These pseudo-dendritic lesions (Figure 6.31) are often confused with *herpes simplex* keratitis (refer later). *H. simplex* should be considered with caution as the primary infection (diagnosis) in a red eye in a contact lens wearer. In addition, the pain is unexpectedly severe for the examination findings.

B) Radial keratoneuritis is another early sign (Figure 6.32), and a classic finding, due to amoeboid locomotion along the corneal nerve together with unusual infiltrates, which occur in the mid-stroma; they begin paracentrally and extend to the limbus in a radial pattern (Figure 6.33). The overlying epithelium remains intact [18].

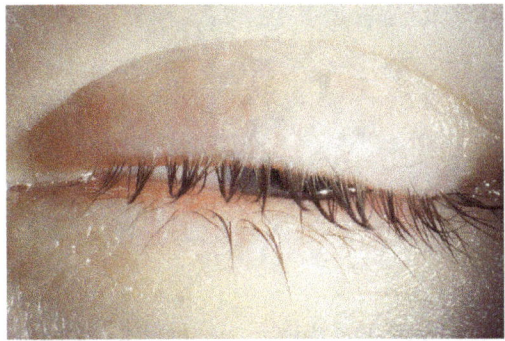

FIGURE 6.29 Swollen lids with a painful eye.

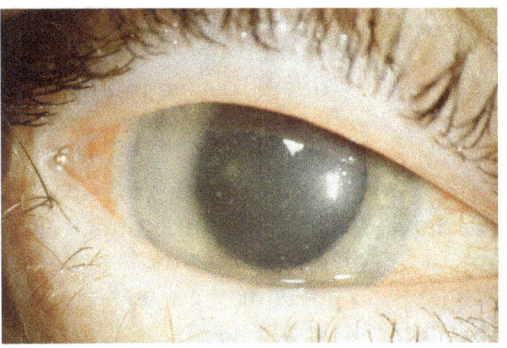

FIGURE 6.30 Diffuse irregular epitheliopathy due to *Acanthamoeba* trophozoites.

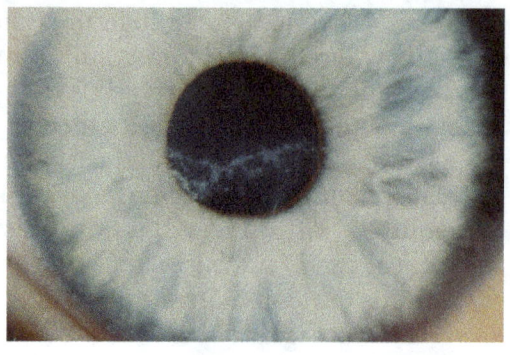

FIGURE 6.31 Early *Acanthamoeba* pseudo-dendrite and corneal nerve below.

Source: (Seal D, Pleyer U. Ocular Infection, 2nd Edition 2007)

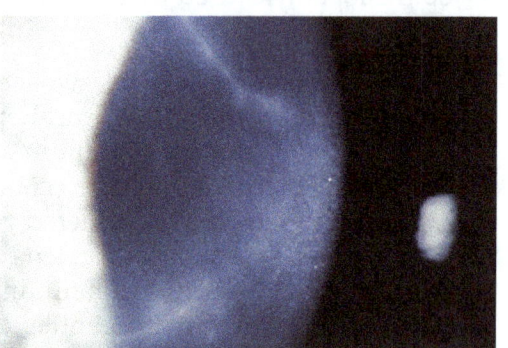

FIGURE 6.32 Typical radial keratoneuritis of *Acanthamoeba* infection.

Source: (Seal D, Pleyer U. Ocular Infection, 2nd Edition 2007)

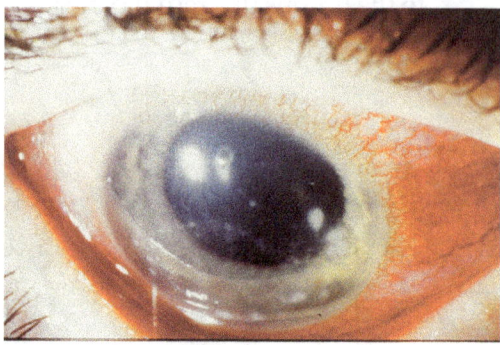

FIGURE 6.33 Typical epitheliopathy and keratoneuritis with early ring abscess formation of *Acanthamoeba* infection (contaminated contact lens storage case shown in Chapter 9).

Source: (Seal D, Pleyer U. Ocular Infection, 2nd Edition 2007)

C) After six to ten weeks, there is epithelial breakdown with defects and stromal inflammation. Deep stromal infiltrates appear, due to penetration of the amoeba, as a paracentral, partial or complete circle with a clear central cornea (Figure 6.34). These infiltrates may also be disciform or nummular with satellite lesions and associated anterior chamber inflammation with a hypopyon. Unbearable pain is pathognomonic and is usually due to perineural infiltration. If left untreated, the amoeba invades all layers of the cornea, forming a ring abscess, which may end with perforation.

D) Late presentation with a cloudy cornea, deep ring infiltrate, 360 degrees of neovascularization, a hypopyon and associated uveitis, limbitis and conjunctivitis. This situation is reached by failed therapy or misdiagnosis. At this stage, *a corneal biopsy is useful to identify the amoeba* when scrapings may be negative and the infection is primarily intrastromal (Figures 6.35 and 6.36).

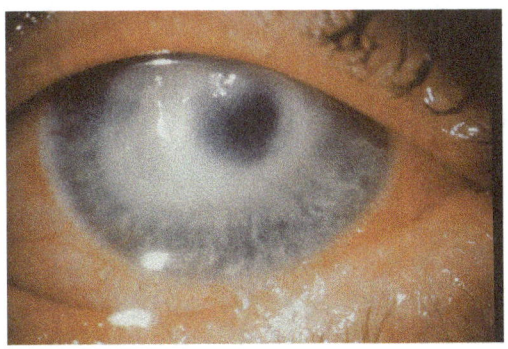

FIGURE 6.34 Deep stromal infiltrates in a complete circle with a clearer central cornea.

Source: (Seal D, Pleyer U. Ocular Infection, 2nd Edition 2007)

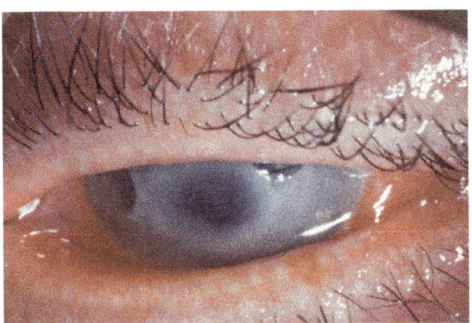

FIGURE 6.35 Corneal biopsy for late presentation of a deep ring abscess.

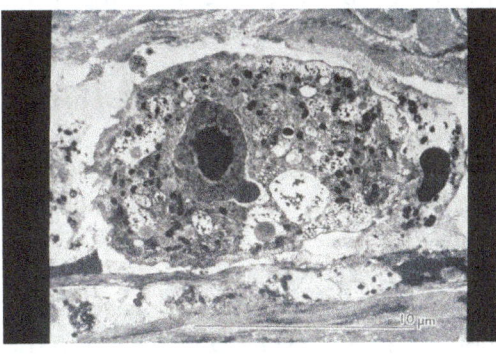

FIGURE 6.36 Transmission electron micrograph of *Acanthamoeba* within the corneal stroma.

E) Occasionally, *Acanthamoeba* infection occurs without contact lens wear, when there is pre-existing damage to the corneal epithelium, such as trachoma—refer to Chapter 7 (Figure 7.2).

F) *Wessely rings*, also known as corneal immune rings, are non-infectious ring-shaped stromal infiltrates that can form in various corneal infections as well as non-infectious disease processes (Figure 6.37). They represent an immune reaction between antigen in the cornea and antibody diffusing into it from the limbus. Wessely rings are an uncommon initial presentation in *Acanthamoeba* keratitis and, while they can appear in the first month, typically appear later, often after inappropriate treatment. They may appear late in successfully treated patients with residual *Acanthamoeba* antigens released from the scarred cornea. In addition, immune inflammatory reactions can occur within the scar (Figure 6.38).

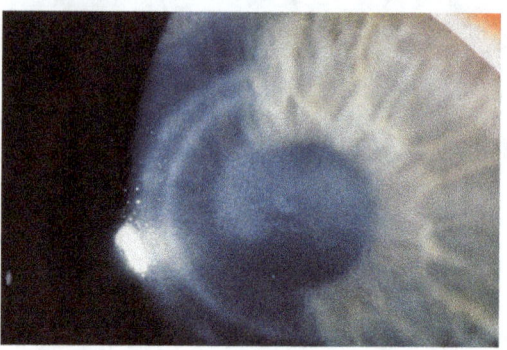

FIGURE 6.37 Wessely rings around a healed scar from an *Acanthamoeba* infection.

Source: (Seal D, Pleyer U. Ocular Infection, 2nd Edition 2007)

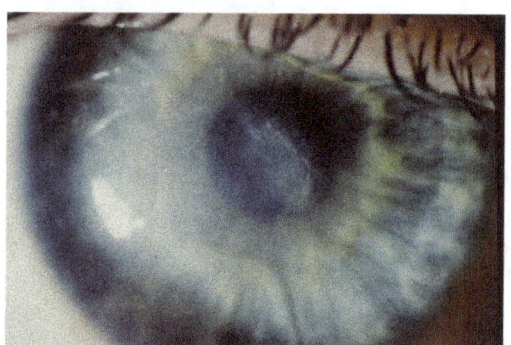

FIGURE 6.38 Immune inflammatory reaction within a healed scar from an *Acanthamoeba* infection, responsive to corticosteroids.

Therapy is best started early, ideally within 14 days of onset of symptoms when the infection is still intra-epithelial. *THIS REQUIRES EARLY RECOGNITION AT PRIMARY CARE.* Patients should be referred urgently to specialist centres, where diagnosis will be confirmed by histology and culture or by PCR. Therapy consists of topical biguanides, with either the bis-biguanide chlorhexidine (0.02% to 0.2%) [19] or the polymeric biguanide (40 polyguanidine units) polyhexamethylene biguanide (PHMB) (0.02 to 0.08%) [20] *combined with* a diamidine, either propamidine isethionate 0.1% or hexamidine 0.1%.

The biguanides are effective against both the trophozoite and cyst stages; the diamidines are only effective against the trophozoites, and recurrence occurs with monotherapy. Initial treatment is given every one hour for the first 24 hours, followed by every hour while awake and then titrated to disease response [13].

Chlorhexidine monotherapy has been used successfully in 31 patients, but combination therapy with a diamidine is preferred [16]. Some biguanide resistance has been reported for which combinations of both chlorhexidine and PHMB have been used successfully [21].

Therapy for late presentation of infection is prolonged and complicated; the average time for expected treatment is five months, with complications of central corneal scarring, secondary glaucoma, cataract development and sometimes iris atrophy, possibly due to biguanide toxicity. The use of corticosteroids is controversial but is used to suppress inflammation starting two weeks after anti-amoebic therapy and has been claimed to produce a better visual outcome [22].

The antifungal drug voriconazole, an imidazole available commercially in both drop and oral formulation, has been found effective recently as monotherapy treatment, and its use is currently evolving [23]. It is effective against both the trophozoite and cyst stages as opposed to earlier imidazoles that were only effective against the trophozoites [14]. It also has the advantage that it penetrates into the corneal stroma and is relatively nontoxic.

Infection by *Acanthamoeba* continues to be reported globally from all five continents [13, 23]. Prevention is better than cure, but it needs continuous education, especially for those wearing cosmetic as well as refractive contact lenses.

Trachoma due to *Chlamydia trachomatis*.

Refer to Chapter 7.

Fungi (yeast and mycelial)—for types, risk factors and clinical manifestations of fungal keratitis, refer to Chapter 7; for therapy, refer to Appendix 6.

Viral Keratitis

Adenovirus Keratoconjunctivitis

Adenovirus is a common cause of acute conjunctivitis, presenting either in association with an upper respiratory tract infection, fever and malaise (pharyngo-conjunctival fever) or as part of an outbreak of moderate (Figure 6.39) or severe keratoconjunctivitis (epidemic keratoconjunctivitis). There are 47 serotypes of adenovirus of which half cause ocular infection, due to serotypes 3, 4, 7, 8, 10, (15/29), 19 and 37.

Epidemic keratoconjunctivitis (EKC) is caused mainly by adenoviruses 8, 19 and 37 and gives rise to epidemics within the community; it is transmitted within the (eye) hospital or clinics. Onset of conjunctivitis in one eye is followed by signs in the fellow eye within two to seven days; patients will complain of redness, discomfort, watering and eyelid swelling. A punctate epithelial keratitis, about four days after onset, is succeeded by a coarse punctate keratitis at one week and then, between the first and second week *(later than day nine)*, by a multifocal, subepithelial keratitis considered to reflect an immune reaction to viral antigen. The keratitis is responsible for symptoms of pain, glare, photophobia and visual loss if the central cornea is involved. A pre-auricular lymphadenopathy may be present. Although the condition may resolve within four weeks, it may give rise to disability for over a year, sometimes with recurrent episodes of papillary conjunctivitis. Viral shedding has usually subsided by two weeks.

Antiviral agents, interferon and antibiotics have not been shown to affect the course of adenoviral keratoconjunctivitis, but some amelioration of symptoms has been observed in patients treated with trifluorothymidine.

In early infection (< 2 weeks), corticosteroids are not indicated. Topical corticosteroids can suppress the symptoms and signs in adenovirus keratoconjunctivitis,

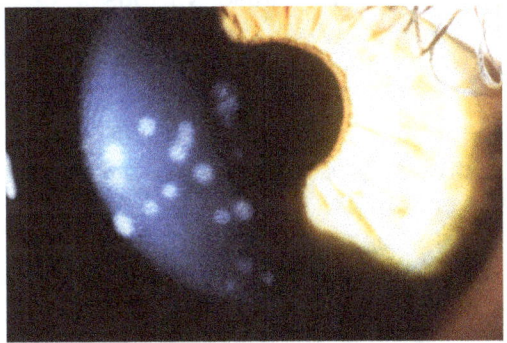

FIGURE 6.39 Punctate epitheliopathy due to adenovirus.

but their use may be followed by a rebound keratitis, and they must be used judiciously. Resolution of the infection occurs in most patients within three weeks.

While adenovirus infection occurs in the young contact lens wearer, the differential diagnosis for both punctate epitheliopathy and early nummular stromal infiltration is *Acanthamoeba* keratitis, *particularly when the infiltration occurs on or before day eight.* Thygeson keratitis is another differential diagnosis but with unknown aetiology. Prevention and control of infection is considered in Appendix 2. Spread of infection is by person-to-person, eye contact and occasionally by the fecal-oral route.

Prophylaxis is particularly important in ophthalmic practices since its role as a vector for spreading the virus is well documented. Hygienic hand rub is an important measure to control adenoviral infection. Unfortunately, most alcoholic or povidone-iodine–based solutions that are commonly used in ophthalmic practices are not able to eradicate the virus (Appendix 2). Therefore, it is recommended to use gloves when examining patients suspected to be infected with adenovirus.

Herpes simplex virus and adenovirus account for 1% of all acute conjunctivitis in an ophthalmic casualty department. Antiviral agents are available for the treatment of *H. simplex* and *H. zoster* infections but not for adenovirus infection. A number of other ocular viral infections occur for which there is no specific antiviral therapy, but topical antibiotics are often prescribed to reduce the risk of secondary bacterial infection.

Herpes Simplex Eye Disease

Humans are the only natural reservoir for *herpes simplex*. Primary ocular infection occurs when a non-immune individual comes into close contact with someone who is shedding virus. Skin or mucosal entry on the face results in zosteriform spread along Vth cranial nerve axons with establishment of latency in the trigeminal ganglion. Latency can follow asymptomatic infection within the territory of the first division of the Vth nerve dermatome or inoculations of the neighboring second and third divisions. Virus may be grown from keratitis specimens in culture, and viral particles have been demonstrated within keratocytes, suggesting the existence of a non-neuronal latency.

Establishment of latency by a given strain of HSV 1 greatly reduces the likelihood of further HSV 1 infection, and recurrences are due to the same strain. While patients who have been infected by HSV 2 usually show resistance to HSV 1 infection, the reverse is not the case; patients who show immunity to HSV 1 may still be susceptible to oculogenital infection by HSV 2. Rarely, both HSV 1 and 2 are isolated from the same cornea. Eighty percent of genital herpes is caused by HSV 2, which causes a small proportion of herpes keratitis. Neonatal ocular infection occurs in about 1:100,000 deliveries and causes various serious complications.

Most ocular HSV disease is caused by HSV 1. Primary infection manifests with gingivostomatitis, pharyngitis, rhinitis or tonsillitis with fevers, chills, myalgias, lymphadenopathy and vesicular eruptions that clear in seven to ten days without scar. Initial episodes involve lid or conjunctiva in 54% (Figure 6.40), superficial cornea in 63%, deeper cornea in 6% and uveitis in 4%. There may be a vesicular blepharitis, follicular or pseudomembranous conjunctivitis and a punctate or dendritic keratitis. HSV-specific antibodies are found in tears at a greater concentration than in saliva, suggesting local production.

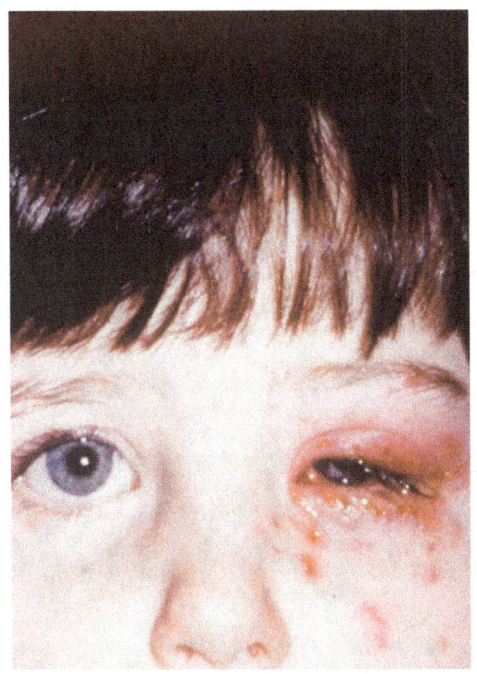

FIGURE 6.40 Herpes simplex infection of lid, conjunctiva and face.

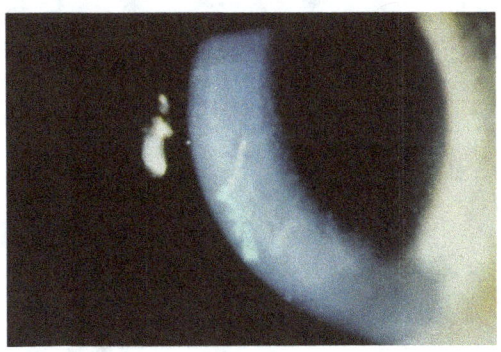

FIGURE 6.41 Dendritic ulcer due to herpes simplex viewed with a slit lamp.

Source: (Seal D, Pleyer U. Ocular Infection, 2nd Edition 2007)

Reactivation of latent virus in immune subjects causes ocular disease associated with peripheral viral shedding and is termed 'recurrent herpetic eye disease.' It includes epithelial keratitis (punctate lesions which coalesce into a dendriform pattern) (Figure 6.41), subepithelial lesions (Figure 6.42), endothelial (disciform) keratitis (epithelial oedema overlying stromal thickening, folds in Descemet's membrane, raised IOP, uveitis and keratic precipitates) (Figure 6.43), trabeculitis and, rarely, acute retinal necrosis. Not all primary eye disease is followed by recurrent disease, and not all recurrent disease is unilateral (2% of cases are bilateral). It is favoured by atopy and systemic diseases, such as pulmonary tuberculosis, malaria or malnutrition with vitamin A deficiency. In Africa, a severe herpes keratitis may be bilateral in children with measles causing blindness. Bilateral disease is more common in those with atopy (25–40%) and in the immunosuppressed patient [24] (refer to College of Optometrists' CMGs for—Herpes simplex keratitis (HSK)).

Dendritic ulcer is due to replication of virus within the corneal epithelium, giving rise to cell lysis and the characteristic branching lesions with terminal

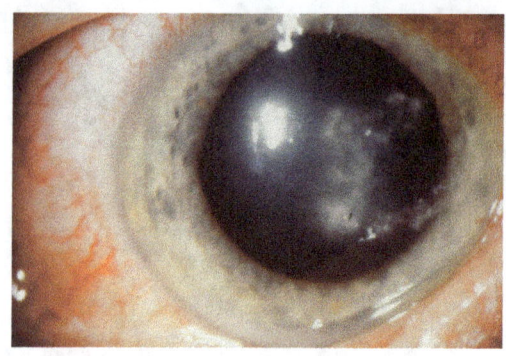

FIGURE 6.42 Subepithelial lesion due to herpes simplex (do NOT use corticosteroids).

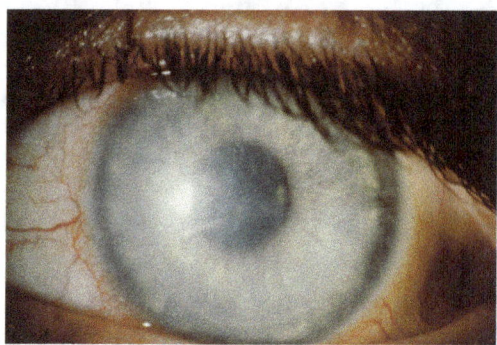

FIGURE 6.43 Disciform herpetic keratitis.

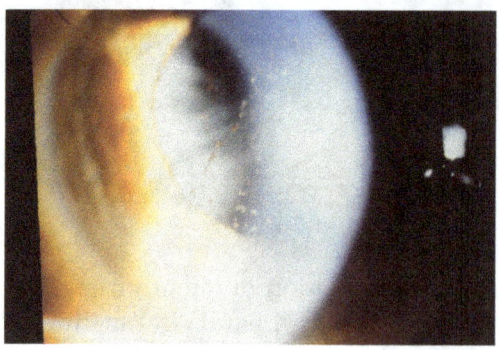

FIGURE 6.44 Stromal herpetic keratitis as seen on a slit lamp.

bulbs. Inadvertent corticosteroid use may broaden this into a geographic ulcer. Disciform keratitis is due to a corneal endotheliitis, with an additional delayed-type hypersensitivity, which explains its inflammatory features, including iritis. Stromal keratitis (Figure 6.44), often with ulceration, is due to an immune response to viral antigens, and the severity of the host stromal response depends partly on the strain of virus and partly on host genetic factors.

Additional photographs of progressive herpetic disease are shown Supplementary Chapter S6.

Therapy of Herpetic Eye Disease

Aciclovir is phosphorylated by viral thymidine kinase and converted to the active triphosphate by host cell enzymes (Appendix 1). The triphosphate is a potent inhibitor of DNA polymerase and acts as a chain terminator to the growing viral DNA strand. Such drugs are more inhibitory to herpetic than cellular DNA polymerase and preferentially inhibit viral DNA synthesis. Aciclovir is highly effective against the dendritic ulcer and as equally effective as trifluorothymidine (F3T). Since aciclovir is less toxic, it is the treatment of choice for dendritic ulcer. While dendritic keratitis may be self-limiting, with about 26% of placebo-treated cases resolving within two to three weeks, antiviral therapy, combined with a minimal wiping debridement, using a cotton-tipped applicator, will produce a clinical cure in 76% to 100% and shorten the median healing time. Where prolonged use is needed, aciclovir is preferable because of its low toxicity. Ganciclovir is available as a topical preparation and demonstrates a similar or superior therapeutic effect, faster treatment response and less irritation for dendritic ulceration.

In disciform keratitis and various forms of stromal keratitis, antivirals are given prophylactically to prevent dendritic lesions, while the inflammatory features of the disorder are suppressed with corticosteroids. Disciform keratitis is treated with a combination of aciclovir or F3T, with a tapering dose of topical corticosteroid. A suitable regime is prednisone 0.5% q.d.s., reducing to 0.3%, 0.1%, 0.03% and 0.01%, according to the response, and weaning finally to a topical nonsteroidal anti-inflammatory drug (NSAID), such as flurbiprofen. Initial therapy with prednisone acetate 1.0% may be required for severe keratouveitis. IOP should be monitored during treatment due to the risk of steroid-induced ocular hypertension [25] (refer to College of Optometrists' CMGs for—see Steroid-related ocular hypertension and glaucoma).

Indolent (metaherpetic) ulcers are not due to active viral disease but to an epithelial surface defect. They are treated by lubricants and anti-collagenases, withdrawal of antivirals and preservatives.

Antiviral Prophylaxis Against Herpetic Disease of the Anterior Segment
The risk of recurrence is increased after corticosteroid use, and for this reason, it is usual to use topical antivirals prophylactically whenever topical corticosteroids are in use in any but the lowest concentration. Weaning of topical corticosteroids should be carried out in a stepwise fashion under ophthalmic supervision. As the intervals between visits increase, it is worth stepping down the dose one week before a planned visit to anticipate rebound inflammation prior to further weaning. Of course, there is also the risk of steroid-related ocular hypertension and glaucoma due to the use of glucocorticoids [26] (refer to College of Optometrists' CMGs for—Steroid-related ocular hypertension and glaucoma).

In addition to their use during the treatment of disciform and stromal keratitis, keratouveitis, trabeculitis and glaucoma, topical corticosteroids are used in patients undergoing keratoplasty for herpetic keratitis. Topical aciclovir (ACV) can be used for a graft on a long-term basis without toxicity, but the incidence of spontaneous epithelial recurrence during the first postoperative year is low, and evidence of benefit is small. Antiviral cover is particularly useful as prophylaxis during the intensive use of topical corticosteroids for allograft rejection, when herpetic recurrence rates can rise from 15% to 32%.

ACV will reach effective aqueous levels within the intact eye after topical use (1.69 mg/mL; range: 0.38–4.87) and has been recommended for treatment of uveitis, limbitis and secondary glaucoma. ACV levels of 1.03 mmol/L can be achieved in human aqueous during oral ACV therapy with lower levels (0.31 mmol/L) in the cornea. F3T does not penetrate intact epithelium, but effective concentrations may penetrate in the presence of an epithelial defect. It is current practice to treat patients undergoing keratoplasty for herpetic disease with a full oral dose of aciclovir (800 mg five times daily) over the operative period and for two weeks thereafter, followed by a maintenance dose of 400 mg twice daily for six to twelve months.

Prophylactic antivirals are also used in patients receiving topical corticosteroids to suppress the inflammatory features of herpetic keratouveitis. Similar considerations to those in corneal graft prophylaxis apply, and risks of antiviral drug toxicity again arise because of the prolonged period (weeks or months) of immunosuppressive therapy. No form of treatment will reduce the frequency of clinical recurrences.

Famciclovir is available to treat *H. simplex* virus types 1 and 2 and *H. zoster*. It is converted in vivo to the triphosphate by virus-induced thymidine kinase and has been shown to be active against aciclovir-resistant *H. simplex*, which has an altered DNA polymerase.

Herpes Zoster Ophthalmicus (HZO)

Involvement of the first division of the Vth cranial nerve by *H. zoster* virus is associated with many ocular complications from involvement of the lids in the primary infection (Figure 6.45) to persistent conjunctivitis, keratouveitis, glaucoma, papillitis, ocular nerve palsy and deep ocular pain [27] (refer to College of Optometrists' CMGs for—Herpes zoster ophthalmicus (HZO)). Although the use of topical ocular corticosteroids to suppress the inflammation does not have the dire consequences seen with *herpes simplex* eye disease (e.g. induction of dendritic or geographic ulceration), studies have suggested that outcome in those treated with ACV alone is better than in those receiving corticosteroids alone (ACV 3%

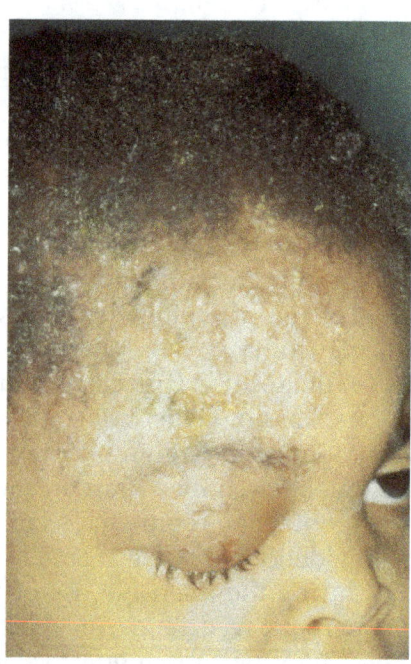

FIGURE 6.45 *Herpes zoster* ophthalmicus.

Source: (Seal D, Pleyer U. Ocular Infection, 2nd Edition 2007)

ointment versus betamethasone 0.1% ointment, five times daily). No recurrence occurred in the ACV-treated group, whereas the recurrence rate was 63% in the corticosteroid-only group. Such recurrences were more difficult to suppress than the initial disease features. Corneal epithelial disease healed significantly more quickly in the ACV patients. ACV has been used intravenously in doses of 5 mg/kg eight-hourly or greater and has been shown in some studies to be effective in improving the healing time of the rash and diminishing the pain associated with the early phase of the disease. However, post-herpetic neuralgia has not been helped, and non-dermatological features of the eye disease have not been suppressed.

There is clinical benefit from oral administration of ACV given at 600 mg five times a day. It is well tolerated and reduces the incidence and severity of dendritiform keratopathy, stromal keratitis and uveitis. Treatment within 72 hours of the onset of skin lesions reduces pain in the acute phase of the disease but not post-herpetic neuralgia. Studies have indicated that doses of 800 mg five times a day are well tolerated and produce higher serum levels. Vaccination with the recombinant zoster vaccine (Shingrix) is recommended for adults aged 50 and older to prevent herpes zoster and its complications, while antiviral prophylaxis may be considered in immunocompromised individuals or those with significant exposure to varicella-zoster virus.

Measles

Conjunctivitis with a mild epithelial keratitis that resolves without sequelae occurs typically in the West. Refer to Chapter 7 for serious complications in the East.

Mumps

Mumps causes dacryoadenitis and conjunctivitis, but keratitis is rare. It may cause superficial punctate epitheliopathy, nummular anterior stromal keratitis and unilateral central interstitial keratitis. This is a distinct syndrome, presenting as a profound drop in visual acuity one week after the onset of parotitis; clearing takes place from the periphery within one month, leaving minimal scars and no vascularization. *Successful mumps immunisation* has effectively reduced the incidence of this infection and its ocular complications.

Epstein–Barr Virus

Epstein–Barr virus causes infectious mononucleosis, a common disease among teenagers (the 'kissing' disease), when follicular conjunctivitis commonly occurs and can be the presenting sign. It has been implicated as a cause of both epithelial and stromal keratitis. It presents with pleomorphic, multifocal and anterior stromal infiltrates with ring opacities in young adults. Treatment has involved topical aciclovir and trifluridine, which have some antiviral activity against Epstein–Barr virus but not as effectively as against *H. simplex*, while epithelial keratitis has resolved with topical corticosteroids [28] (refer to College of Optometrists' CMGs for—noting, Steroid-related ocular hypertension and glaucoma), suggesting the disease has an underlying immunopathological component.

REFERENCES

1. College of Optometrists. Clinical Management Guidelines. Cellulitis, Preseptal and Orbital 2025. Accessed 03/09/25.

2. National Institute of Biomedical Imaging and Engineering. Magnetic Resonance Imaging (MRI) 2025. Accessed 18/08/25 (https://www.nibib.nih.gov/science-education/science-topics/magnetic-resonance-imaging-mri).

3. Ficker L et al. Am J Ophthalmol 1991. PMID: 2012150 (https://doi.org/10.1016/s0002-9394(14)72383-9).

4. Seal DV et al. Immunology and Therapy of Marginal Ulceration as a Complication of Chronic Blepharitis Due to *S. aureus*. In: J Lass (ed.). Advances in Corneal Research. Selected Abstracts of the World Congress on the Cornea IV. New York: Plenum Press 1997, pp 19–25.

5. College of Optometrists. Clinical Management Guidelines. Blepharitis (Lid Margin Disease) 2025. Accessed 18/08/25 (https://www.college-optometrists.org/clinical-guidance/clinical-management-guidelines/blepharitis_lidmargindisease).

6. College of Optometrists. Clinical Management Guidelines. Conjunctivitis (Bacterial) 2025. Accessed 18/08/25.

7. College of Optometrists. Clinical Management Guidelines. Conjunctivitis, Chlamydial 2025. Accessed 18/08/25.

8. College of Optometrists. Clinical Management Guidelines. Ophthalmia Neonatorum 2025. Accessed 18/08/25.

9 Manasseh G et al. BMJ 2022. PMID: 35321902 (https://doi.org/10.1136/bmj-2021-068023).

10. College of Optometrists. Clinical Management Guidelines. Ophthalmia Conjunctivitis (Viral, Non-Herpetic) 2025. Accessed 18/08/25.

11. College of Optometrists. Clinical Management Guidelines. Microbial Keratitis (Bacterial, Fungal) 2025. Accessed 18/08/25.

12. Hoffmann J et al. Comm Eye Health J 2024. PMID: 40115630 (https://cehjournal.org/articles/820).

13. Linaburg T et al. Inf Dis Clinics N Amer 2024. PMID: 39271302 (https://doi.org/10.1016/j.idc.2024.07.010).

14. Seal D. Eye 2003. PMID: 14631394 (https://doi.org/10.1038/sj.eye.6700563).

15. Stapleton F et al. Clin Inf Dis 1991. PMID: 2047670 (https://doi.org/10.1093/clind/13.Supplement_5.S392).

16. Rahimi F et al. J Ophthalmic Vis Res 2015. PMID: 26425310 (https://pmc.ncbi.nlm.nih.gov/articles/PMC4568605/).

17. College of Optometrists. Clinical Management Guidelines. Microbial Keratitis (Acanthamoeba sp.) 2025. Accessed 18/08/25.

18. Alphawaz A. Middle East Afr J Ophthalmol 2011. PMID: 21887085 (https://10.4103/0974-9233.84062).

19. Seal D et al. Eye 1996. PMID: 8944089 (https://doi.org/10.1038/eye.1996.92).

20. Duguid I et al. Ophthalmol 1997. PMID: 9331195 (https://www.aaojournal.org/article/S0161-6420(97)30092-X/pdf).

21. Ferrari G et al. Case Rep Ophthalmol 2011. PMID: 22174703 (https:/10.1159/000334270).

22. Carnt N et al. Ophthalmology 2016. PMID: 26952591 (https:/doi/10.1016/j.ophtha.2016.01.020).

23. Bagga B et al. Eye 2021. PMID: 32719525 (https://www.nature.com/articles/s41433-020-1109-4#citeas).

24. College of Optometrists. Clinical Management Guidelines. Herpes Simplex Keratitis (HSK) 2025. Accessed 18/08/25.

25. College of Optometrists. Clinical Management Guidelines. Steroid-Related Ocular Hypertension and Glaucoma 2025. Accessed 03/09/25.

26. Clinical Management Guidelines. Steroid-Related Ocular Hypertension and Glaucoma 2025. Accessed 03/09/25.

27. College of Optometrists. Clinical Management Guidelines. Herpes Zoster Ophthalmicus (HZO) 2025. Accessed 03/09/25.

28. College of Optometrists. Clinical Management Guidelines. Steroid-Related Ocular Hypertension and Glaucoma 2025. Accessed 03/09/25.

7: Tropical Public Health and Global Eye Care

Infectious Diseases Resulting in Blindness

CORE MESSAGES

This chapter reviews infections frequently found in the tropics as they affect the eye. Some causes local disease, viz. trachoma, while others are systemically-sourced, such as microfilariae of onchocerciasis.

There are successful eradication programs for trachoma and onchocerciasis, but none are 100% successful, and much work remains to maintain their eradication. This is because the particular type of organism, often a parasite from an insect bite, cannot be eliminated in the same way as some virus diseases with immunisation, viz. measles, and even that needs constant attention.

Microbial keratitis remains a particular and frequent problem, especially in rural workers, often due to a mixed bacterial and fungal aetiology. Some countries, viz. India, have made good progress by managing the problem with rural eye care workers and basic laboratories along with a supply of affordable drops, produced in India, of antibiotics against both bacteria and fungi.

MAJOR CHALLENGES

Trachoma

Trachoma is the leading infectious cause of blindness worldwide, causing chronic conjunctivitis with scarring, entropion, trichiasis and multiple episodes of keratitis resulting in a scarred cornea. *Chlamydia trachomatis* is transmitted directly or indirectly from ocular and nasal discharges of infected children, who are the principal reservoir of infection. Flies spread the infectious discharges repeatedly from person to person in poor communities without running water or sanitation. In hyperendemic states, 30 to 50% of the population has active disease, and 10% exhibit blinding sequelae. Active trachomatous inflammation is common among preschool children, with prevalence rates as high as 60–90%; infection becomes less frequent and shorter in duration with increasing age when complications emerge of entropion, trichiasis, secondary keratitis (bacterial, fungal or *Acanthamoeba*) and corneal scarring.

Trachoma is caused by the obligate intracellular bacterium *Chlamydia trachomatis* serotypes A, B, Ba or C. It has no peptidoglycan in its cell wall and cannot be grown on agar. It is visualised as inclusion bodies in a scrape of epithelial cells using Giemsa stain and a UV light source (Figure 7.1).

Chlamydia is grown in McCoy or HEp-2 cells at 37°C in 5% CO_2 with detection after 72 hours by direct fluorescent antibody staining. It is easier and quicker

DOI: 10.1201/9781003606789-8

to use a PCR test, which is highly sensitive and specific. GeneProof offers a *Chlamydia trachomatis* polymerase chain reaction (PCR) kit, available in two packaging options: 25 reactions and 100 reactions. Both kits use real-time PCR technology [1].

In trachoma, the superior tarsal conjunctiva shows more severe follicular reaction than the inferior and is the only type of conjunctivitis that exhibits Herbert's pits. The 'pits' on the limbus are the sequelae of sloughed limbal follicles that cicatrize (Figure 7.2).

The WHO has defined a grading scheme for the amount of superior tarsal inflammation with four categories (Figures 7.3–7.6) *(Courtesy of Dr. G. Johnson, ICEH, London).*

Treatment of the early inflammatory stage is highly effective with a single *oral* dose of azithromycin, due to the high intracellular concentration that it achieves (Chapter 5), and it is the treatment of choice. Topical treatment with tetracycline or erythromycin eye ointment, or quinolone drops, must be given three times

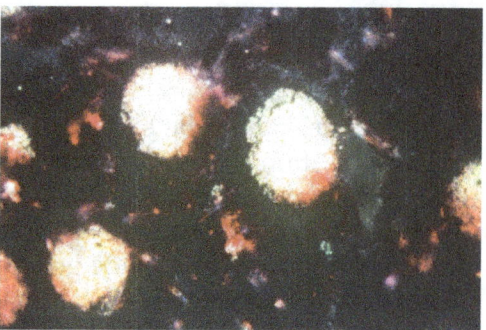

FIGURE 7.1 Chlamydial inclusion bodies in epithelial cells—Giemsa stain + UV light.

Source: (Seal D, Pleyer U. Ocular Infection, 2nd Edition 2007)

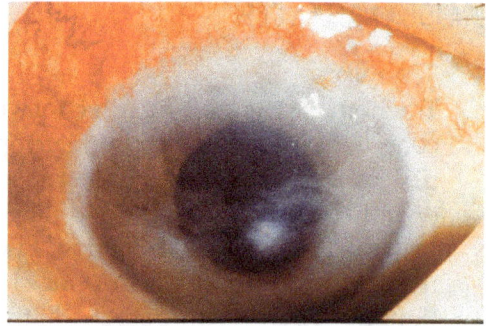

FIGURE 7.2 Herbert's pits (old limbal follicles) from trachoma with secondary corneal infection (epithelial and stromal infiltrates) due to *Acanthamoeba* (St. John's Hospital, Jerusalem).

Source: (Seal D, Pleyer U. Ocular Infection, 2nd Edition 2007)

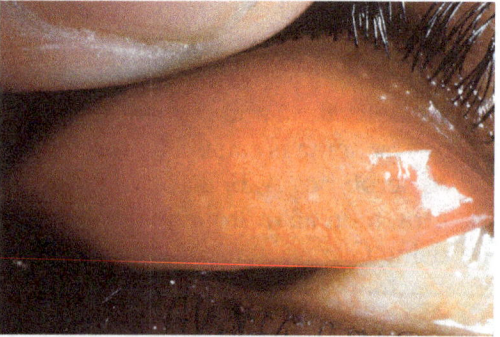

FIGURE 7.3 Follicular (TF)—the presence of five or more follicles.

Source: (Seal D, Pleyer U. Ocular Infection, 2nd Edition 2007)

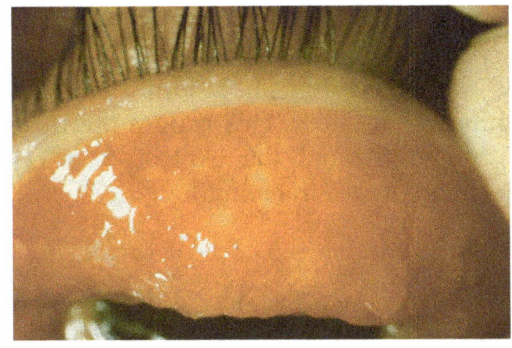

FIGURE 7.4 Intense inflammation (TI)—with thickening of the tarsal conjunctiva.

Source: (Seal D, Pleyer U. Ocular Infection, 2nd Edition 2007)

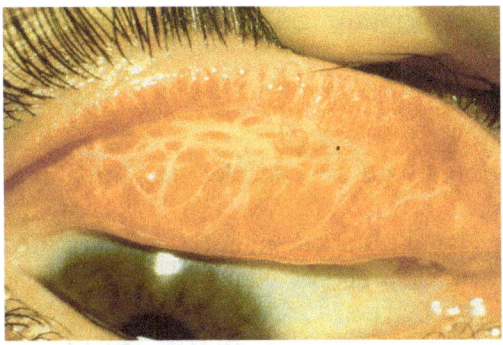

FIGURE 7.5 Scarring (TS)—the presence of conjunctival scarring.

Source: (Seal D, Pleyer U. Ocular Infection, 2nd Edition 2007)

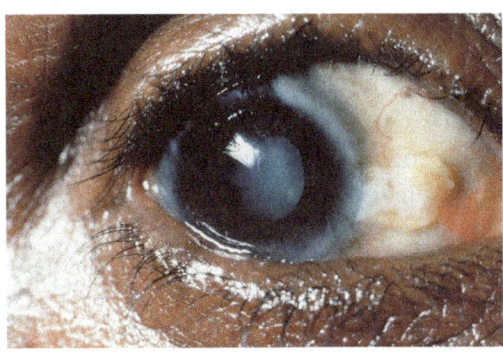

FIGURE 7.6 Trichiasis (TT)—the eyelashes rub on the ocular surface with entropion to cause repeated keratitis.

Source: (Seal D, Pleyer U. Ocular Infection, 2nd Edition 2007)

daily for five weeks and is considered second choice. Treatment of other family members, or whole villages, is needed to prevent re-infection. Keratitis is treated with antibiotics. Surgery is needed to correct the entropion.

Trachoma can still be found in 39 countries, mostly in Africa, the Middle East and a few in the Americas and Asia; it has been eliminated from India, a great success story from recent endemicity [2]. Globally, 103.2 million people are still at risk for trachoma, which represents an 11% reduction from 115.7 million in 2023. However, 1.5 million are still at immediate risk for blindness from trachomatous trichiasis (TT). The Carter Center works to control and prevent blinding trachoma in Ethiopia, Niger, South Sudan and Sudan. Ethiopia has the highest known burden of active trachoma infection in the world. The Carter Center supports Ethiopia's (and thus the world's) most affected region, Amhara; it has funded the construction of more than 3.6 million household latrines to reduce breeding sites for flies [3] (https://www.cartercenter.org/health/trachoma/index.html).

The World Health Organization (WHO) launched the Global Elimination of Blinding Trachoma by 2020 (GET2020) initiative in 1998. This program aimed to eliminate trachoma as a public health problem through the SAFE strategy [4] (https://www.who.int/news-room/fact-sheets/detail/trachoma):

- Surgery: for trichiasis [5] when the eyelashes scratch the corneal surface followed by secondary bacterial infection.
- Antibiotics: use of azithromycin in whole villages to eradicate *Chlamydia trachomatis*.
- Facial cleanliness: to reduce spread of the bacterium.
- Environmental improvement: to provide fresh running water and sanitation to reduce breeding grounds for flies.

Onchocerciasis

Onchocerciasis (also known as river blindness) is the second leading infectious cause of blindness. It is classified as a neglected tropical disease (NTD). It causes intense itching, rashes, skin discoloration, visual impairment and ocular disease leading to permanent blindness. The parasite is spread by bites of infected black flies (*Simulium sp.*) that breed in rapidly flowing rivers.

The life cycle of *Onchocerca volvulus* involves two hosts: humans and black flies of the genus *Simulium*. When a female fly bites an infected human, it ingests microfilariae (immature worms) circulating in the blood. The microfilariae develop into infective third-stage larvae (L3) within the fly over a period of one to three weeks. This development occurs in the thoracic flight muscles and the proboscis. When the infected fly bites another human, the L3 larvae are transmitted into the new host's skin through its proboscis. *Onchocerca volvulus* is a parasite that is maintained almost entirely by the human host; there is no animal involvement.

Within the human host, the L3 larvae migrate to subcutaneous tissues, where they develop into adult worms over six to twelve months. They form fibrous nodules under the skin, where they can live for up to 15 years. Males are smaller and more mobile, moving between nodules to mate with females. Female nematodes (roundworms) in the nodules produce microfilariae, which can live up to two years in the host's skin and circulate via the bloodstream. Microfilariae invade the eye from the skin by direct penetration through the conjunctiva and sclera, with a sucker in one extremity. They penetrate under the conjunctival epithelium to the superficial layers of the cornea (Figure 7.7), Descemet's membrane, the ciliary body, lens, the choroid and retina, causing localised cumulative mechanical damage.

The inflammatory reaction that occurs is due to a cell-mediated immune response to dead microfilariae. In the cornea, microfilariae can be seen with the slit lamp, generally deep to Bowman's membrane and moving slowly at the centre of ill-defined opacities representing a sequence of inflammation and scarring.

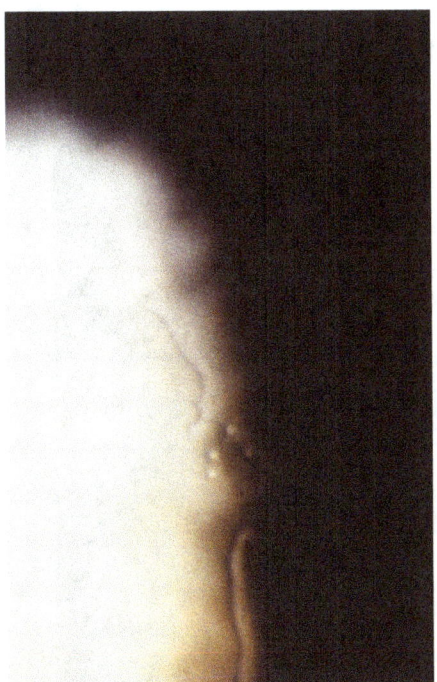

FIGURE 7.7 Microfilariae of *Onchocerca volvulus* viewed under the conjunctival epithelium.

Source: (Seal D, Pleyer U. Ocular Infection, 2nd Edition 2007)

Ocular manifestations include keratitis (Figure 7.8), anterior uveitis, glaucoma, chorioretinitis (Figure 7.9) and optic neuritis.

Treatment is given with ivermectin, 150 mcg/kg, as a single oral dose once or twice per year for 10 to 15 years, corresponding to the life span of the adult worm, or as long as there is evidence of active infection (Appendix 6) in the eye or skin; it is effective in killing microfilariae but does not affect adult worms. In addition, doxycycline (200 mg orally daily for six weeks) can be used to target the endosymbiotic bacteria *Wolbachia*, which are crucial for the survival of adult worms, leading to their death. Management of the retinitis is difficult and associated with immuno-inflammatory effects, especially with a high count of microfilariae.

Progression of the corneal infection without treatment is shown in different patients earlier. For patients co-infected with *Loa loa*, supportive precautions must be taken due to the risk of severe adverse effects from the ivermectin.

Globally, at least 244 million people in 31 countries suffer from this debilitating and painful disease. Africa is home to 99% of people at risk; the remaining 1% live on the border between Brazil and Venezuela.

ONCHOCERCIASIS CONTROL AND ERADICATION PROGRAM

The Onchocerciasis Control Programme (OCP) was conceived in 1969 and launched 50 years ago in 1974 by the WHO and the World Bank. The OCP originally covered Benin, Burkina Faso, Côte d'Ivoire, Ghana, Mali, Niger and Togo. By 1986, the OCP expanded its operations to four more countries—Guinea, Guinea-Bissau, Senegal and Sierra Leone—and has been successful in controlling the disease.

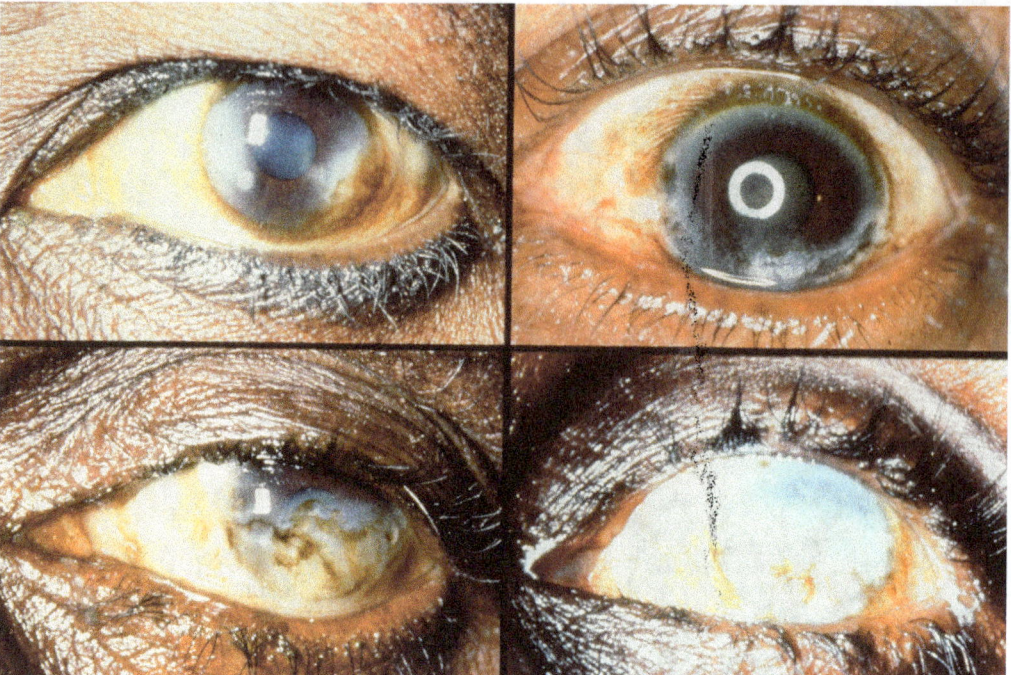

FIGURE 7.8 Progression of keratitis in different patients due to *Onchocerca volvulus* in the eye.

Source: (Courtesy of Gordon Johnson, International Centre of Eye Health, London)

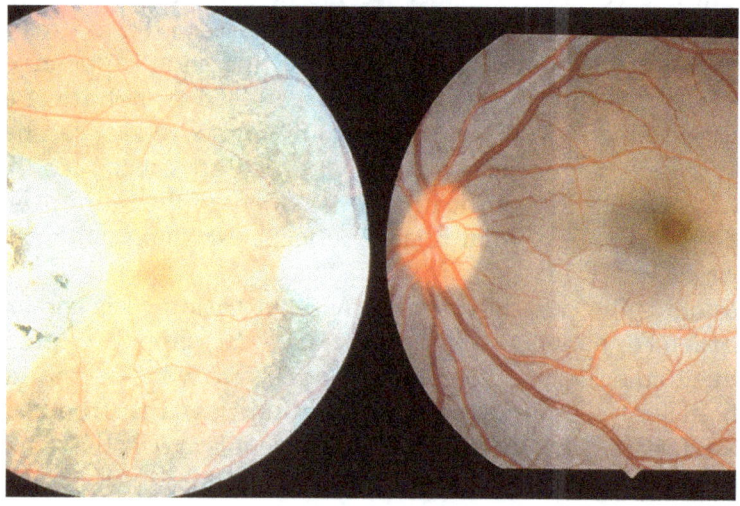

FIGURE 7.9 Severe chorioretinitis in the right eye from onchocerciasis (left eye normal).

The program has utilised larvicide spraying into fast-flowing rivers to control black fly populations and the use of oral ivermectin to treat infected people starting from 1988. The OCP covered 30 million people in Benin, Burkina Faso, Côte d'Ivoire, Ghana, Togo, Mali and Niger.

The African Programme for Onchocerciasis Control (APOC) has been making progress towards the elimination of onchocerciasis but faces many challenges.

Elimination has been possible in some areas, with some countries meeting criteria for stopping treatment, others close to elimination and some still facing challenges.

As of January 31, 2025, *Niger* is the first African country to eliminate onchocerciasis:

- In *Burundi*, the program has seen mixed results. For example, in the Cibitoke Bubanza region, some areas like North Tchollire and Cross River have shown positive trends, while others like Kwara and Oyo have not.
- In *Nigeria*, the program faces challenges in Enugu and Anambra, where progress is slower compared to other areas like Cross River.
- In *Uganda*, the program has seen progress in Kasese, but challenges persist in Adjumani Mojo.
- In *Cameroon* and *Congo*, efforts to control and eliminate the disease continue.

In the Americas, the Onchocerciasis Elimination Program for the Americas (OEPA) was launched in 1993. It made significant progress in eliminating onchocerciasis, with transmission interrupted in 11 of the 13 foci in the region. The OEPA's strategy involved mass drug administration of ivermectin, donated by Merck & Co., Inc., with at least 85% coverage of eligible populations.

As a result of these efforts, four countries have achieved the elimination of onchocerciasis: Colombia in 2013, Ecuador in 2014, Mexico in 2015 and Guatemala in 2016. The OCP shifted its focus from control to elimination in 2002, and the success of the OEPA has influenced programs in Africa, leading some countries to move from a control to an elimination strategy. However, caution is needed, especially in Africa, as onchocerciasis can recur without annual dosing with ivermectin [7].

Luckily, optimism persists when more than 150 onchocerciasis partners gathered in November 2023 in Mbour, Senegal, for the first meeting of the new Global Onchocerciasis Elimination Network (GONE) to strengthen collaboration among countries and partners [8].

Loiasis

Loa loa—meaning the 'worm worm', but known as the *eye worm*, is a roundworm that migrates throughout the body, including the eye. It is found in West Africa and is transmitted by horseflies (intermediate larval host) of the genus *Chrysops* (deer flies, yellow flies), including the species *C. dimidiata* and *C. silacea*, which bite humans who are the definitive host. After bites, the unique microfilariae reside in the peripheral blood during the day and migrate into the lungs at night. The microfilariae develop into worms in the host's blood within five to six months and can survive up to 17 years.

The *L. loa* adult worm (20 to 34 mm long by 350 to 430 µm wide) travels under the skin, causing inflammations known as Calabar swellings. They move to any site in the body and also invade the eye under the sclera to cause occasional blindness from the inflammatory reaction. They can be seen in the slit lamp, partially paralysed by local anesthetic and attempted removal made with forceps but can also escape! Specialist treatment is needed with ivermectin or DEC (Appendix 6) [9].

Bacterial Keratitis

Refer to Chapter 6.

Fungal Keratitis

Fungi are a common cause of keratitis in tropical climates, especially in rural workers and those living near a cement factory. Patients with compromised corneas are also more susceptible. Fungal keratitis often shows an infiltration with a serrated margin and raised profile with or without a hypopyon [10].

Whenever possible, a corneal scrape should be performed for staining and culture (Appendix 5) [11].

Candida albicans commonly infects immune-compromised patients, including the eye (Figure 7.10).

The corneal scrape (Figure 7.11) shows pseudohyphae of *C. albicans* in a wet prep and a Grocott silver stain; the latter shows the characteristic black elongated yeast cells giving the false appearance of hyphae.

Corneal injuries are also prone to fungal infection, especially if associated with agriculture. They may present with a localised infiltrate, with serrated margin, without hypopyon (Figure 7.12).

The corneal scrape showed filamentous septate hyphae using a Grocott silver stain (Figure 7.13).

Fungal keratitis may also present with an infiltrate and hypopyon (Figure 7.14). Presentation can be late in the tropics when the fungal infection has advanced.

There is a dense infiltrate with a serrated margin and a hypopyon present. A Gram's stain of a corneal scrape shows septate hyphae typical of *Curvularia sp.* (Figure 7.15).

The patient responded to treatment with antifungal antibiotics.

Fungal keratitis due to *Fusarium sp.* is often aggressive with a serrated margin, raised profile, deep stromal infiltration, hypopyon and uveitis (Figure 7.16). Urgent investigation and treatment, both medical and surgical, is required, or

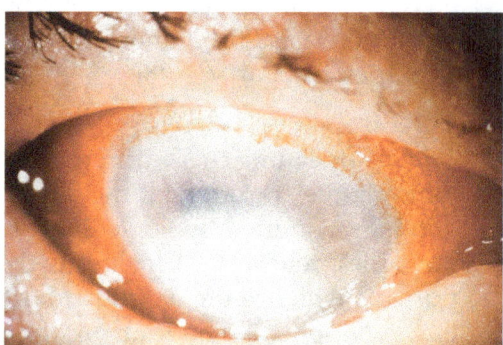

FIGURE 7.10 Corneal perforation due to *C. albicans* in a neuroparalytic eye.

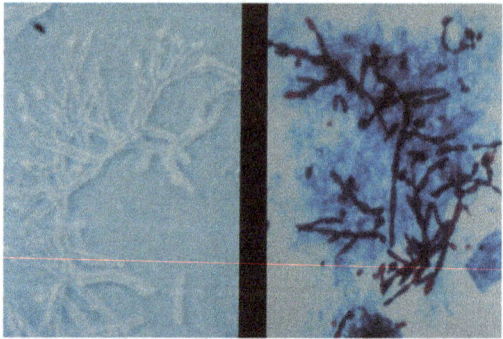

FIGURE 7.11 (L) Wet prep and (R) Grocott silver stain of *Candida albicans* (yeast cells and pseudohyphae).

Source: (Seal D, Pleyer U. Ocular Infection, 2nd Edition 2007)

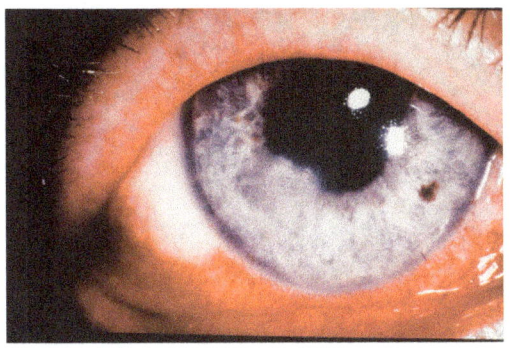

FIGURE 7.12 Dry fungal keratitis from horse manure injury.

Source: (Seal D, Pleyer U. Ocular Infection, 2nd Edition 2007)

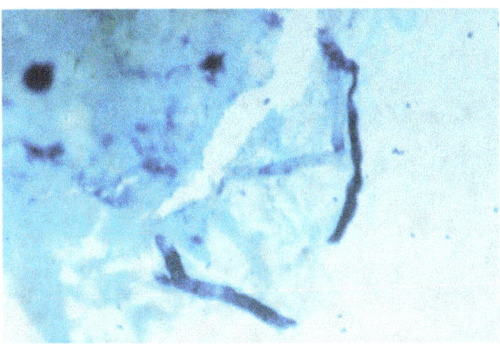

FIGURE 7.13 Grocott (silver) stain of filamentous septate hyphae in the corneal scrape.

Source: (Seal D, Pleyer U. Ocular Infection, 2nd Edition 2007)

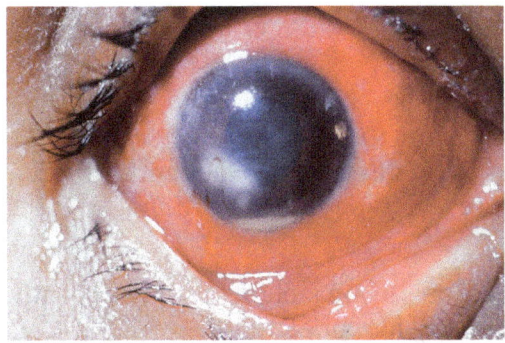

FIGURE 7.14 Fungal keratitis due to *Curvularia sp.* pre-treatment in Bangladesh.

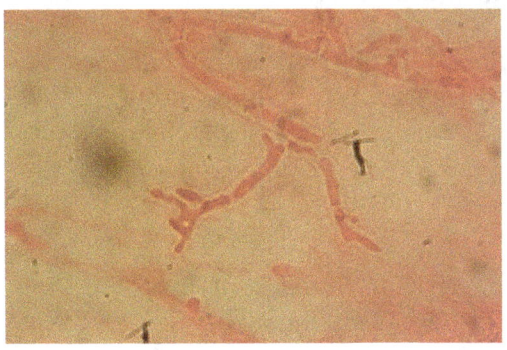

FIGURE 7.15 Gram stain of corneal scrape showing septate hyphae.

the infection can progress to an endophthalmitis. Referral is needed for intensive therapy, or the eye may be lost within six weeks.

The corneal scrape showed septate hyphae stained with PAS (periodic acid–Schiff) stain (Figure 7.17) and *Fusarium* was cultured. The hyphae could also have been stained with lactophenol blue or Gram's stain.

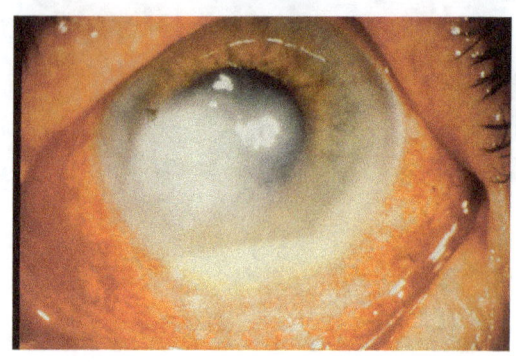

FIGURE 7.16 Fungal keratitis due to *Fusarium sp.*

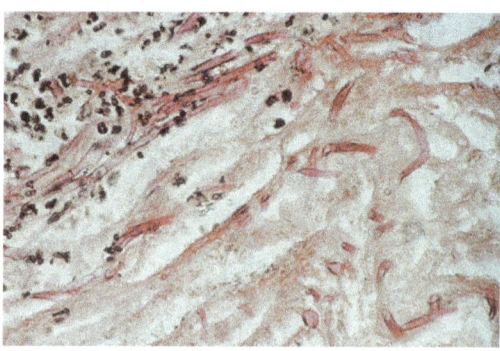

FIGURE 7.17 PAS (periodic acid–Schiff) stain of corneal scrape showing filamentous, septate hyphae.

Management and Treatment

It is important to identify the type of fungus, *particularly between a yeast or a filamentous fungus*, as soon as possible. Practically, this is quick to identify from a corneal scraping (Appendix 5), as it influences the type of therapy. *Appendix 6 lists all antifungal therapies.*

For unknown fungal infection, use ketoconazole or voriconazole drops 1% frequently and oral tablets 200–600 mg/day (200 mg/day for voriconazole).

For Candida albicans (or another yeast) infection, use fluconazole drops 1% and oral tablets 100 mg/day.

For filamentous fungal infection, use natamycin 5% drops frequently. There is experimental and clinical trial evidence for use of topical chlorhexidine 0.2% as alternative antifungal therapy, but it was not found to be as effective as topical natamycin [12].

MIXED BACTERIAL AND FUNGAL INFECTIONS

Some patients have keratitis due to both bacteria and fungi as a mixed infection and even with *Acanthamoeba* or other protozoa as well; it may be difficult to distinguish between the primary and secondary pathogens.

Both pathogens may be seen on microscopy or found on culture [13]; if possible, distinction is made between commensals and pathogens. If required, antifungal therapy is combined with antibiotics, viz. moxifloxacin, or with anti-amoebic therapy (Appendix 6).

MEASLES KERATITIS

Most cases of measles are associated with conjunctivitis. In the West, it causes a mild epithelial keratitis that resolves without sequelae. In the East, keratitis occurs in 67 to 100% of cases and is a major cause of blindness in developing nations. It presents as a stromal disease with ulceration, when secondary infection from traditional eye medicines and vitamin A deficiency are compounding factors. Although no specific antiviral drug available, topical antibiotics and systemic vitamin A supplements will help prevent secondary bacterial disease. *Measles immunisation has an important role to play in developing countries for preventing blindness.*

DEFICIENCY OF VITAMIN A (XEROPHTHALMIA)

Ocular signs and symptoms associated with vitamin A deficiency include conjunctival and corneal xerosis (xerophthalmia), Bitot's spots, keratomalacia, nyctalopia and retinopathy. Vitamin A deficiency is a major problem in developing countries and a leading cause of preventable blindness; it contributes to increased morbidity and mortality and adversely effects the child's growth. These children are also particularly susceptible to measles virus-associated keratitis (Figure 7.18).

EMERGING VIRAL DISEASES

For West Nile fever, dengue and chikungunya virus infections, refer to Supplementary Chapter S7.

NEGLECTED TROPICAL DISEASES (NTD)

Microbial keratitis is responsible for over 2 million cases of monocular blindness annually in Africa and Asia. It can result in significant morbidity, including stigma and pain. Recently, there have been calls for microbial keratitis to be recognised as a *neglected tropical disease* by the WHO [10].

Rationale and main challenges for developing eradication investment cases for onchocerciasis, lymphatic filariasis and human African trypanosomiasis are considered in the following link: https://doi.org/10.1371/journal.pntd.0002446 [14].

PROPHYLAXIS OF ENDOPHTHALMITIS AFTER CATARACT SURGERY

Refer to Chapter 8 (1b) for the European Society of Cataract and Refractive surgeons (ESCRS) placebo-controlled trial demonstrating a fivefold reduction in

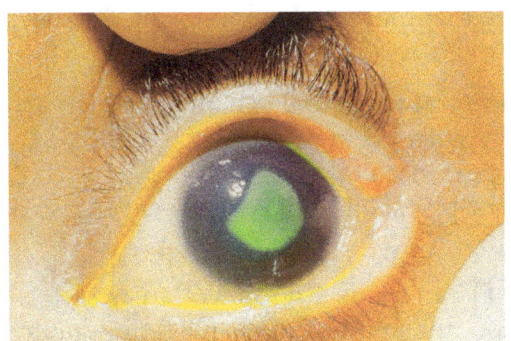

FIGURE 7.18 Keratitis associated with measles and xerophthalmia.

Source: (Seal D, Pleyer U. Ocular Infection, 2nd Edition 2007)

postoperative endophthalmitis with the use of intracameral cefuroxime (1.0 mg in 0.1 ml) *at the time of surgery*. Refer to Supplementary Chapter S7 and Appendix 6 for more details. Subsequent work in retrospective studies has shown that both cefuroxime and moxifloxacin are suitable antibiotics.

Thea Pharmaceuticals (Clermont-Ferrand, France) produces a single-use product (Aprokam) as a powder dissolved in 0.9% sterile saline available in Europe (not the USA). It is cost-saving for hospitals and has minimal risk of dilution error. Each vial contains 50 mg of cefuroxime (as 52.6 mg of cefuroxime sodium). After reconstitution with 5 ml of saline, a 0.1 ml solution contains 1 mg of cefuroxime. This is considered highly effective and free of toxicity.

Alcon Laboratories (Fort Worth, Texas, USA) produces a single-use vial of moxifloxacin at 5 mg/ml (use 0.1 ml containing 0.5 mg [500 micrograms]); it is available from Imprimis Pharmaceuticals, San Diego, USA.

Aurolab (www.aurolab.com) produces unpreserved sterile vials of moxifloxacin 0.5% w/v (Auromox), each containing 1 ml, for routine intracameral injection of *0.1 ml* (containing 0.5 mg [500 micrograms]) of moxifloxacin at the time of cataract surgery, as a prophylactic antibiotic to prevent postoperative endophthalmitis. This is considered highly effective and free of toxicity.

PROPHYLAXIS OF MALARIA

Hydroxychloroquine retinopathy is more common than previously reported. The prevalence in long-term users appears to be around 7.5% and, depending on dose and duration of therapy, can increase to 20–50% after 20 years of therapy. Risk increases for patients taking more than 5 mg/kg/day. This is important, as the only intervention to prevent further damage is stopping the drug. The risk is increased for patients taking more than 5 mg/kg/day, those also taking tamoxifen and those with renal impairment.

RETINAL TOXICITY DUE TO CHLOROQUINE

Chloroquine and hydroxychloroquine are both 4-aminoquinoline compounds and share similar mechanisms of action and potential toxicities, including cardiomyopathy, cardiac conduction defects and retinal toxicity. Hydroxychloroquine (Plaquenil) is used to treat lupus and rheumatoid arthritis while chloroquine is primarily used to treat malaria. Both drugs can cause similar adverse effects, but hydroxychloroquine is considered less toxic. Chloroquine toxicity occurs with an overdose or prolonged use and causes cardiac arrhythmias, vision loss with macula damage and other sequelae.

Individuals on chloroquine therapy need regular yearly monitoring to detect early signs of retinal toxicity as follows:

Visual field testing: to identify any paracentral or central scotomas, which are characteristic of chloroquine retinopathy with a HVF 10-2 chart.
Fundus photography: to document the appearance of the retina.
OCT: to assess the integrity of retinal layers, particularly the parafoveal ellipsoid zone, which is often disrupted early.

In addition, fundus autofluorescence (FAF) can be used to detect areas of retinal pigment epithelium (RPE) dysfunction and multifocal electroretinography (mfERG) to evaluate retinal function.

If two of these tests show abnormalities consistent with chloroquine toxicity, it indicates definite signs of retinopathy. The degree of retinopathy is classified as mild, moderate or severe. If retinopathy is detected, the patient needs to reduce the dose or discontinue the chloroquine and be monitored closely. Early detection is crucial, as cessation of the drug can arrest progression, but cellular damage may continue for a while. Hydroxychloroquine is less toxic to the retina [15] (screeninghttps://www.rcophth.ac.uk/news-views/hydroxychloroquine-and-chloroquine-retinopathy/).

GLOBAL BURDEN OF OCULAR DISEASES

Estimates on the number of people blind or visually impaired—(Vision Loss Expert Group of the Global Burden of Disease Study, the GBD 2019 Blindness and Vision Impairment Collaborators)—refer to Chapter 3.

Glaucoma—Global estimates on the number of people blind or visually impaired by glaucoma: A meta-analysis from 2000 to 2020 [16].

Diabetic retinopathy—Global estimates on the number of people blind or visually impaired by diabetic retinopathy: a meta-analysis from 2000 to 2020 [17].

Age-related macular degeneration—Global estimates on the number of people blind or visually impaired by AMD: a meta-analysis from 2000 to 2020 [18].

Cataract—Global estimates on the number of people blind or visually impaired by cataract: a meta-analysis from 2000 to 2020 [19].

COMMUNITY EYE HEALTH

Community Eye Health Journal (https://cehjournal.org/)

The *Community Eye Health Journal* (CEHJ) provides practical, peer-reviewed educational information and guidance to eye care providers, managers and policy-makers in low-resource settings for free. A printed copy has been sent free of charge to eye care health workers around the world for the last 30 years. It is published by the International Centre for Eye Health (https://iceh.lshtm.ac.uk/), based at the London School of Hygiene and Tropical Medicine, and provides information, education and insight to eye care and public health professionals in 126 countries. The CEHJ is now available as an app for smartphones and tablets and can be downloaded free of charge from the App Store (iOS devices) and Google Play. Users with intermittent internet access, or expensive mobile data charges, benefit from the app's offline access with bookmarking and a personal library to store and organise content.

a) Development of 'Telemedicine' Eye Care and Treatment in the Tropics

For instructions on how to use the ophthalmoscope to view the retina, and types of disease, go to the Moorfields Eye Hospital educational video on 'YouTube' [20].

Instructions on how to use the mobile telephone to photograph the retina with an indirect lens are given in a 'YouTube' video together with advice on how to create still clips for record purposes [21] (https://www.youtube.com/watch?v=iMut5iMbgIE&t=1s). Use of new mobile telephone apps for photographic identification of disease, including retinal photographs, are also available [22] (https://doi.org/10.1016/j.preteyeres.2020.100900).

b) Cost-Effective Ophthalmic Products

Aurolab (Aravind Eye Hospital) manufactures a wide range of ophthalmic consumables, including intraocular lenses; pharmaceutical products, including eye drops; and surgical adjuncts. *Aurolab* products are exported to 160 countries around the world and account for 9% of intraocular lenses globally [23] (www.aurolab.com).

REFERENCES

1. GeneProof (2025). GeneProof Chlamydia trachomatis PCR Kit. Accessed 18/8/25 (https://www.geneproof.com/geneproof-chlamydia-trachomatis-pcr-kit/p1073).
2. Noopur G et al. Indian J Ophthalmol 2022. PMID: 36018099 (https://doi.org/10.4103/ijo.IJO_503_22).
3. The Carter Center. Health Programs. 2025. Accessed 18/8/25 (https://www.cartercenter.org/health/index.html).
4. Word Health Organization. Trachoma 2025. Accessed 18/8/25 (https://www.who.int/news-room/fact-sheets/detail/trachoma).
5. College of Optometrists. Clinical Management Guidelines (Trichiasis) 2025. Accessed 03/09/25.
6. College of Optometrists. Clinical Management Guidelines (Entropion) 2025. Accessed 03/09/25.
7. Babalola O. Clin Ophthalmol 2011. PMID: 22069350 (https://doi.org/10.2147/OPTH.S8372).
8. World Health Organization. Global Onchocerciasis Network for Elimination (GONE) 2025. Accessed 18/08/25 (https://www.who.int/initiatives/global-onchocerciasis-network-for-elimination).
9. US Centers for Disease Control and Prevention. Clinical Treatment of Loiasis 2024. Accessed 18/08/25 (https://www.cdc.gov/filarial-worms/hcp/clinical-care/loiasis.html).
10. Hoffman J et al. J Fungi (Basel) 2022. PMID: 35205955 (https://pubmed.ncbi.nlm.nih.gov/35205955/).
11. Leck AK et al. Comm Eye Health J 2025. PMID: 40115629 (https://cehjournal.org/articles/818).
12. Yadav R et al. Ophthalmol 2022. PMID: 34896126 (https://doi.org/10.1016/j.ophtha.2021.12.004).
13. Clare G et al. Eye 2024. PMID: 3835567 (https://doi.org/10.1038/s41433-024-02966-w).
14. Tediosi F et al. D. PLoS Negl Trop Dis. 2013. PMID: 24244762 (https://doi.org/10.1371/journal.pntd.0002446. eCollection 2013 Nov).
15. Royal College of Ophthalmologists. Hydroxychloroquine and Chloroquine Retinopathy: Recommendations on Monitoring 2020. Accessed 18/8/25 (https://www.rcophth.ac.uk/news-views/hydroxychloroquine-and-chloroquine-retinopathy/).
16. Vision Loss Expert Group. Eye 2024. PMID: 38565601 (https://doi.org/10.1038/s41433-024-02995-5).
17. Vision Loss Expert Group. Eye 2024. PMID: 38937557 (https://doi.org/10.1038/s41433-024-03101-5).
18. Vision Loss Expert Group. Eye 2024. PMID: 38965321 (https://doi.org/10.1038/s41433-024-03050-z).
19. Vision Loss Expert Group. Eye 2024. PMID: 38461217 (https://doi.org/10.1038/s41433-024-02961-1).
20. Okhravi N et al. Direct Ophthalmolscopy 2025. Accessed 18/8/25 (https://www.youtube.com/watch?v=7lhvhKvK_iM).
21. Espinosa J. Retinal Photography with Smartphone 2025. Accessed 18/8/25 (https://www.youtube.com/watch?v=iMut5iMbgIE&t=1s).
22. Li JO et al. Prog Retin Eye Res. 2021. PMID: 32898686 (https://doi.org/10.1016/j.preteyeres.2020.100900. Epub 2020 Sep 6).
23. Aurolab. Our Products 2025. Accessed 18/8/25 (www.aurolab.com).

8: Epidemiological Surveys and Basic Statistics—Pitfalls and Solutions

CORE MESSAGES

In order to investigate risk factors for disease, a basic understanding of epidemiological methods is required. This is important to avoid misinterpretation when comparing the results of one study with another. For example, crude rates should not be used to compare populations of different structures without definition. Similarly, it is not appropriate to draw population-based conclusions from studies of limited size and power; this is always dangerous.

EPIDEMIOLOGY AND STATISTICS

Questionnaire reporting surveys are popular today and often used to compare results of surgical techniques, medical management or drug use in clinical practice; surveys are made within one unit or within and between multiple units. However, a response rate of less than 66% is often found giving rise to non-response bias, considered later.

Epidemiology—The study of disease in relation to a defined population and requires study of both diseased and healthy persons. The measurement of incidence and prevalence rates form the basis for comparison between defined population groups.

- Clinical appearances determine decisions about individual patients.
- Epidemiological observations determine decisions about groups and are the basis for preventive medicine.

Incidence—The proportion (1 in 1,000), or percentage (%), with *new* disease in a defined group occurring within a given time period. It is annualised unless otherwise expressed but maybe stated over any time period.

Prevalence—The proportion or percentage with disease, including both *old* and *new* cases, of a defined group occurring at or over a specific time. This may take place over a day, week or month and so on.

Error—In epidemiology, statistical inference is valid only if the sample is truly representative of the population, and thus random, accepting that each individual has defined criteria. In addition, the control group/s must have no inherent bias. Because it is impossible to sample the whole population, a selection has to be made, and this is where error frequently arises.

- In *random* error, individuals may be wrongly assessed or misclassified. This is serious in clinical practice but not so much in epidemiology which is concerned with group decisions.

DOI: 10.1201/9781003606789-9

- In *biased* error, the wrong groups are selected, usually the controls, which then distort comparisons—*an epidemiological disaster that cannot be corrected by statistics*. Using hospital-based controls, instead of community-based controls, for patients admitted to the hospital from the community often causes bias and should be avoided.

In epidemiology, computed information is usually used. This can have errors from the following:

Imprecision—Information correctly entered into the computer but the data is wrong.
Unreliability—Correct data entered into the computer incorrectly.

Disease outcome has to be assessed accurately. Clinical experience alone cannot predict prognosis and outcome. Important causes of bias that frequently occur are in the selection of cases, in the choice of medical therapy or surgical technique and in incomplete follow-up with unconfirmed assumptions about final outcomes.

Within a drug trial, sources of error to avoid include misallocation of interventions, wrong drug given to the wrong person and poor compliance with drop administration. These two sources of error should be prevented by careful study design and protocol enforcement; otherwise, the expected effect will not be realised.

RETROSPECTIVE AND PROSPECTIVE STUDIES

1(a) Observational Retrospective Study

An observational study of community or hospital experience can be a useful start to investigate a particular problem but does not record the incidence or prevalence in the population at large. The assessment of risk factors is open to bias by the population attending the particular hospital and/or the medical or surgical techniques used; the sample is not representative of the population at large. However, this type of study does provide a useful basis on which to plan a case-control or cohort study. It is also cheap to perform. If the population is known, from whom cases have been collected, it may be possible to calculate an approximate incidence figure from a large retrospective study. The accuracy of such studies can be increased by analysing a group of similar studies in a meta-analysis (refer to Chapter 7, Global Burden of Ocular Disease).

A meta-analysis is a statistical process that combines the results of multiple studies to draw conclusions that are stronger than the individual studies. Meta-analyses are often used to perform the following:

- establish statistical significance when individual studies have conflicting results
- estimate the magnitude of an effect
- analyse the safety, benefits and harms of a treatment
- examine subgroups that are not statistically significant

Meta-analyses increase precision by combining data and can help resolve controversies that arise from conflicting claims. However, meta-analyses can also be misleading if certain factors are not carefully considered, such as study design, biases and variation across and between studies; not all studies are suitable to be combined into a meta-analysis.

1(b) Analytical Prospective Study

The ESCRS set up a large prospective, randomised, double-blind, placebo-controlled study for the use of *intracameral (IC) antibiotics to prevent postoperative endophthalmitis following cataract surgery* within eight European countries in 2002, which took five years to complete and involved 16,603 operations [1]. This study followed a retrospective study of IC cefuroxime (1 mg in 0.1 ml) at the time of cataract surgery, between 1996 and 2000, giving a low postoperative endophthalmitis rate of 0.06% (20/32,180 surgeries) [2, 3]. The prospective study confirmed the retrospective study results with an infection rate of 0.05% (2/4,052) in those receiving IC cefuroxime and of 0.35% (12/4,054) (nearly seven times higher) in those without IC cefuroxime.

Further retrospective studies have been conducted to add confirmatory data, for use of both IC cefuroxime and IC moxifloxacin (Appendices 1 and 6[S]), but each has limitations of historic controls, changes of surgical technique as well as surgeons and types and material used for intraocular lenses. While moxifloxacin, with a broader antibacterial spectrum, was not available for the ESCRS study, the principle established—a large reduction in postoperative endophthalmitis following the use of an intracameral antibiotic *at the time of cataract surgery*—holds true and relevant for the future. The use of intracameral antibiotics at the end of cataract surgery is now adopted worldwide.

2. Case-Control Study

A case-control study compares those with and without disease who are suitably matched. The study should include only incident cases of disease—i.e. new cases that develop during the study—and not chronic cases of long duration before the study started. Case-control studies are usually prospective but maybe retrospective as well. Diagnostic criteria must be well defined and, for infection, should include a positive Gram or other stain, positive culture or antigen recognition by antibody or PCR tests (Chapter 6 and Appendix 5). Patients who have developed an infection, such as postoperative endophthalmitis, are compared with controls who have not developed infection when risk factors can be identified reliably. A case-control study permits estimation of odds ratio statistics but not the population attributable risk.

Allowance must be made for potential confounding factors. Care must be taken that the controls match the patients so that if the patients enter the hospital from a countrywide community, then the controls *must be selected* likewise and not from the hospital or local area. Controls are best matched to each patient for age, sex and location of residence. However, some studies, such as those of contact lens wearers, require controls to be matched as well for educational status, income and type of housing.

Case-control studies are effective for investigating different risk factors within a defined group. However, they do not identify the incidence (frequency of the disease in the population) nor the prevalence (proportion present at any time).

A case-control study is best conducted prospectively with random selection of patients and controls.

3. Longitudinal and Cohort Studies

A longitudinal study examines the associations between exposure to suspected causes of disease and morbidity—the actual disease. The simplest type of longitudinal study is the prospective cohort study; subjects exposed to one or a number of risk factors, and those not exposed, are followed up prospectively in a defined community-based population study over a period of time. This method measures the *incidence* of disease in each group in the community and can, therefore, measure the relative risk of the different exposures, together with the population attributable risk.

Cohort studies are time-consuming and costly and, therefore, reserved for testing precisely formulated hypotheses that have been previously explored by descriptive and case-control studies, which are used for initial exploratory investigations.

4. Cross-Sectional Study

A cross-sectional study measures the prevalence of any disease, condition, functional impairment or health outcome in a population at a point in time or over a short period. The *prevalence* rate is the proportion afflicted by that defined clinical state at one point in time. Prevalence is estimated using sample surveys, which can introduce bias, as discussed later.

- The cross-sectional study considers *existing* disease as contrasted with the *development* of disease in a cohort study.
- Care is required in detecting known existing cases.
- Sampling involves selection of a representative fraction of the population.
- Cases of chronic disease of long duration are over-represented in a cross-sectional study.

A cross-sectional study may be used to initiate a cohort study by defining the population at risk, such as the type of contact lens worn or ocular trauma suffered prior to the development of microbial keratitis; it does not replace the cohort study, which measures the *incidence* and risk factors of *new* cases of the disease under study.

5. Questionnaire Reporting Surveys

Questionnaire surveys distributed by post do not usually provide a response rate above 66%, although ideally, a minimum response rate should be obtained of 80%. The danger with a low response rate, where the sample surveyed has been carefully chosen to be representative of the population under study, is that it may introduce non-response bias. Without some check of the likely effect of the non-response bias, the results of such surveys will remain 'questionable' in many cases.

One way to validate such a survey is to choose a manageably small but representative sample of all those surveyed, who failed to respond initially, and to coax responses from them. An estimate of the non-response bias can then be obtained from this exercise, such as the difference in participation by senior and junior staff or trained and untrained health workers; the difference may influence the outcome of decision making. The chi-squared test can be used to establish if there is a significant difference between the two groups, such as a higher participation by senior or trained staff in the response group.

https://www.mathsisfun.com/math-tools.html

https://www.bmj.com/about-bmj/resources-readers/publications/statistics-square-one/8-chi-squared-tests*

Another way to investigate the significance of the non-response bias is to use logistic regression equations, but this is complicated and needs the help of a statistician; it is always best to plan the study together in advance. Guidelines are given later:

If a maximum response rate of 66% is obtained from an uncorrected survey, then a 99% significance level ($p < 0.01$) should be considered the minimum for statistical significance*.

ASSESSMENT OF STATISTICAL ASSOCIATIONS

When a significant result is obtained, the following questions should always be considered:

- Is there bias in the selection of the controls?
- Have the wrong controls been selected?
- Have hospital controls been used for community patients?
- Is there bias in patient selection or in patient referral to hospital?
- In a questionnaire study, is there a non-response bias?
- Could the result be due to chance? The confidence intervals should be calculated and the degree of statistical significance considered. Statistics define the degree of chance but do not abolish it altogether.
- Does the significance level calculated represent a real effect for a risk factor or a confounding effect that may be associated with the disease or infection but is not the primary cause of it?
- Have the correct statistical methods been used?
- Should the data have been stratified before analysis?
- Is there a better statistical model by which to analyse the results of the study?

PITFALLS AND SOLUTIONS

Pitfalls are easily made and hard to rectify afterwards, especially with questionnaire surveys, many of which are published with misleading results.

Solutions involve the following:

- Plan and develop a specific research question prior to design and deployment.
- Consider the population under study, their numbers and the problem to solve. It is best to involve a statistician, in particular to advise on the numbers of people to poll in order to achieve a significant result.
- Include questions only if their responses will directly contribute to answering the problem.
- When designing a questionnaire, consider the layout, length and general presentation.
- Surveys should be concise, well organized and easy to read, understand and complete; in addition, the survey should be as brief as possible to gain the required information.

Further methods are recommended [4, 5].

REFERENCES

1. Endophthalmitis Study Group, European Society of Cataract & Refractive Surgeons. J Cataract Refract Surg. 2007. PMID: 17531690 (https:doi.org/10.1016/j.jcrs.2007.02.032).
2. Montan PG et al. J Cataract Refract Surg 2002. PMID: 12036640 (http://doi.org/10.1016/s0886-3350(01)01270-6).
3. Montan PG et al. J Cataract Refract Surg 2002. PMID: 12036639 (http://doi.org/10.1016/s0886-3350(01)01269-x).
4. Safdar N et al. Infect Control Hosp Epidemiol 2016. PMID: 27514583 (https://doi.org/10.1017/ice.2016.171).
5. Fowler FJ. Survey Research Methods. 5th ed. Los Angeles: SAGE 2014. (https://www.google.co.uk/books/edition/Survey_Research_Methods/WM11AwAAQBAJ?hl=en&gbpv=1&printsec=frontcover).

9: Refractive Error, Myopia Control and Contact Lenses

CORE MESSAGES

Refractive error is the leading cause of visual impairment globally: 153 million people suffer from visual impairment due to uncorrected refractive errors. The impact affects individuals' quality of life, limiting educational and employment opportunities leading to economic losses estimated at $202 billion annually due to lost productivity.

The myopia 'epidemic' in children (*particularly in Asia*) is progressive and currently the subject of many studies, which are reviewed later. The increase in myopia is thought to be due to children spending more time in front of screens and less time outdoors with other factors considered as well. Work is ongoing towards changes in lifestyle as well as use of specialist spectacles and contact lenses to reduce peripheral defocus.

Contact lenses are an alternative to spectacles, but in some cases, they are essential for improvement in vision beyond the ability of a spectacle lens.

Complex or medical contact lens fittings improve patients' lives and give them the ability to function in everyday life. However, as well as fitting lenses, maintenance and ongoing ocular health assessments are required to ensure safe wear of these medical devices.

Uncorrected Refractive Error

Refractive error remains one of the leading causes of visual impairment globally. A recent comprehensive analysis of global and regional estimates of effective refractive error coverage (eREC) assessed progress towards the WHO global target of achieving a 40% increase in eREC by 2030 [1].

The study revealed that the global eREC for distance vision correction in adults is significantly below the WHO's target, indicating that a substantial portion of the adult population with refractive error does not have access to effective corrective measures. There are also notable disparities in eREC across different regions. High-income countries generally exhibit higher eREC levels, while low- and middle-income countries lag behind, highlighting inequalities in access to eye care services. The current trajectory suggests that without significant interventions, many regions will not meet the WHO's 2030 target for eREC. This underscores the need for enhanced strategies to improve access to refractive error correction services globally. Furthermore, there is a global epidemic of both myopia and high myopia, particularly in East/Southeast Asia.

DOI: 10.1201/9781003606789-10

Myopia Epidemic in Asian Children

The myopia epidemic in Asia is particularly severe, with high prevalence rates among schoolchildren. In East Asia, studies show exceptionally high myopia prevalence rates, reaching up to 73% in some regions [2, 3]. In China, the prevalence among 15–19-year-olds is now 69%, with 10% having high myopia [4]. Rates in China, Korea and Taiwan are higher compared to Europe, the USA and the Middle East.

Risk factors for myopia in schoolchildren in Asia include low outdoor time, excessive near work, dim light exposure, use of LED lamps for homework, low sleeping hours, reading distance of less than 25 cm and living in an urban environment. Spending more time outdoors has been shown to reduce myopia incidence by 64%. There is a clear generational difference with younger populations exhibiting higher rates of myopia. *This increase may be due to children spending more time in front of screens and less time outdoors.*

Public health strategies are needed to tackle and reduce myopia progression in children, including the use of myopia control spectacles and contact lenses [5, 6].

Myopia control in children is important, as there is up to a 70% chance of slowing the progression, thus reducing the axial length growth and future pathology. No procedure prevents it. Some of the myopic control treatments involve 0.01% atropine, spectacles and contact lenses.

Recommendations for managing myopia control and using atropine and/or contact lenses/spectacle designs are given by the UK College of Optometrists [7] and supported by evidence from a recent Cochrane review [8]:

A myopia calculator, found on the BHVI (Brien Holden Vision Institute) website, will help practitioners with myopia management options, demonstrating the benefits over time of treating myopia progression [9]. A management protocol has been produced by the French Myopia Institute (02/06/2025) [10].

Unwanted Eye Growth Leading to Increased Myopic Prescriptions

Peripheral light rays that fall beyond the retina may establish a growth signal and lead to the lengthening of the eye. The result of ongoing correction with traditional contact lenses may be continued eye growth (Figures 9.1–9.4).

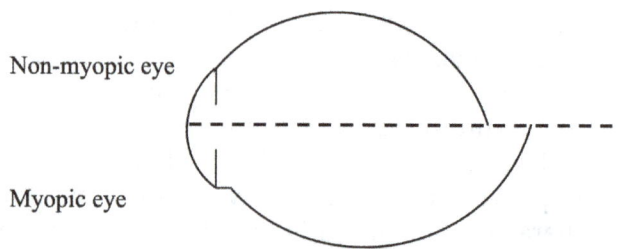

Non-myopic eye

Myopic eye

FIGURE 9.1 Continued eye growth in the myopic eye.

Uncorrected myopia

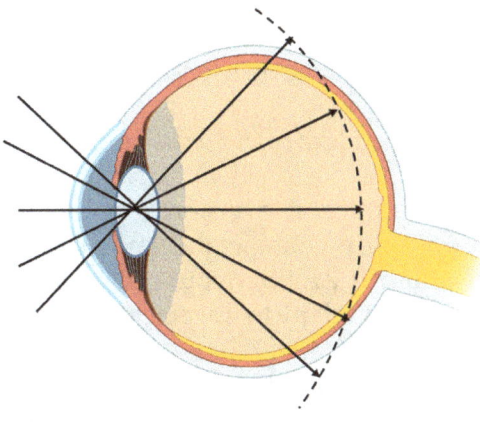

FIGURE 9.2 In uncorrected myopia, the central light rays fall short of the retina centrally and beyond the retina peripherally.

Traditional correction

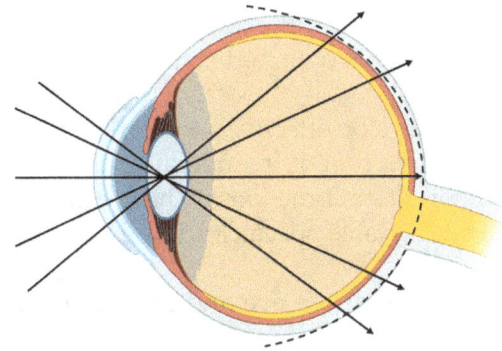

FIGURE 9.3 Traditional spherical minus power contact lenses correct myopia by moving central light rays to the central retina but do not correct peripheral images that fall beyond the retina.

Optimal correction

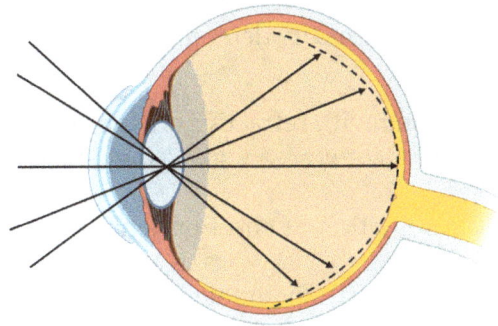

FIGURE 9.4 The light rays fall on the retina centrally but focus peripheral light rays in front of the retina to remove peripheral hyperopic defocus.

Myopia Control with Spectacles

Myopia management in children using spectacle lenses has evolved with the development of innovative designs aimed at slowing the progression of myopia, such as the ZEISS MyoCare, Hoya MiYOSMART spectacle lenses and Essilor Stellest lenses for myopia.

ZEISS MyoCare: These lenses incorporate patented microstructures called cylindrical annular refractive elements, which are designed to slow the elongation of the eyeball while providing clear, comfortable vision. The design includes a central zone for clear vision and alternating management and correction zones to balance effectiveness and wearability. ZEISS MyoCare lenses are tailored to consider children's varying abilities to adapt to spectacle lenses at different ages.

Hoya MiYOSMART: Utilizing defocus incorporated multiple segments technology, the MiYOSMART lens consists of a central clear zone for distance vision and honeycomb-like segments that introduce controlled myopic blur on the peripheral retina. This design has been shown to slow myopia progression compared to standard single vision lenses and has sustained benefits over six years.

Essilor Stellest lenses use highly aspherical lenslet target (HALT) technology; a network of small aspherical 'lenslets' are spread across the lens surface to create a defocus signal to reduce growth. Clear vision is obtained centrally so that children can still see for distance and near tasks.

Spectacle lenses are part of a broader effort to develop effective and non-invasive solutions for myopia. In all cases of spectacle correction, it is imperative that the spectacles sit well on the child's face and do not tilt or come loose. The 'treatment zones' of these spectacles rely on well-fitting and stable spectacles in order to be effective [11].

Contact lenses have the advantage of moving with the eye and maintain the correct positioning needed for maximum treatment.

Myopia Control with Contact Lenses

Specialist Contact Lenses for Myopia Control

MiSight 1 day (Coopervision) [12] (https://coopervision.co.uk/our-products)

The mechanism for myopia control is simultaneous defocus. Wearers of this lens are instructed to wear the lenses six days a week for ten hours, which has been shown to produce the best results. Chamberlain *et al.* in 2019 demonstrated the following [13]:

- Axial elongation that underlies, and is correlated with refractive error progression, was significantly less with the MiSight lens compared with a single-vision soft contact lens.
- No safety concerns were evident for this population of children who started daily disposable soft contact lens wear between 8 and 12 years of age.
- The high subject retention, long wearing time and favourable subjective ratings demonstrated that contact lens acceptance was sustained across three years, supporting previous findings that soft contact lenses are well accepted by children. Children as young as 8 years old were able to achieve full-time wear, handle the lenses confidently soon after initial fitting and achieve good comfort.

Positive Impact/Vtivision [14]
Menicon Bloom Day EDOF design
Milo SCL monthly EDOF reusable

The mechanism for these lenses is peripheral defocus. Neurofocus Optics®, NaturalVue® Multifocal contact lenses and EDOF (extended depth of focus) lenses focus peripheral light rays in front of the retina to remove peripheral hyperopic defocus.

Ongoing studies show that the NaturalVue® (etafilcon A) Enhanced Multifocal 1 Day™ contact lens produces a delay in progression of myopia (global.vtivision.com/protect-study/). The PROTECT Study is a three-year, multinational, double-masked, randomised controlled trial (RCT) that started in 2024. So far, the study has found that NaturalVue® Multifocal lenses significantly reduced myopia progression compared to a control group.

ORTHO K

Johnson & Johnson—ACUVUE® Abiliti™ [15]
These lenses are not yet available in the UK.

ACUVUE® Abiliti™ Overnight Therapeutic (silicone hydrogel tisilfocon A) Contact Lenses (FDA approved) are indicated for use in the management of myopia. They are orthokeratology lenses worn during sleep, requiring disinfection afterwards with a chemical disinfection system. They temporarily reshape the cornea, allowing clear vision during the day typically without the need for vision correction.

UK-based companies, such as Menicon and Coopervision, produce Menicon Bloom night Ortho K lenses for myopic control, as well as Coopervision's Dream Night lenses.

CONTACT LENSES

a) Contact Lens Types

Awareness of types of lenses, materials, replacement schedules and cleaning regimes are important when assessing the patient in a primary care setting.

A detailed history allows a differential diagnosis to be considered of ocular infection, discomfort or poor vision.

i) Types of Lenses

- Soft hydrogel (of variable water content and materials) was introduced in 1971, and later, in 2002, silicone hydrogel (SiH) lenses were first marketed.
- Rigid gas permeable lenses (RGP) are made from a combination of silicone and fluoropolymers, which allows oxygen to pass through the lens material to the corneal surface. These are hard to the touch and can vary in size from as small as 8 mm *corneal lenses* to large, mini and full *scleral lenses* of 15–23+ mm.
- Hybrid lenses. A combination of a small corneal RGP with a soft skirt made from hydrogel or silicone hydrogel material. Lenses are approximately 14–15 mm in total diameter.

ii) Replacement Schedules

Soft contact lenses (SCLs) became available in a daily disposable form in the 1980s.

This means they are used for a one-time-only wear and should be discarded after each use.

Still available today, however, are monthly lenses (30-day disposables) as well as 3 monthly, 6 monthly and 12 monthly lenses.

When a lens is being reused, it is important to find out from the patient how old it is, as well as the age of their contact lens storage case, and to ensure that the patient is complying with the replacement schedule and cleaning regime.

RGP lenses are made to be replaced, in most cases, every 12–18 months, as recommended by the manufacturers.

In Ortho K treatment lenses, due to the night-time wear of these lenses, they are recommended to be replaced every six months.

Before gas permeable materials, PMMA was used, and these lenses lasted 5–10 years in some cases!

iii) Lens Materials

It is important to consider the lens material of the contact lens being worn by the patient.

The oxygen permeability, tear exchange and thickness of the lens on the eye will affect the overall ocular health. Lens materials have improved with time, and the introduction of SIH has increased the overall DK/t (oxygen permeability) of the lens. Hydrogel lenses will range from 30% to 77% water content.

Silicone Hydrogel Contact Lenses

The biggest advantage of using SiH contact lenses over regular hydrogel lenses is increased oxygen permeability. Allowing oxygen to permeate to the cornea reduces symptoms, such as dryness, redness, blurred vision, discomfort and corneal swelling [16] and [17].

Silicone hydrogel contact lenses have a gel-like consistency that makes them extremely flexible. There are approximately 15 different types of SiH materials available at present, including senofilcon, galyfilcon, efrofilcon and delefilcon. Each material has a varying amount of water content, oxygen permeability and other properties so that they vary in their comfort and adaptability [18]. The oxygen permeability level of a contact lens depends directly on its water content [19]; the lower the water content, the higher the oxygen transmissibility and vice versa.

Studies have shown that wearers of SiH lenses report significantly higher levels of comfort, both during the day and at the end of the day, compared to conventional hydrogel lenses. Because of the increased oxygen permeability, SiH contact lenses are useful for people who develop dry eyes, need to wear thicker lenses because of higher prescriptions, experience end-of-day discomfort and dryness, work in dry air-conditioned environments or wear contact lenses for more than 12 hours a day.

Silicone hydrogel lenses attract less protein, particularly lysozyme, than pHEMA-based materials, with < 10 μg/lens for non-ionic and up to 34 μg/lens for ionic materials, but denatured proteins can adhere more frequently as 'deposits' [20]. This leads to discomfort and the need to replace lenses more frequently.

Silicone hydrogel lenses must not be disinfected or stored in solutions manufactured for use with RGP lenses.

Staining of the cornea can occur with PHMB contained in some MPS (refer to table later). If this occurs with a particular MPS, and causes problems, then another MPS should be substituted instead using an alternative chemical [21].

iv) Contact Lens Cleaning Solutions

Contact lens cleaning (rinse and rub) is essential for comfortable contact lens wear. It has been shown that deposits on a lens' surface reduce wettability and, therefore, comfort [22]. As well as being essential, cleaning physically removes microbes, enhancing the effect of disinfecting solutions and so reducing the risk of infection. Both these functions have to occur without causing epithelial harm.

Solutions Methods

- MPS (multipurpose solutions) are produced as one bottle solutions for 'rinse and rub', disinfection, wetting, conditioning and storing (Table 9.1). The disinfecting chemical is often polyhexamethylene biguanide (PHMB) or polyquaternium (polyquad) [21]. Various MPS are produced, including the following:

Menicare (RGP)
B&L Boston Simplus RGP
Quattro (for SCL and RGP)
Regard (for SCL and RGP)
B&L Biotrue, Renu (SCL)
Superdrug Stores UK All in One (manufactured by Stericon Pharma, Bangalore, India) (SCL)

TABLE 9.1 Contact Lens Multipurpose Solutions (MPS)

Manufacturer	Solution Name (MPS)	Preservatives
ALCON	OptiFree PureMoist	Polyquad (polyquaternium) 0.001% Aldox* 0.0005%
	OptiFree Replenish	Polyquad (polyquaternium) 0.001% Aldox* 0.0005%
	OptiFree Express	Polyquad (polyquaternium) 0.001% Aldox* 0.0005%
	ClearCare ClearCare with HydraGlide	Non-preserved sterile micro-filtered hydrogen peroxide 3%
Johnson & Johnson Vision (AMO)	Acuvue Revitalens	Alexidine** 0.00016% Polyquad (polyquaternium) 0.0003%
	Complete Moisture (Comfort) Plus MPS	Polyhexamethylene biguanide (PHMB) 0.0001%
	Oxysept UltraCare	Non-preserved sterile hydrogen peroxide 3%
Bausch + Lomb	Renu Advanced Formula	Polyhexamethylene biguanide (PHMB) 0.0001% Polyquaternium 0.001% Alexidine** 0.00016%
	Renu Multiplus	Polyaminopropyl biguanide 0.0001% (DYMED)
	Renu MoistureLoc	Alexidine** 0.00045%
	Biotrue	Polyaminopropyl biguanide 0.00013% Polyquaternium 0.0001%
CooperVision	Refine 1-Step	Non-preserved sterile hydrogen peroxide 3%
CIBA Vision	SOLOCare Plus	Polyhexamethylene biguanide (PHMB) 0.0001%
	AOSept	Non-preserved sterile hydrogen peroxide 3%
Ophtecs	Cleadew	Povidone-iodine
Menicon	MeniCare Soft	Polyhexamethylene biguanide 0.0001%

* Aldox—myristamidopropyldimethylamine ** Alexidine—alexidine dihydrochloride 0.00016%

Source: 2021 [21]

Rossmann Germany 'bestview' (manufactured by Schalcon, Rome, Italy) (SCL)
Ote: Sensation and Fine

• Two-step systems

These involve a separate cleaner, which should not come into contact with the eye, and a wetting/conditioning solution.
Some examples of separate cleaning solutions:

Boston Advance
Ote Clean
Menicon Spray and clean
Progent
Protein Tablets

Hydrogen peroxide cleaners:
These use hydrogen peroxide to clean and remove all organisms, such as *Acanthamoeba,* and are considered the most effective. If not neutralised, these methods can cause epithelial damage [23] (refer to College of Optometrists' CMGs for—Please see Trauma (chemical)). The peroxide is neutralised with tablets or discs at the bottom of the cases.
They include EasySept, AoSept and Oxysept.
Povidone-iodine cleaner: Cleadew.

v) Contact Lens Storage Case Hygiene

The storage case is best cleaned each week with the multipurpose solution (MPS) and air dried. The storage case must *NOT* be cleaned with tap water unless the water has been previously boiled and cooled. The storage case should be renewed each time that a new bottle of MPS is opened and the old case thrown away. The lens should be rubbed and rinsed with MPS before being placed in fresh MPS in the storage case. When the lens is next used, the storage solution in the case must be thrown away and the storage case air dried before it is used again.

Polyquad (0.001%) and PHMB (0.0001%) were found to be equally effective against bacteria, minimally effective against fungi and had *NO* effect against *Acanthamoeba at the concentrations used in most MPS* [21]; the concentration of PHMB used in MPS is 200 times lower than that used in therapy (0.02%). However, chlorhexidine, as used in MPS at 0.005%—50 times the concentration of PHMB at 0.0001%—will be effective against *Acanthamoeba,* as the concentration is only four times lower than that used in therapy (0.02%).

Hydrogen peroxide is effective against both trophozoites and cysts of *Acanthamoeba.* Povidone-iodine (PI) has greater activity against *Acanthamoeba* and lacks toxicity for the corneal epithelium [24]; in addition, PI is effective against bacteria within a storage case biofilm.

Cleaning of the lens (rub and rinse) and storage in a MPS, which lowers the bacterial count within the storage case ideally towards zero, can be expected to reduce numbers of *Acanthamoebae* by physical removal and destruction of the amoeba's food source, which is bacteria. However, this process is not amoebicidal, and a recent study has found that *Acanthamoeba castellanii* and *Pseudomonas aeruginosa* can survive together in low-nutrient conditions preferably at 22°C (room temperature) with a bacteria-to-amoeba ratio below 100:1 [25].

vi) Companies Producing General and Specialist Contact Lenses

Menicon, Positive Impact, Marc Ennovy
Scleral lenses from Scott Lenses, B&L, Menicon, Wave and Eaglet Eye
Johnson & Johnson
Cooper Vision
Alcon
Bausch and Lomb
Individual companies that produce specialist lenses, e.g. Rose K2 design and RGP Menicon,
   Ultravison and Cantor and Barnard (Originally Cantor and Nissel) Northern Lenses

vii) Patient Lens Choices

The type of lens a patient wears is often dictated by their prescription and corneal condition. Another consideration is cost. A monthly lens in a non-complex prescription is often less expensive than a daily lens, even with the solution costs.

A 'hard or rigid' RGP lens is used for a corneal condition, such as keratoconus, PMD or post-graft eye. RGPs are also fitted in high myopia and Ortho K treatment lenses.

Scleral lenses are prescribed for corneal dystrophies, such as keratoconus, post-graft, ectasia, dry eye or high astigmatism. With improvement of the lens materials and mini-scleral lenses, however, more patients with presbyopia and high prescriptions are favouring these lenses to a more uncomfortable corneal lens. The DK of mini sclerals using Boston XO2 has also helped with wearing times.

b) Contact Lens–Related Complications

CLARE (Contact Lens–Associated Red Eye)

Contact lens–associated red eye is often associated with extended wear lenses or patients who 'nap' in their contact lenses. Overnight wear of the contact lens, with corneal hypoxia, and poor storage case hygiene, in particular, the use of tap water, are the main risk factors of CLARE.

Hypoxia produced by extended wear lenses, or sleeping in hydrogel lenses, can cause corneal swelling and infiltrates seen with the slit lamp; they are grey in colour and do not or minimally stain with fluorescein. The conjunctival vessels and limbal vessels will swell in order to enhance oxygen supply to the cornea.

Symptoms of mild photophobia, irritation and epiphora can be alleviated by ceasing contact lens wear until symptoms and signs resolve. In cases of mild staining, an ocular lubricant can be given, and some practitioners will prescribe a broad-spectrum antibiotic as well.

It's imperative to differentiate CLARE from conditions such as microbial keratitis, infiltrative keratitis and contact lens peripheral ulcers (CLPUs). The patient should be seen after 24 hours to ensure the correct diagnosis has been made.

Contact lens wear increases the risk of microbial keratitis, with an incidence of 2 to 20 cases per 10,000 wearers annually. Bacteria, including *Pseudomonas aeruginosa*, are primarily responsible. While only causing about 5% of overall cases, the tap water–associated protozoa *Acanthamoeba* causes a particularly painful and difficult-to-treat infection with an incidence ranging from 0.15 per million in the USA to 1.4 per million in the UK, nearly ten times higher. *Acanthamoeba infection needs to be diagnosed early* and is now recognised in many countries. These infections are described in detail in Chapter 6. Presentation includes *rapid onset of ocular pain, redness, tearing and vision loss*. A corneal scrape should be collected for microscopy and culture, together with the contact lens and storage case—refer later and Appendix 5. Correct hygiene practice is described earlier. Further information is given in [26].

Contact Lens–Associated Peripheral Ulcer (CLPU)

A CLPU is a single, small, circular, mid-peripheral or peripheral gray/white lesion in the anterior stroma. This can be seen often using retro-illumination with a slit lamp and will stain with fluorescein. There should be no anterior chamber activity of cells or flare. It is an inflammatory and/or hypersensitivity response to exotoxins released by Gram-positive bacteria (usually) and is often termed a sterile ulcer.

It presents with symptoms of mild to moderate pain, lacrimation and mild photophobia. It is important to differentiate this from microbial keratitis, which is a more serious condition, classified as an ocular emergency; symptoms are more severe pain, lacrimation, photophobia and hyperemia (Chapter 6). Marginal keratitis should also be differentiated.

With CLPU, prophylactic drops (such as ciprofloxacin) can be given as well as lubricants. Symptoms should resolve quickly, and the patient should be seen the next day to confirm the diagnosis and check if signs and symptoms are resolving. Patients are often left with a residual scar, which can be seen many months afterwards.

Limbal pannus/neovascularization

This can present as a superficial pannus, commonly at the superior limbus under the upper lid due to hypoxia induced by contact lenses often associated with extended wear (Figure 9.5).

Switching to rigid gas-permeable lenses or higher DK dailies or monthly or discontinuing contact lens wear has been shown to regress vascularization in many cases.

Tight Fit Lens Syndrome

This can occur with lenses made of any material. The signs (Figure 9.6) may represent a differential diagnosis of early *Acanthamoeba* infection (see Chapter 6), *but the eye is NOT painful,* which is an important distinction. Removal of the lens and lubricants resolves the problem, but the patient should be followed up. A tight lens may need refitting.

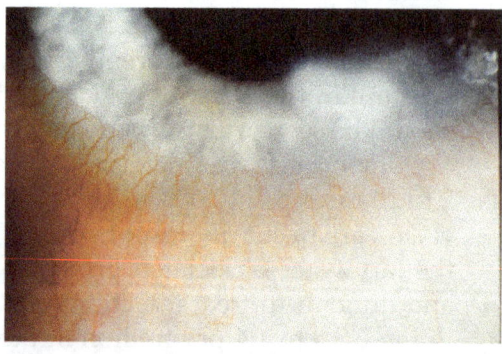

FIGURE 9.5 Pannus with sterile infiltrate from contact lens wear.

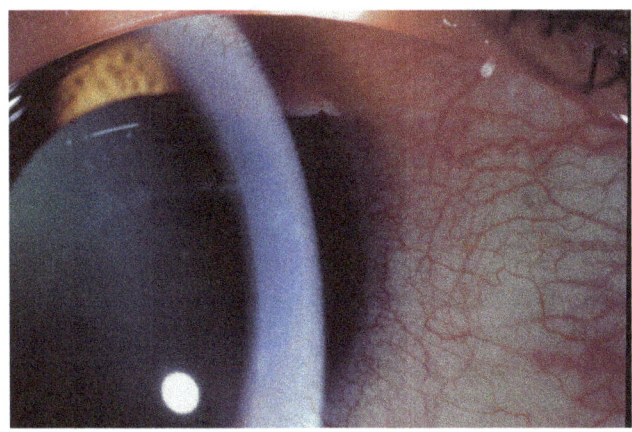

FIGURE 9.6 Tight fit lens syndrome in a wearer of a hydrogel lens.

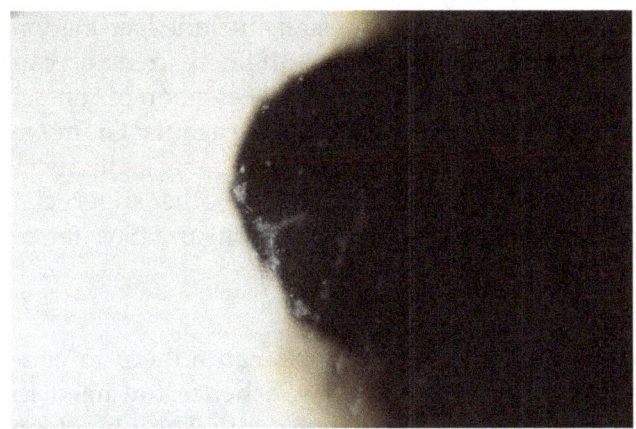

FIGURE 9.7 Epitheliopathy due to oedema.

Sterile Infiltrates

These can occur with wearing a hydrogel contact lens, especially if used for extended wear (Figure 9.7).

Limbal Stem Cell Deficiency

This occurs when the limbal stem cells, which maintain the corneal epithelium, become damaged or lost due to prolonged contact lens wear. Scleral lens limbal landing zones need to be managed for this. This can lead to persistent epithelial defects, corneal conjunctivalisation, neovascularization and scarring.

Toxic Epitheliopathy from Cleaning and Disinfecting Solutions

This can occur due to an allergic or toxic reaction to the active ingredients, the vehicle or preservatives in the solution. Symptoms include eye irritation, redness and blurred vision. Signs include epitheliopathy, conjunctival and limbal hyperaemia and corneal staining. The contact lenses should be removed until the inflammation has resolved, and an alternative cleaning/disinfecting solution containing different chemicals should be used instead (Table 9.1) [21].

Contact Lens–Associated Papillary Conjunctivitis/Giant Papillary Conjunctivitis

Contact lens–associated papillary conjunctivitis (CLAPC)/giant papillary conjunctivitis (GPC) is often an immunological complication of wearing contact lenses along with mechanical factors. Protein deposits on the lens may act as antigens and initiate an allergic condition [27], which disappears when the lens is discontinued.

Both Type 1 and Type IV hypersensitivity reactions are involved, and the risk of CLAPC increases with duration of contact lens wear. It is more common in reusable soft lens wear compared to disposable soft or rigid lens wear. The condition is nearly always bilateral, with localised or generalised papillae and hyperaemia with stringy mucus in the tear film. Treatment options include removal of lens deposits (or replacing the lens), reducing wearing time and mast cell stabilisers [28] (refer to College of Optometrists' CMGs for—CL-associated papillary conjunctivitis (CLAPC), giant papillary conjunctivitis (GPC)).

Corneal Abrasions and Erosions

A foreign body under a lens can concur with all types of lenses, causing erosion of the superficial epithelium. Patients may complain of sudden onset of pain (sometimes out of proportion to clinical findings), and signs include lacrimation and redness. Corneal epithelial defects will be best seen with fluorescein and can appear as scratches on the corneal surface. Treatment will be cessation of contact lens wear, lubricants and use of prophylactic antibiotic effective against Gram -ve organisms; use levofloxacin, moxifloxacin or an aminoglycoside, e.g. gentamicin [29–31] (refer to College of Optometrists' CMGs for—Corneal (or other superficial ocular) foreign body—College of Optometrists/Corneal abrasion) and (Sub-tarsal foreign body [STFB]).

c) Biofilms

Bacteria, fungi and *Acanthamoeba* trophozoites and cysts can adhere to contact lens materials within a biofilm (Figures 9.8 and 9.9), hence the need to clean and disinfect both the lens and its storage case repeatedly. The advantage of the daily wear lens, that is worn properly as daily wear and disposed of nightly, is simplification with a fresh sterile lens inserted into the eye each day; this is the ideal arrangement to avoid any infection from contamination with overnight storage.

The formation of a biofilm (Figures 9.8 and 9.9), made up of bacteria, fungi and trophozoites, and cysts of *Acanthamoeba*, on the surface of contact lenses and storage cases (Figure 9.10) plays a role in pathogenesis; in addition, bacterial cells within a biofilm show increased resistance to antimicrobial agents. Biguanidebased (PHMB) contact lens solutions have been shown to have no effect against

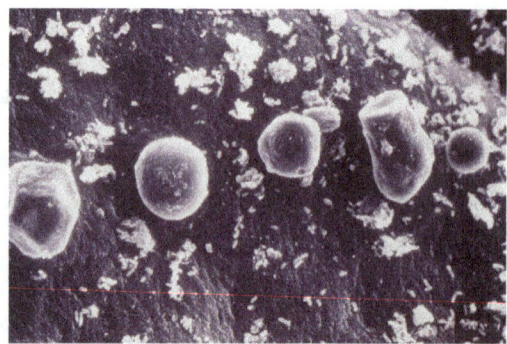

FIGURE 9.8 Scanning electron micrograph of bacteria and *Acanthamoeba* (rounded-up trophozoites and cysts) adhering to a contact lens.

Source: (Seal D, Pleyer U. Ocular Infection, 2nd Edition 2007)

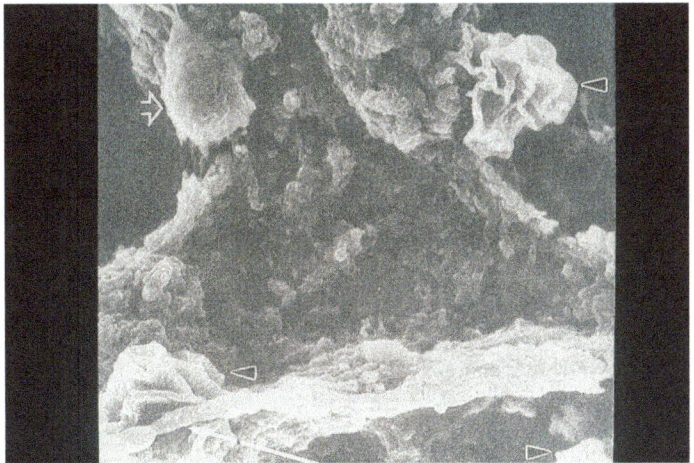

FIGURE 9.9 Scanning electron micrograph of biofilm from a contact lens storage case (later) showing *Acanthamoeba* trophozoites (open arrow) and cysts (closed arrow) with various bacteria and a septate fungal mycelium.

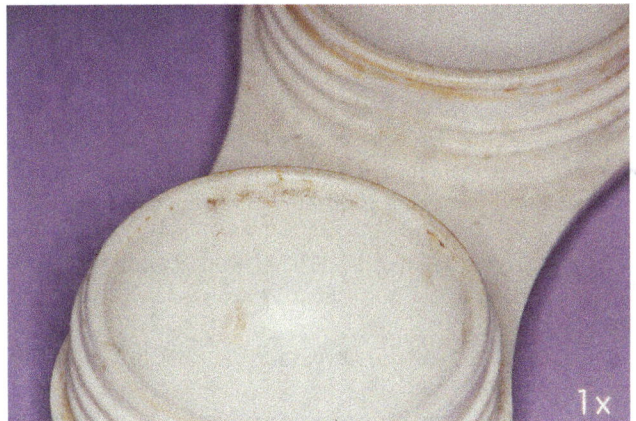

FIGURE 9.10 Storage case of a patient presenting early with *Acanthamoeba* keratitis (Chapter 6).

biofilms of *Serratia marcescens*, *Staphylococcus aureus* and *Pseudomonas aeruginosa* formed on silicone hydrogel lenses [26].

d) Patient Education

In a study of 'Patient Compliance During Contact Lens Wear: Perceptions, Awareness, and Behavior' [32], Bui et al. found the following:

> Perceived compliance is not an indicator for appropriate patient behavior. A large proportion of patients remain non-compliant despite awareness of risk. Education alone is not a sufficient strategy to improve behavior; newer approaches aimed at improving compliance with lens care practices are urgently needed.

The problem of non-compliance can also be a problem of the patient not listening. There is an art both in listening to the patient and persuading your patient to listen to you [33].

Patient education regarding contact lenses is available from the UK Association of Optometrists [34] (https://www.aop.org.uk/advice-and-support/for-patients/contact-lens-advice/soft-lenses).

FURTHER INFORMATION ON FITTING CONTACT LENSES

Elliott DB Clinical Procedures in Primary Eye Care. 5th Edition 2020 ISBN: 9780702077890. https://www.asia.elsevierhealth.com/clinical-procedures-in-primary-eye-care–9780702077890.html.

Bennett E S, Vinita A H. Clinical Manual of Contact Lenses. 2019. ISBN: 9781496397805. *https://www.lww.co.uk/9781496397799/clinical-manual-of-contact-lenses/.* This has a good section on scleral lenses.

REFERENCES

1. Bourne R et al. Lancet Glob Health 22/05/2025:S2214-109X(25)00194-9. PMID: 40414243 (https://www.thelancet.com/journals/langlo/article/PIIS2214-109X%2825%2900194-9/fulltext).

2. Grzybowski A et al. BMC Ophthalmol 2020. PMID: 31937276 (http://doi.org/10.1186/s12886-019-1220-0).

3. Pan W et al. Lancet Reg Health Wes Pac 2025. PMID: 39931228 (http://doi.org/10.1016/j.lanwpc.2025.101484).

4. National Eye Institute. Global Perspectives on Childhood Myopia: Addressing the Rising Epidemic 2024. Accessed 18/08/25 (https://www.nei.nih.gov/about/news-and-events/news/global-perspectives-childhood-myopia-addressing-rising-epidemic).

5. Nucci P et al. Eye 2023. PMID: 37142779 (http://doi.org/10.1038/s41433-023-02558-0).

6. Lawrenson JG et al. Cochrane Database Syst Rev 2025. PMID: 39945354 (http://doi.org/10.1002/14651858.CD014758.pub3).

7. College of Optometrists. Guidance for Professional Practice. Assessing and Managing Children with Myopia 2025. Accessed 18/08/25 (https://www.college-optometrists.org/clinical-guidance/guidance/knowledge,-skills-and-performance/assessing-and-managing-children-with-myopia/principles-of-managing-children-with-myopia).

8. Lawrenson JG. Cochrane Database Syst.Rev. PMID: 39945354 (http://doi: 10.1002/14651858.CD014758.pub3.)

9. Brien Holden Vision Institute. New and Improved BHVI Myopia Calculator 2025. Accessed 18/8/25 (https://bhvi.org/myopia-calculator-resources/).

10. Bijon J et al. Eye 2025 Online. Published 02/06/2025. Accessed 02/06/2025 (https://doi.org/10.1038/s41433-025-03858-3).

11. Paudel N. Review of Myopia Management 2023. PMID: none (https://reviewofmm.com/next-gen-spectacle-designs-for-myopia-management-what-we-know-now/).

12. CooperVision. MiSight 1 Day 2025. Accessed 18/08/25 (https://coopervision.co.uk/contact-lenses/brilliant-futures-misight-1-day/misight-1-day).

13. Chamberlain P et al. A 3-Year Randomized Clinical Trial of MiSight Lenses for Myopia Control. Optom Vis Sci 2019. PMID: 31343513 (https://doi.org/10.1097/opx.0000000000001410).

14. Visioneering Technologies Inc. Give Children the Clearest Path Forward to Reach Success 2025. Accessed 18/8/25 (https://vtivision.com/practitioner/myopia/).

15. Johnson and Johnson. Myopia Management 2025. Accessed 18/08/25 (https://www.jnjvisionpro.com/en-us/myopia-management/).

16. CooperVision. The Benefits of Silicone Hydrogel Daily Disposable Lenses 2025. Accessed 18/08/25 https://coopervision.com.sg/practitioner/fitting-tips-and-tools/benefits-of-silicone-hydrogel-lenses).

17. Morgan P et al. Cont Lens Anterior Eye 2021. PMID: 33775377 (https://doi.org/10.1016/j.clae.2021.02.006).

18. Tighe B. Eye & Contact Lens 2013. PMID: 23292050 (https://doi.org/10.1097/ICL.0b013e318275452b).

19. Lentiamo. Hydrogel vs. Silicone Hydrogel Contact Lenses: Pros and Cons 2025. Accessed 18/08/25 (https://www.lentiamo.co.uk/blog/hydrogel-vs-silicone-hydrogel-lenses.html).

20. Luensmann D. Cont Lens Anterior Eye 2012. PMID: 22326604 (https://www.contactlensjournal.com/article/S1367-0484(11)00180-9/abstract).

21. Bradley C et al. Clin Optom (Auckl) 07/09/2021;13:271–285. PMID: 34522149. Accessed 02/06/2025 (https://doi.org/10.2147/OPTO.S235679).

22. Benjamin W et al. International Contact Lens Clinic 1989. PMID: none (https://www.sciencedirect.com/science/article/abs/pii/0892896789900059?via%3Dihub).

23. College of Optometrists. Clinical Management Guidelines. Trauma (Chemical) 2025. Accessed 18/08/25.

24. Kilvington S. Cont Lens Anterior Eye 2004. PMID: none (https://www.contactlensjournal.com/article/S1367-0484(04)00069-4/abstract).

25. Rhiannon C et al. PLoS One 24/06/2024. PMID: 3891368. Accessed 28/05/2025 (https://doi.org/10.1371/journal.pone.0305973).

26. Lingburg T et al. Inf Dis Clin N America 2024. PMID: 39271302 (https://www.sciencedirect.com/science/article/pii/S0891552024000618).

27. Mondino B et al. Surv Ophthalmol 1982. PMID: 6810487 (http://doi.10.1016/0039-6257(82)90126-6).

28. College of Optometrists. Clinical Management Guidelines. CL-Associated Papillary Conjunctivitis (CLAPC), Giant Papillary Conjunctivitis (GPC) 2025. Accessed 18/08/25.

29. College of Optometrists. Clinical Management Guidelines. Corneal Abrasions 2025. Accessed 03/09/25.

30. College of Optometrists. Clinical Management Guidelines. Corneal (or Other Superficial Ocular) Foreign Body 2025. Accessed 03/09/25.

31. College of Optometrists. Clinical Management Guidelines. Sub-Tarsal Foreign Body (STFB) 2025. Accessed 03/09/25.

32. Bui H et al. Eye & Contact Lens 2010. PMID: 20935569 (https://doi.org/10.1097/ICL.0b013e3181f579f7).

33. Murphy K. What You're Missing & Why It Matters. In: You're Not Listening. Vintage 2021. ISBN 978-1-784-70940-2 (penguin.co.uk/vintage).

34. Association of Optometrists. Contact Lens Advice 2025. Accessed 18/08/25 (https://www.aop.org.uk/advice-and-support/for-patients/contact-lens-advice/).

ADDENDUM

The Medicine & Healthcare products Regulatory Agency (MHRA) approved the first licensed, low-dose atropine (LDA) treatment for slowing the progression of childhood myopia on 10th November 2025. Ryjunea® (low-dose atropine 0.1 mg/ml), licensed by Santen, is indicated for children aged 3–14 years with myopia between –0.50 DS and –6.00 DS and a progression rate of 0.50 DS or more per year. The product is only available by private prescription and not from the NHS, where it is still undergoing assessment. Its use must be considered against findings from a recent (2023) randomised, placebo-controlled, double-blind trial in the USA, in which the results did not support use of low-dose atropine in USA children, as no difference existed in either myopia control or axial elongation between children receiving atropine or placebo drops at night [Repka M. JAMA 2023. PMID: 37440213] (http://doi.org/10.1001/jamaophthalmol.2023.2855). For use and possible adverse reactions refer to College of Optometrists Clinical Management Guidelines.

10: Pathogenesis of Infection and the Ocular Immune Response

CORE MESSAGES

Understanding the immunology of the eye is essential to understanding the basis of disease within it and how to manage treatment. The eye is unique for the immune deviation that occurs within it, in both the anterior and posterior segments, allowing some pathogens, in particular herpes and cytomegalovirus, to survive and multiply without a cell-mediated immune reaction to neutralize them. While this mechanism of immune tolerance has developed to prevent unwanted inflammation, and its subsequent damage, it has unwanted side effects. The mode of action of anti-inflammatory drugs is explained, and when to use them, in conjunction with Appendix 1.

Surface Protection of the Eye

The normal conjunctiva and cornea are protected by a triple-layered tear film comprising an outer oily layer from the meibomian glands, an aqueous layer from lacrimal glands and an inner layer of mucus derived chiefly from conjunctival goblet cells. Blinking maintains the integrity of this protective layer. The goblet cells and subsurface vesicles of the conjunctiva create the deep mucus layer of the tear film, which is anchored to the ocular surface glycocalyx.

Tears produced by the lacrimal gland have a high concentration of immunoglobulin A (IgA) (0.6g/L), lysozyme (1G/L) and lactoferrin (1.2g/L), which have an antimicrobial action. This occurs from the coating of bacteria by tear IgA, growth inhibition by lactoferrin iron chelation and the action of lysozyme. Lysozyme (acetylmuramidase) splits the bond between acetylmuramic acid and acetylglucosamine in the peptidoglycan of the bacterial cell wall with a direct lytic action on *Micrococcus lysodeikticus*. Synergy with immunoglobulin and complement is required for lysis of other bacteria. Immunoglobulin G (IgG) (0.05 g/L) and complement are found in low concentration in tears but leak through inflamed conjunctiva vessels and are important for causing cell wall lysis by the complement cascade. IgA binds to bacteria to initiate attachment and phagocytosis by neutrophils migrating out of inflamed conjunctival vessels.

From age 40 onwards, tear volume and the concentration of lacrimal proteins (lysozyme, lactoferrin, and IgA) decrease due to reduced lacrimal gland function [1, 2, 3]. Interestingly, the eye does not become infected more frequently unless there is concomitant development of a severely dry eye. This emphasizes the beneficial effect of constant tear flow, removing bacteria and other debris from the ocular surface, although the moderately dry eye

DOI: 10.1201/9781003606789-11

develops a compensatory antibacterial mechanism based on leakage of IgG and complement.

The corneal epithelium consists of five layers, is transparent and rests on Bowman's membrane. It is generated by the limbal stem cells. The epithelium can resurface an epithelial defect within 24–48 hours. Its surface cells are linked by tight junctions, and it provides an important barrier to the invasion of the corneal stroma by microbes. This is well demonstrated by the increased frequency of microbial keratitis in certain soft contact lens wearers with a compromised, hypoxic epithelium, especially those using extended wear lenses. Similarly, while bacterial keratitis is rarely found in an eye with a normal epithelium, it is more common in patients with recurrent epithelial defects, such as those due to chronic herpetic virus infection.

In order to cause infection, the organism has to penetrate into the eye. This can be facilitated by an epithelial defect following an abrasion, or as in recurrent epithelial erosion syndrome [4], corneal trauma or a contaminated contact lens. Penetration of the posterior segment by a contaminated, high-velocity fragment, such as a hammer-and-chisel injury or shrapnel, can cause bacterial endophthalmitis, although the metal fragment is often hot and sterile [5]. The blood-borne route (bacteraemia) must always be considered for endophthalmitis when there is no history of accidental or surgical trauma, particularly the possibility of endocarditis. Intravenous drug addicts are more likely to develop endophthalmitis, particularly with *Candida albicans*.

For invasion of the corneal stroma to occur, the organism must first adhere to the epithelium. *Pseudomonas aeruginosa* is particularly adept at invading the compromised epithelium from a superficial source, often from contaminated contact lenses or eye drops. For the contact lens wearer, the initial problem involves bacterial, amoebal or polymicrobial contamination of the storage case with adherence of bacteria, or adsorption of *Acanthamoeba*, to the lens. The storage case is often coated with a biofilm protecting the organisms from the disinfecting solution (Chapter 9). The contact lens then acts as a mechanical vector, transferring the microbes to the corneal epithelium. The situation is exacerbated by the sequestration of tear fluid behind the lens.

Penetration alone by an organism is not sufficient to cause infection; it must proliferate to establish sufficient numbers of cells to overcome host defenses. The importance of bacterial load is emphasized by the finding that while up to 25% of intraoperative aqueous samples at cataract surgery contain bacteria, the rate of postoperative endophthalmitis following cataract surgery is low, at 0.1% to 0.7%. In most cases, the bacterial inoculum is insufficient to result in multiplication, the cells being inactivated by antibacterial substances present in the anterior chamber (AC) or by antibiotics given intraoperatively. In a few patients, bacterial proliferation does occur, along with adhesion to the intraocular lens, and a devastating endophthalmitis results (Chapter 7).

The virulence of the organism also dictates the outcome for the patient. This usually relates to the production of lethal toxins by the bacterium, which causes tissue necrosis, such as the exotoxins and proteases liberated by *P. aeruginosa*. *Streptococcus pyogenes* is highly virulent for the eye, producing exotoxin A and needing only a small inoculum, possibly as low as ten cells, to cause necrotizing fasciitis of the lids or a fulminant endophthalmitis within 24 hours of cataract surgery. While this situation applies to all tissues of the body, it is different for *P. aeruginosa*, which is highly pathogenic for the cornea but not for the skin. The cornea is unique in that it is both avascular and lacks professional antigen-processing cells except in the peripheral epithelium. Its ability to mount an immediate immunological reaction to trauma is therefore limited. This is unusual in other vascularized sites in the body. The posterior segment also possesses immune-privileged compartments and provides an excellent environment for bacterial multiplication.

Local Corneal Surface Immunity

This depends on IgA, IgM, C1 complement and Langerhans cells (LCs), all of which are found in the peripheral but not the central, corneal epithelial sheet in the normal non-inflamed eye. Irritation of the central cornea, such as with herpes virus infection, can result in centripetal migration of the Langerhans dendritic cells to promote an immuno-inflammatory response.

Langerhans cell migration also occurs centrally with age. LCs are professional antigen-processing cells and are the only corneal cells to express the major histocompatibility complex (MHC) class II antigens without prior inducement by cytokines. IgG diffuses into the stroma from the limbus, achieving 50% of the serum concentration.

LCs take up antigens by pinocytosis or endocytosis. Upon exposure to antigen, LCs and other antigen-presenting cells (APCs), such as corneal epithelial cells and macrophages, undergo functional maturation and gain the ability to present the antigen to CD4 T helper (Th) lymphocyte cells attracted to the area by cytokines. Antigens taken up into APCs are enzymatically degraded to oligopeptides, with an unfolded secondary structure, which are expressed at their surface as antigenic peptides bound to MHC (major histocompatibility complex) molecules. These cells interact with B lymphocytes to produce IgM and/or IgG antibodies. The B lymphocytes then prime plasma cells for clonal antibody production or transformation to memory cells, which quickly produce new antibodies when exposed to similar processed antigen months or years later (Figure 10.1).

For the role of IgA antibody, refer to mucosa-associated lymphoid tissue (MALT) (Supplementary Chapter S10).

Macrophages can be transformed into APCs by interleukin-1 (IL-1) released from corneal epithelial cells, which induces the expression of MHC class II molecules at their surface. These APCs then process antigenic peptides to form a binary complex with MHC class II molecules. Macrophages can also process particulate antigens, including whole bacteria, such as staphylococci, and free-living amoebae, such as *Acanthamoeba*; however, they more effectively process soluble antigens, such as protein A of *St. aureus*, internalized in endocytic vesicles. This is in contrast to Langerhans cells, which only process soluble antigen.

T lymphocytes exert their local effector function by secreting cytokines in tissues that act directly on target cells. Interferon (IFN)-gamma induces the expression of MHC class II molecules in keratinocytes, epithelial cells, endothelial cells and fibroblasts, which can all, to a variable degree, act as APCs that process and present immunogenic peptides complexed with MHC class II molecules. They can

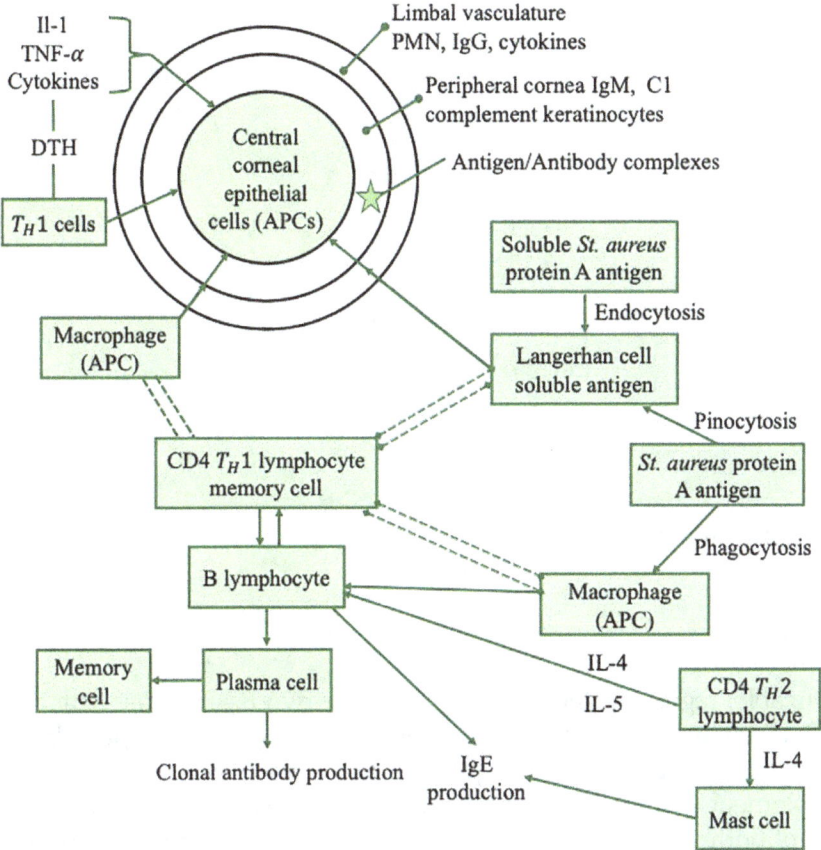

FIGURE 10.1 Factors determining the immunity of the cornea using *Staphylococcus aureus* protein A as an example of a bacterial antigen. APC: antigen-presenting cells. DTH: delayed-type hypersensitivity (cell-mediated immunity). PMN: polymorphonuclear (pus) cells. Also refer to Appendices 3 and 4.

all process and present immunogenic peptides but differ in capacity to produce costimulatory signals and do not stimulate resting T cells, which require IL-2 to become activated. The expression of ICAM-1-b2 integrin is needed to attract neutrophils to the site, as part of the inflammatory process, and will attract activated Th1 lymphocytes as well.

Immune complex activation occurs by stimulation of either the C1 complement component, with a resulting cascade to C5a that acts chemotactically for polymorphonuclear leukocytes (PMNs) and causes release of cytokines, or activation of the alternative pathway (Appendix 4).

Humoral Immunity

This is mediated by antibodies produced by the B lymphocytes, plasma and memory cells (Figures 10.1 and 10.2). An antibody is a Y-shaped molecule consisting of two heavy chains and two light chains, connected by disulfide bonds. The heavy chains are larger polypeptides while the light chains are smaller. These chains fold into specific configurations that allow them to interact with each other and form the functional antibody molecule.

The structure of an antibody is divided into two main regions: the two F_{ab} (fragment antigen-binding) regions, at each end of the 'Y' arms, and the F_c (fragment

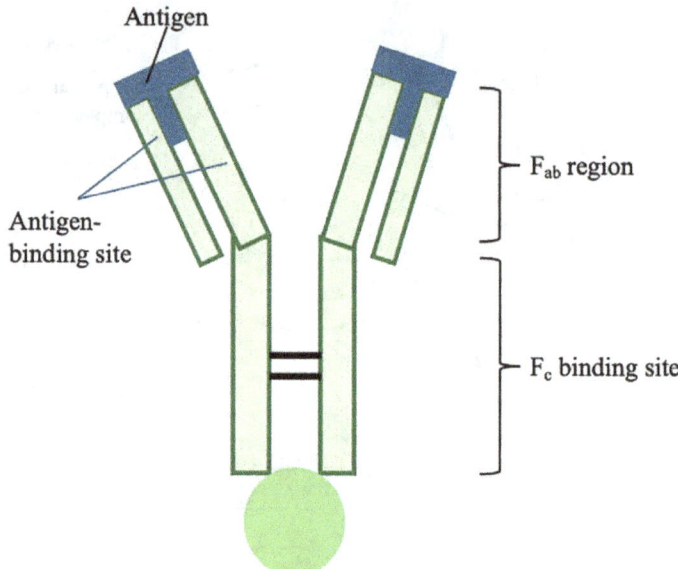

Antigen

Antigen-
binding site

F$_{ab}$ region

F$_c$ binding site

FIGURE 10.2 Structure of the antibody molecule.

crystallizable) region, at the opposite end. The two F$_{ab}$ regions, which include the variable domains of both the heavy and light chains, are responsible for *binding to antigens*. The single F$_c$ region (green circle) is involved in *effector functions*, such as complement fixation and interaction with cell surface receptors. The variable regions of both chains determine the specificity of the antigen binding site, while the constant regions of the heavy chains determine which antibody class the antibody belongs to. The various antibody classes are found in different compartments of the body.

Immediate Hypersensitivity (IgE) Reaction
In sites such as the conjunctiva, CD4 Th2 lymphocytes play a key role in immediate hypersensitivity reactions. They produce IL-4 and IL-5, which stimulate B lymphocytes to switch to IgE production and to express IgE receptors. Furthermore, IL-4 induces mast cell proliferation and IgE production. CD4 Th2 cells are found in the conjunctiva of children with vernal disease.

Adult patients with severe allergic keratoconjunctivitis, who have very high systemic IgE antibodies associated with IL-5 induction of eosinophils, may have lids colonized by *Staphylococcus aureus* but lack DTH to *Staphylococcus aureus* protein A [6] (Chapter 4).

Delayed-Type Hypersensitivity (DTH) Due to Cell-Mediated Immunity (CMI)
DTH is induced by bacteria, such as *Mycobacterium tuberculosis* and, in some people, protein A of *Staphylococcus aureus*, as well as microfilariae of the roundworm *Onchocerca volvulus*, which can excite a cell-mediated immune (CMI) reaction, expressed by the Th1 lymphocyte cells and mediated by cytokines. It has been proposed as a mechanism to explain episodes of marginal ulceration consequent to recurrent blepharitis caused by *St. aureus* (Chapter 6) [7]. This is discussed later, and illustrated in Figure 10.1, as an example of immune mechanisms operating in the peripheral cornea.

St. aureus repeatedly colonizes the lid margins of both the normal population (at approximately 10%) and those that are atopic (at approximately 50%). It is likely that diffusible cell wall antigens from *St. aureus*, especially protein A but also ribitol teichoic acid, reach the antigen-presenting cells (APC) of the corneal epithelium across the tear film. In the peripheral cornea and also the conjunctiva, these antigens are processed by dendritic Langerhans cells (LCs). The LCs have receptors for the F_c portion of the antibody molecule, which assists endocytosis of antigens, such as protein A, by the binding of specific antibodies. In the latter case, there can also be cross-linking between specific (F_{ab}) and non-specific (F_c) sites both found on protein A (Appendix 3).

The CD4 Th1 lymphocyte is responsible for most DTH reactions. The Th1 subtype (as opposed to the Th2 subtype) mediates DTH by a cascade of cytokines produced by T-cell clones. Th1 cells produce IL-2 and IFN-g responsible in part for the induration response of the DTH reaction found in the skin 48 hours after exposure to the antigen. CD4 Th1 and Th2 lymphocytes regulate the actions of each other on antibody production; IFN-g produced by the Th1 cell inhibits the stimulatory effect of IL-4, produced by the Th2 cell, on antibody production by B lymphocytes. This may be the mechanism for the clinical observation that a strong DTH response is associated with a weak antibody response and vice versa.

Activated CD4 Th1 cells secrete IFN-gamma at the site of antigen entry and induce MHC class II expression on 'nonprofessional' APCs, thereby activating them. The recognition of the MHC-peptide complex of the APC by a T-cell receptor initiates an intracellular signal transduction pathway via the p56 and p59 tyrosine kinases. The molecules that are then produced increase binding of Th cells to APCs and are called adhesion molecules (ADMs); for CD4 cells, this includes the 55 kd monomeric transmembrane glycoprotein belonging to the Ig gene superfamily and for CD8 T lymphocyte cytotoxic cells (CTC), two 34 kd alpha chain molecules.

The cellular response is regulated by expression of adhesion molecules (ADMs) on inflammatory cells and vascular endothelium, which in turn is controlled by cytokines, which can also act as chemotactic factors for polymorphonuclear cells (PMNs). These ADMs cause the adhesion of PMNs and lymphocytes to the local limbal vascular endothelium when they bind to it and migrate to the site of activated lymphocytes in the peripheral cornea.

Memory Th lymphocytes will also migrate to this site if the patient has undergone systemic enhancement of CMI to the particular antigen, in this example, *St. aureus* protein A. The expression of integrins (b1, b2, b3) attracts these activated Th1 lymphocytes to the inflammatory site. The expression of b1 is upregulated on the surface of activated memory cells, which bind to the counter receptor on vascular endothelium (very late antigen-4 [VLA-4], a member of the Ig superfamily), resulting in extravasation into the site (peripheral cornea) of the processed antigen (in this example protein A).

The CD4 T helper cell (Th) is responsible for most DTH reactions. The Th1 subtype mediates DTH, not given by the Th2 subtype, based on an array of cytokines produced by T-cell clones including IL-2, IFN-gamma and TNF-alpha (Appendix 3). The Th2 subtype stimulates B lymphocytes with IL-4, IL-5, IL-10 and IL-13 cytokines to produce an antibody response. Other cytokines, not characterized as either Th1 or Th2, include IL-12, which promotes IFN-gamma and TNF-alpha production and hence a Th1 response. Polymorphonuclear cells, macrophages, and dendritic cells can produce both Th1 and Th2 cytokines, but ocular APCs cannot produce the Th1-inducing cytokine IL–12.

DTH is thought to be responsible for the underlying pathogenic mechanisms of trachoma, HSV stromal keratitis and some forms of idiopathic uveitis. Anterior chamber-associated immune deviation (ACAID—refer later) is believed to be a mechanism that prevents the trivial activation of the DTH arm of the immune response as a method for sustaining immune-homeostasis in the eye.

Macrophages produce IL-1, which stimulates other macrophages to become APCs and to present antigen to Th1 lymphocytes. IL-1 also regulates macrophage inflammatory protein-2 (MIP-2), which acts as a chemo-attractant for PMN influx and may be susceptible to down regulation to reduce the inflammatory response.

Th1 lymphocytes produce IL-2 and INF-gamma, responsible in part for the induration response of the DTH reaction. Th1 and Th2 cross-regulate each other's activities via cytokine production, with one inhibiting production by the other, e.g. IFN-gamma inhibits the effect of IL-4 on B lymphocytes. Their role in cross-regulating each other and thereby maintaining a balance in the immune response is responsible for the adaptive immunity to various pathogens, e.g. Th1 protects against intracellular pathogens, while Th2 protects against helminths. Novel therapeutic strategies hold promise for modulating the alloimmune response to corneal allografts by either promoting antigen-specific tolerance or redirecting the host's response from a Th1 pathway towards a Th2 pathway to reduce immune rejection.

Ocular Immune Privilege

This has five primary features:

- Blood-ocular barriers (refer to Chapter S11 'Pharmacology and Pharmacokinetics')
- Absence of lymphatic drainage
- Soluble immunomodulatory factors in the aqueous humour
- Immunomodulatory ligands on the surface of ocular parenchymal cells
- Tolerogenic antigen-presenting cells in the anterior and posterior chambers

Immune-privileged sites, such as the eye, have evolved with the mechanisms earlier to *prevent* the induction of inflammation. In addition, neuropeptides constitutively present in ocular tissue are recognized as part of the immune privilege mechanism. Johnson *et al.* [8] first showed in rabbits, which had been immunized subcutaneously with a whole-cell vaccine to develop systemic enhancement (CMI/DTH) to *Staphylococcus aureus*, that there was *tolerance* instead of DTH in the AC. This situation applies similarly to most other organisms able to induce a systemic DTH reaction.

Aqueous humour contains three complement regulatory proteins: membrane cofactor protein (MCP), decay-accelerating factor (DAF) and CD59, as well as a cell surface regulator of complement (Crry) that inhibits its activation to prevent severe inflammation. These proteins are continuously active at a low level in the normal eye but are tightly regulated. The cornea, choroid and retina are particularly susceptible to autoimmune-mediated, immune-complex disease; however, the vitreous and subretinal space are not.

Anterior chamber (ACAID) and Posterior chamber (POCAID)-Associated Immune Deviation

ACAID and POCAID (Figure 10.3) exist to protect the single-cell-layered corneal endothelium, anterior chamber (AC), subretinal space and vitreous from immune-mediated damage by CMI or DTH. This POCAID effect is not present in the retina or choroid but does apply to the immune-privileged retinal pigment epithelium, in which cytomegalovirus can persist.

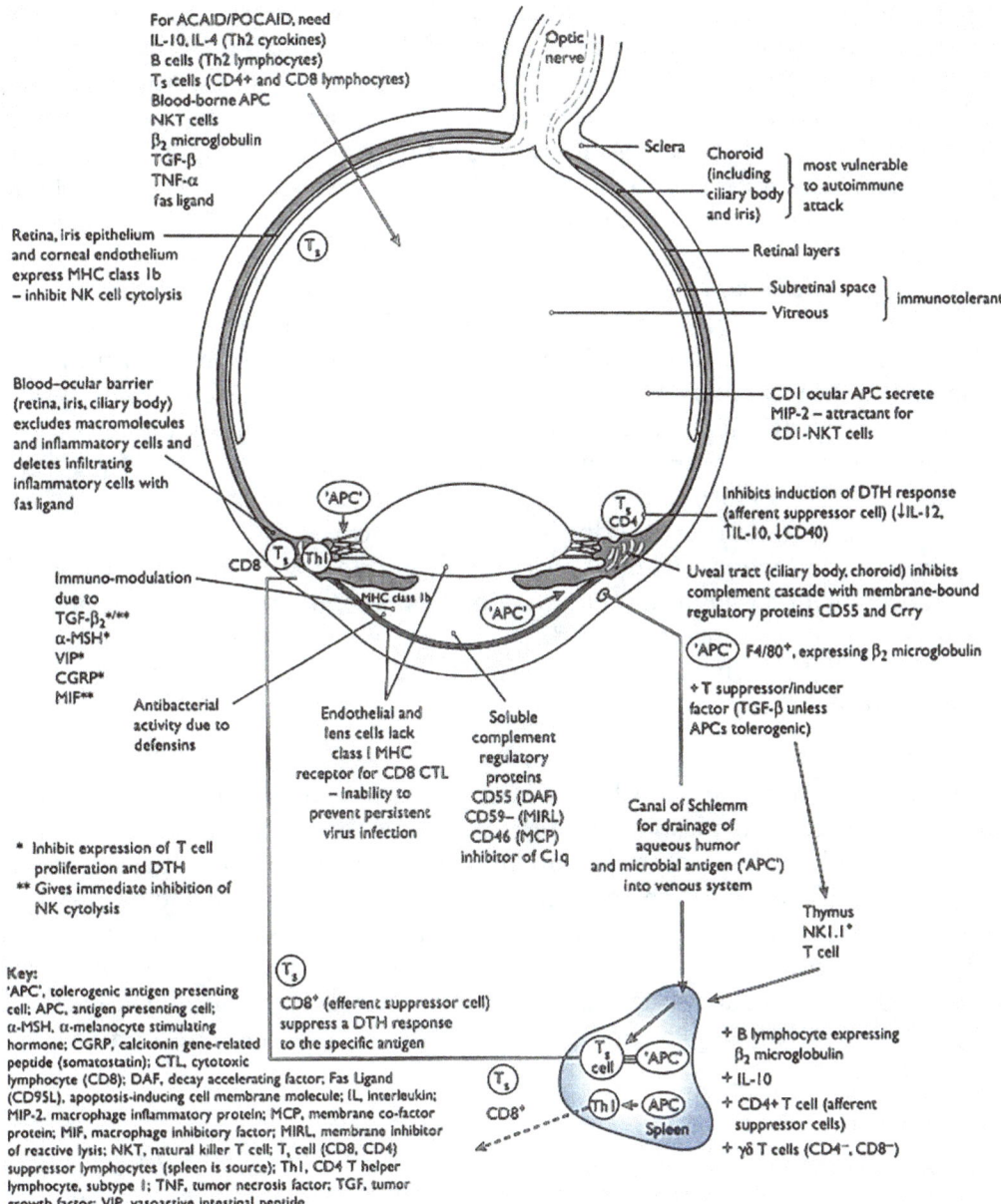

FIGURE 10.3 Anterior (ACAID) and posterior (POCAID) chamber associated immune deviation.

Source: (Seal D, Pleyer U. Ocular Infection, 2nd Edition 2007)

ACAID: Immune deviation is achieved by avoidance of CD8 cytotoxic T lymphocyte (CTL)-mediated cytolysis and inhibition of the CD4 Th1 lymphocyte response in the AC with production of tissue-damaging cytokines. These aims are achieved by an absence of class I MHC expression on endothelial and lens cells, so avoiding lysis by class I restricted CTLs. The problem with this mechanism for the AC endothelium is the inability to prevent persistent viral infection. One explanation proposed for the normally-reduced immune response is engagement of the pro-apoptotic molecule Fas by its ligand (FasL), which leads to apoptosis (programmed cell death) and consequently limits an inflammatory response.

The prevention of a DTH (cell-mediated) immune reaction is gained by the camero-splenic axis (Figure 10.3). Microbial antigen in the AC is discharged in the aqueous to the venous blood flow via the canal of Schlemm, often phagocytosed within 'tolerogenic' APCs, and *go to the spleen* instead of the lymphatics; a small percentage of these APCs reach the submandibular gland but remain inactive, as they cannot produce IL–12. Within the spleen, there is a production of T suppressor (Ts) lymphocytes that migrate back to the AC to inhibit Th1 lymphocytes. These T cells also suppress a DTH response, acting systemically to the specific antigen. This systemic protection is lost if the spleen, which is the source of the Ts cells, is removed. *A functioning spleen has been shown essential for developing and maintaining ACAID.*

TNF-alpha and Th2 cytokine IL-10 are needed within the AC to induce an ACAID response to an antigen. The AC also contains TGF (tumour or transforming growth factor)-beta, which renders local APCs tolerogenic and is another necessary part of ACAID, particularly if the host has systemically enhanced DTH to the specific antigen. However, this mechanism does not prevent the severe inflammatory response to the live and dead microfilariae of *Onchocerca volvulus* (Chapter 7), causing 'river blindness' in West Africa.

Specific production of antibodies occurs within the vitreous and posterior chamber during endophthalmitis. Antibodies recognizing the same antigen in both serum and intraocular fluid differ in the epitopes that are recognized, demonstrating that the intraocular compartment determines its own antibody profile against intraocular pathogens.

Immunopathogenesis

The immune response to a bacterial challenge, such as contamination of the AC with phacoemulsification surgery, influences the outcome together with the numbers and virulence of the organism. The combination of the type of immune response (Th1 or Th2 with relevant cytokines) together with the bacterial virulence factors and toxins, if any, will determine whether there is an acute or chronic inflammatory response or, when the immune response is satisfactory, there is no inflammatory effect at all. A high bacterial count can also influence the outcome overwhelming the host immune response to lead to infection.

Immune Suppression

Immune suppression can be obtained with the drug *ciclosporine*, a polypeptide which *suppresses the activity of the p56 and p59 tyrosine kinases in the Th1 lymphocytes*, when the DTH (CMI reaction) activity cascade is blocked (Appendix 3). This drug also acts on calcineurin, blocking T-cell activation. Ciclosporin acts specifically and reversibly in an immuno-modulating way that inhibits the activation of CD4 T helper cells to produce processed antigen for cytotoxic CD8 T 'killer' cells and induction of inflammatory cytokines.

It does not depress haemopoiesis and has no effect on the function of PMNs. It is a potent immunosuppressive drug and prolongs the survival of allogeneic transplants, including the *cornea*. Ciclosporin prevents and treats rejection and graft-versus-host disease or when there is an immunological pathogenesis.

Fusidic acid is an anti-staphylococcal antibiotic, for which there is a topical preparation (1% viscous eye drop), that also has a similar immunosuppressive action to ciclosporin. This may explain its beneficial effect for treating the blepharitis of rosacea (Chapters 5 and 6).

Immune Modulation and Corticosteroids

Corticosteroids have a specific role inhibiting phospholipase conversion of membrane phospholipids to arachidonic acid (Figure 10.4) and thus preventing its conversion to highly inflammatory prostaglandins. Corticosteroids have both anti-inflammatory and immunosuppressive effects. The anti-inflammatory effects are non-specific to the cause of the disease process and will inhibit the inflammatory reaction to nearly any type of stimulus. The effects include the following:

- Inhibition of increased capillary permeability due to the acute inflammatory reaction and suppression of vasodilation
- Inhibition of degranulation of neutrophils, mast cells and basophils with monocytopenia and eosinopenia
- Reduction of prostaglandin synthesis by inhibiting phospholipase
- Temporary neutrophil leukocytosis four to six hours after administration but with reduced adherence to vascular endothelium

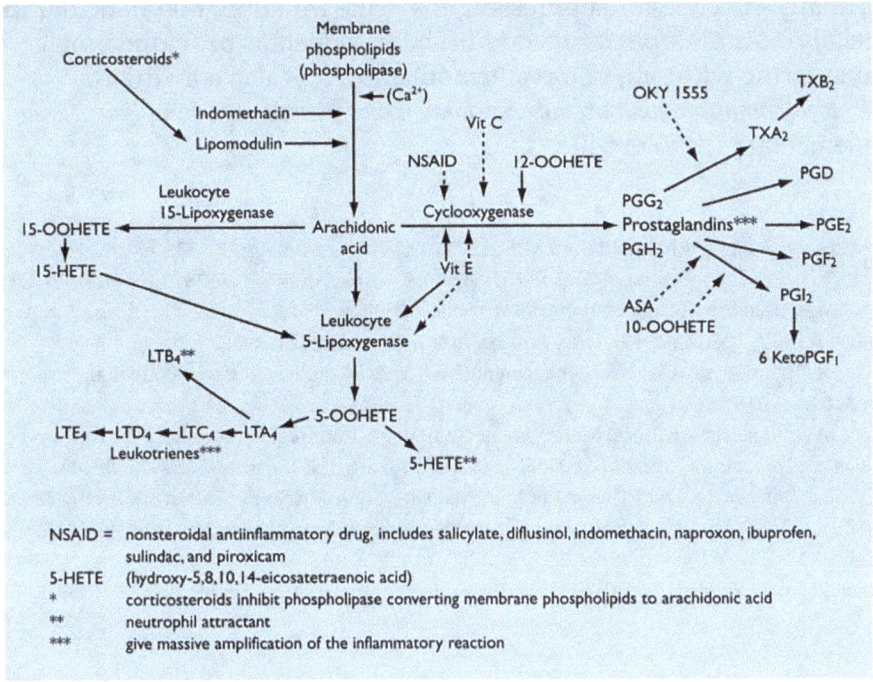

FIGURE 10.4 Arachidonic acid metabolic pathways and sites of blockage by immune-modulating drugs—corticosteroids and NSAIDs.

Source: (Seal D, Pleyer U. Ocular Infection, 2nd Edition 2007)

Effect of an Immuno-Suppressive Drug

There is induction of lymphocytopenia. T lymphocytes are more susceptible than B lymphocytes, so antibody production is not reduced, but DTH/CMI reactions are modified at low concentrations. The following occur:

- Inhibition of migration of macrophages and neutrophils
- Suppression of lymphocyte proliferation
- Suppression of action of cytokines
- Inhibition of DTH/CMI
- Depression of bactericidal activity of monocytes and macrophages

Corticosteroids reduce the activity of macrophages but not necessarily their activation by cytokines. They inhibit cytokine release with additional suppression of PMN activity, explaining progression of fungal, protozoal or parasitic infections in their presence, since it is these latter infections especially that require macrophages as scavenger cells.

The use of corticosteroid therapy in managing endophthalmitis has continued to be a necessary albeit controversial treatment. Intravitreal corticosteroid therapy should be used for bacterial and considered for fungal endophthalmitis BUT should be injected at the same time as the antibiotics.

Nonsteroidal anti-inflammatory drugs (NSAIDs) act by inhibiting the conversion of arachidonic acid to prostaglandins by cyclo-oxygenase (Figure 10.4). NSAIDs such as flurbiprofen have superseded conventional steroid preparations, such as dexamethasone or prednisolone, by removing unwanted side effects. This is particularly so when corticosteroids are introduced systemically for treatment of severe ocular inflammatory disease. Flurbiprofen, given orally, has been found particularly effective for suppressing the acute inflammation of ocular infection, especially keratitis, episcleritis and limbitis, as well as providing analgesia without interfering with satisfactory chemotherapy. It is also a mydriatic.

For local immune complex disease and mucosa-associated lymphoid tissue, refer to Supplementary Chapter S10.

REFERENCES

1. Mackie I et al. Brit J Ophthalmol 1976. PMID: 1268164976 (https://doi.org/10.1136/bjo.60.1.70).
2. Hanstock H et al. Front Immunol 2019. PMID: 31231369 (https://doi.org/10.3389/fimmu.2019.01178).
3. Zahoor M et al. In Vitro Study on the Antimicrobial Activity of Human Tears with Respect to Age. Korean J Clin Lab Sci 2018. PMID: none (https://doi.org/10.15324/kjcls.2018.50.2.93).
4. College of Optometrists. Clinical Management Guidelines. Recurrent Corneal Epithelial Erosion Syndrome 2025. Accessed 03/09/25.
5. College of Optometrists. Clinical Management Guidelines. Trauma (Penetrating) 2025. Accessed 03/09/25.
6. Tuft S et al. Ophthalmol 1992. PMID: 1553205 (https://doi.org/10.1016/s0161-6420(92)31995-5).
7. Seal D et al. Immunology and Therapy of Marginal Ulceration as a Complication of Chronic Blepharitis Due to *St. Aureus*. In: J Lass (ed.). Advances in Corneal Research. Selected Abstracts of the World Congress on the Cornea IV. New York: Plenum Press 1997, pp 19–25. PMID: none.
8. Johnson J et al. J Exp Med 1960. PMID: 19867186 (https://pubmed.ncbi.nlm.nih.gov/19867186/).

PART 2
Supplementary Chapters

S1: Equipment Needed for Domiciliary and Clinic Visits

A) DOMICILIARY VISITS—(THE DOMICILIARY EYE EXAMINATION— COLLEGE OF OPTOMETRISTS)

Minimum Equipment needed to deliver the best optometric care includes the following:

- Amsler grid
- Dispensing equipment and range of spectacle frames
- Distance and near ocular-muscle balance tests, plus suitable targets and occlude
- Focimeter
- A full range of diagnostic drugs
- Illuminated test chart
- Means to examine the external eye, including an appropriate method if using diagnostic stains
- Near chart
- Ophthalmoscope
- Picture tests, as appropriate, for patients with learning disabilities
- Retinoscope
- Means of assessing visual fields other than confrontation
- Tonometer
- Trial case and trial frame

Assessment:

- Carry out tests that are possible to determine patient's needs for vision care for both sight and health.
- Format and content of exam is determined by your professional judgement, patient needs and legal requirements.
- Be flexible about the approach you use as this may be dependent on the environment.
- If carried out under UK General Ophthalmic Services (GOS), then contractor must submit a GOS6 Pre-Visit Notification in line with domiciliary visit regulations.

Typical routine:

- Arrival, introduction and consent
- History and symptoms
- Vision assessment

DOI: 10.1201/9781003606789-13

- Refraction
- Ocular health assessment
- Discussion
- Advice and management (e.g. dispensing, referral)
- Documentation

B) PRACTICE VISITS

Equipment needed:

- Accommodation rule
- Amsler charts
- Tonometer
- Appropriate ophthalmic diagnostic agents and drugs
- Colour vision test
- Selection of condensing lenses for binocular indirect biomicroscopy techniques
- Direct ophthalmoscope
- Distance and near oculomotor balance tests
- Focimeter
- Hand washing facilities and signage where the care is being delivered
- Keratometer
- Letter matching card
- Near vision tests (adult and children)
- Near vision unit
- Pen torch
- Appropriate peripheral visual fields equipment
- Retinoscope
- Slit-lamp biomicroscope
- Internally illuminated or digital visual acuity test chart (adult, children and language agnostic)
- Suitable rule (s) for measuring frames, lenses, PD
- Stereopsis test
- Threshold controlled visual field equipment
- Trial lens, frame and accessories
- Waste disposal facilities, signage and equipment

Optional Additional Equipment

- Autorefractor
- Binocular headset indirect ophthalmoscope
- Children's acuity charts
- Corneal topographer
- Contrast sensitivity chart
- Digital imaging system (e.g. fundus camera, optical coherence topographer, widefield imager, slit-lamp mounted camera)
- Gonioscopy lens
- Equipment for foreign body removal
- Equipment for DED assessment
- Equipment for punctum plug insertion and tear duct syringing

- Indirect ophthalmoscope
- Pachymeter
- Patient management system
- Prism bars
- Supplementary vision charts

Assessment:

- Must carry out such examinations as appear to be necessary to detect signs of injury, disease or abnormality in the eye or surrounding area.
- Use professional judgement to decide format and content of eye examination.
- Record all clinical findings.

Typical routine:

- History and symptoms
- Vision assessment
- Refraction
- Ocular health assessment including ocular muscle balance assessment, internal and external eye examination
- Discussion
- Advice and management (e.g. dispensing, referral)
- Documentation

C) THE WORKING DIAGNOSIS: DEFINITION AND APPLICATION

A working diagnosis refers to a provisional identification of the patient's condition, formed on the basis of current evidence and understanding. It acts as a temporary label that guides immediate decision-making while acknowledging that further refinement may be required as new information emerges. In eye care, it enables prioritisation of differential diagnoses, informs investigation and treatment strategies and provides a basis for communication with patients and other healthcare professionals.

Cognitive Strategies and Dual Process Theory

Clinical reasoning involves both System 1 (fast, intuitive) and System 2 (slow, analytical) thinking. While System 1 aids in recognising common patterns quickly, System 2 is engaged in complex or ambiguous cases. Eye care practitioners (ECPs) must be adept at switching between these cognitive strategies as needed.

Diagnostic Error and Cognitive Bias

Common cognitive biases such as anchoring, confirmation bias and premature closure can lead to diagnostic errors in eye care. These biases may cause practitioners to overlook important signs or alternative explanations. Ainge (2025) recommends structured reflection, use of differential diagnosis lists and peer consultation as safeguards against such biases [1]. Recognising and addressing these errors are key components of developing clinical expertise.

Developing Clinical Reasoning

Techniques such as case-based learning, simulation and reflective practice help develop this skill. Tayade (2021) supports early clinical exposure and feedback as methods to enhance diagnostic skills [2]. Students are encouraged to consider reasoning processes, participate in peer discussions and engage in reflective study.

REFERENCES

1. Ainge LE et al. BMC Medical Education 2025. PMID: 39780160 (https://bmcmededuc.biomedcentral.com/articles/10.1186/s12909-024-06613-6).
2. Tayade MC et al. J Educ Health Promot 2021. PMID: 34084864 (https://www.ncbi.nlm.nih.gov/pmc/articles/PMC8150058/).

S2: Common Scotomas Involving the Optic Nerve and Tract

A lesion involving the right optic nerve (labelled 1 in Figure S2.1) or loss of function of the right optic nerve head, such as a central retinal artery occlusion or end-stage glaucoma, results in uniocular vision loss in the right field of vision.

Pressure on the optic chiasm, such as from a pituitary tumour (often a benign adenoma) lying immediately beneath it, results in loss of vision from both nasal areas of retina, to give a bitemporal hemianopia (labelled 2 in Figure S2.1).

A lesion involving the right optic tract (labelled 3 in Figure S2.1) results in a left homonymous hemianopia with a loss of vision in the left fields of vision, often found with a stroke.

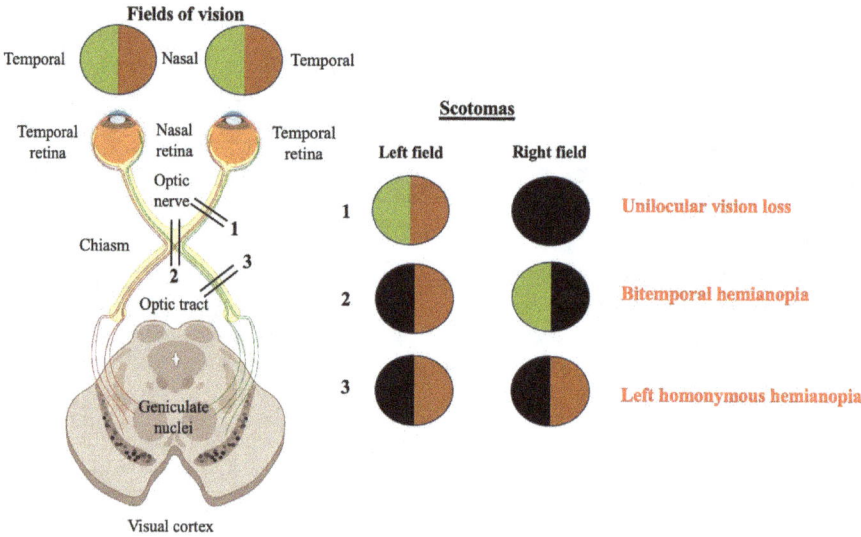

FIGURE S2.1 Common scotomas involving the optic nerve and tract.

Source: (Courtesy of Mr. J.Z. Ong, RUMC, Penang, Malaysia)

DOI: 10.1201/9781003606789-14

S3: Presentation of Common Ocular Conditions

GLAUCOMA

Large (normal) physiological cup (Figure S3.1) with a cup-to-disc ratio of 0.45.

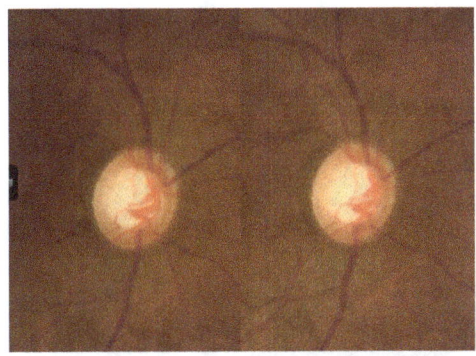

FIGURE S3.1 Large physiological cup.

Source: (Courtesy of Dr. S. Basu, LV Prasad Institute, Hyderabad, India)

Severe Bilateral Glaucoma (Figures S3.2 and S3.3)

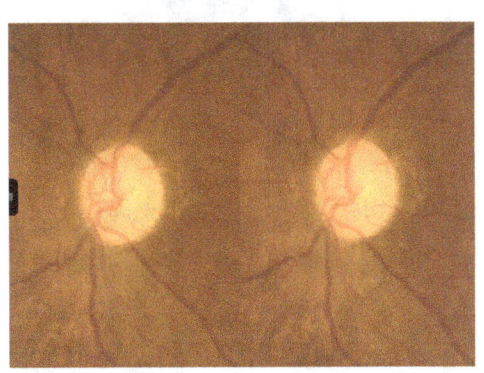

FIGURE S3.2 Severe glaucoma with cup-to-disc ratio of 0.76/0.63 (refer to scan analysis S3.3).

Source: (Courtesy of Dr. S. Basu, LV Prasad Institute, Hyderabad, India)

159

DOI: 10.1201/9781003606789-15

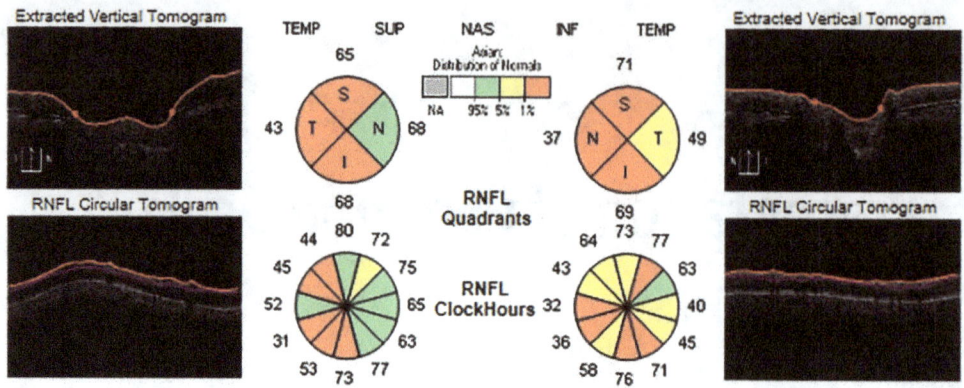

FIGURE S3.3 OCT imaging with RNFL analysis.

Source: (Courtesy of Dr. S. Basu, LV Prasad Institute, Hyderabad, India)

Acute Glaucoma After Corneal Graft Surgery (Figures S3.4 and S3.5)

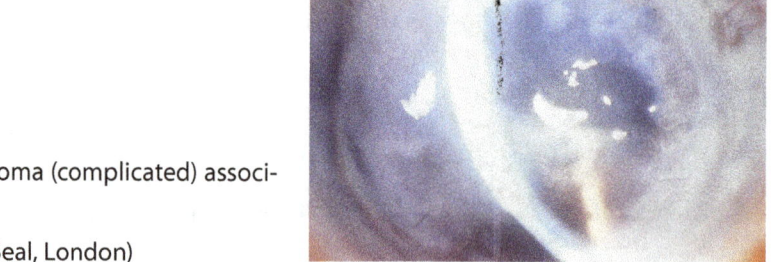

FIGURE S3.4 Acute glaucoma (complicated) associated with a corneal graft.

Source: (Courtesy of Dr. D. Seal, London)

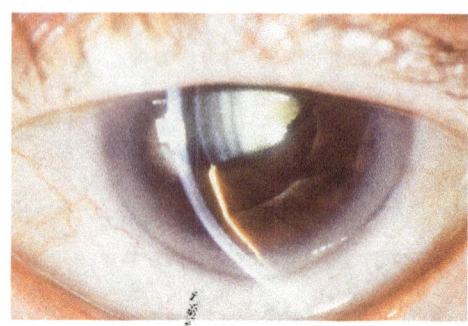

FIGURE S3.5 Other eye (normal) to show the angle.

Source: (Courtesy of Dr. D. Seal, London)

DIABETIC RETINA

Diabetic Proliferative Retinopathy (Figures S3.6–S3.7)

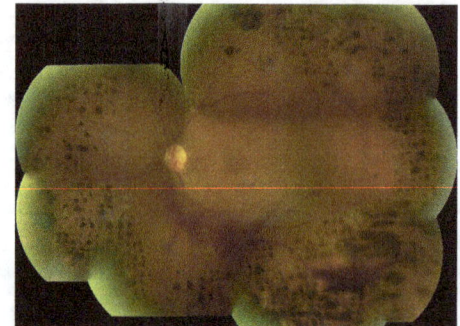

FIGURE S3.6 Composite Retinography showing diabetic proliferative retinopathy managed with laser photocoagulation.

Source: (Courtesy of Dr. Fatima Mesa-Lugo, Hospital Universitario de Canarias, Spain)

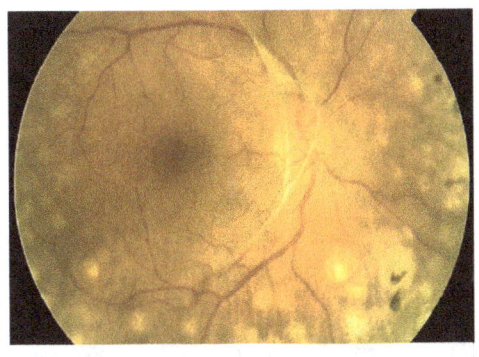

FIGURE S3.7 Regressive diabetic proliferative reti-nopathy managed with photocoagulation.

Source: (Courtesy of Dr. Fatima Mesa-Lugo, Hospital Universitario de Canarias, Spain)

Diabetic Macular Oedema (Figures S3.8–S3.10)

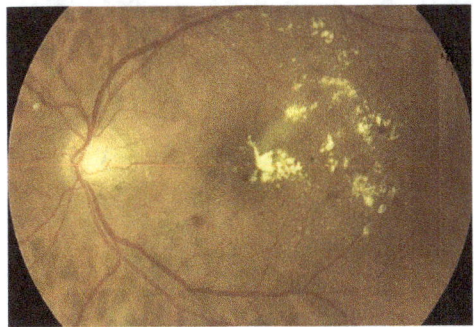

FIGURE S3.8 Diabetic macular oedema with hard exudates (R3A,M1)

Source: (Courtesy of Dr. Fatima Mesa-Lugo, Hospital Universitaro de Canarias, Spain)

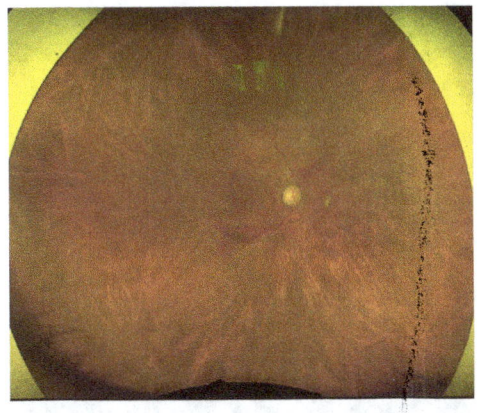

FIGURE S3.9 Diabetic proliferative retinopathy with macular oedema and retrohyaloid haemorrhage due to bleeding from new vessels

Source: (Courtesy of Dr. S. Basu, LV Prasad Eye Institute, Hyderabad, India)

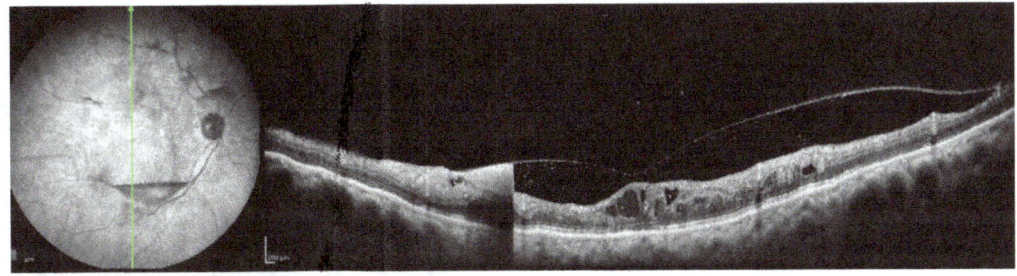

FIGURE S3.10 OCT showing vitreous retraction (posterior vitreous face) as incomplete detach-ment (physiological), and fluid under the retina

Source: (Courtesy of Dr. S. Basu, LV Prasad Eye Institute, Hyderabad, India)

RETINAL DETACHMENT (FIGURES S3.11 AND S3.12)

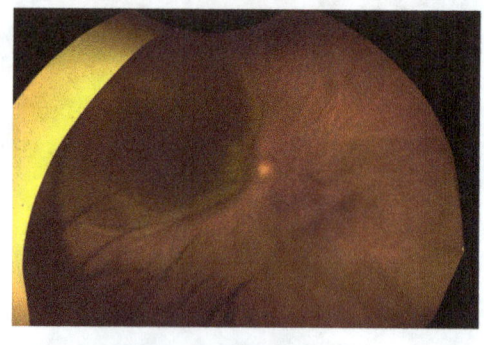

FIGURE S3.11 Retinal detachment.

Source: (Courtesy of Dr. S. Basu, LV Prasad Institute, Hyderabad, India)

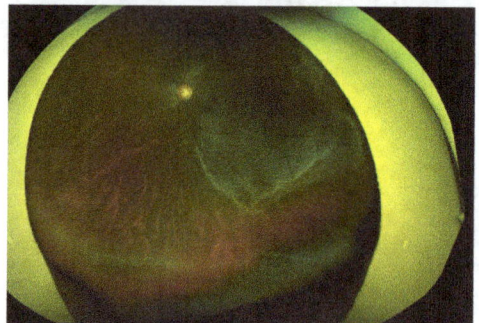

FIGURE S3.12 Retinal detachment.

Source: (Courtesy of Dr. S. Basu, LV Prasad Institute, Hyderabad, India)

HYPERTENSIVE RETINOPATHY (FIGURES S3.13–S3.16)

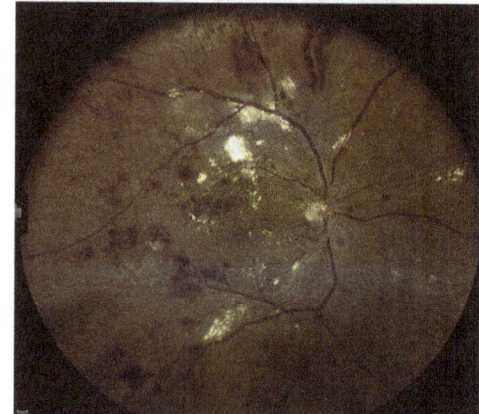

FIGURE S3.13 Severe hypertensive retinopathy in an eye that has also received laser photocoagulation.

Source: (Courtesy of Dr. S. Basu, LV Prasad Eye Institute, Hyderabad, India)

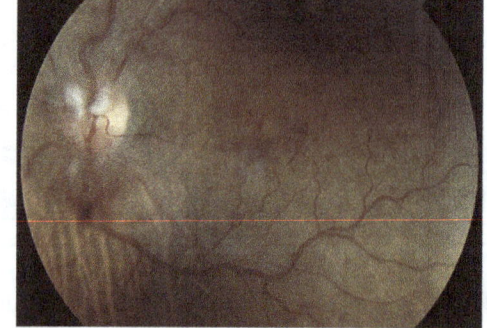

FIGURE S3.14 Hypertensive retinopathy with retinal vein occlusion.

Source: (Courtesy of Drs. Marta Crespo-Rodriguez and Miguel Acosta-Darias, Hospital Universitario de Canarias, Spain)

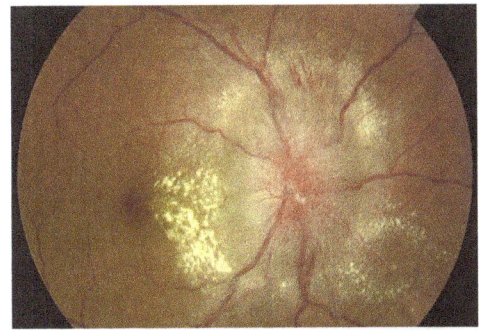

FIGURE S3.15 Severe hypertensive retinopathy with papilloedema.

Source: (Courtesy of Drs. Marta Crespo-Rodriguez and Miguel Acosta-Darias, Hospital Universitario de Canarias, Spain)

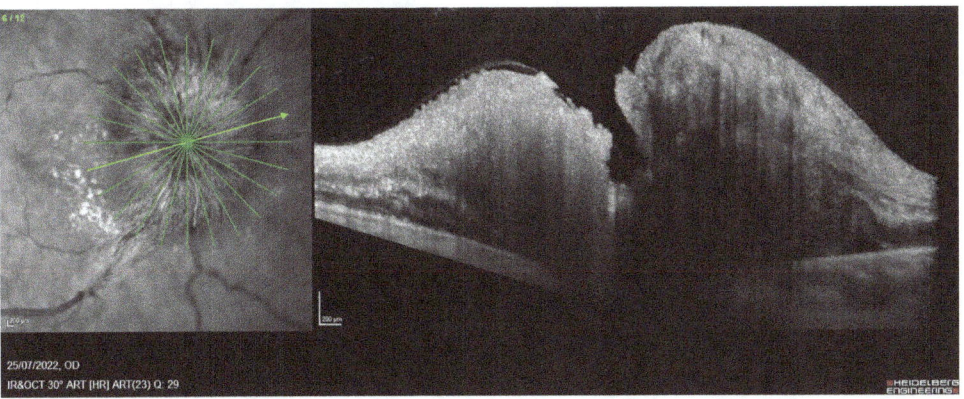

FIGURE S3.16 OCT of optic disc showing swelling due to increased arterial pressure.

Source: (Courtesy of Drs. Marta Crespo-Rodriguez and Miguel Acosta-Darias, Hospital Universitario de Canarias, Spain)

PAPILLOEDEMA (FIGURES S3.17 AND S3.18)

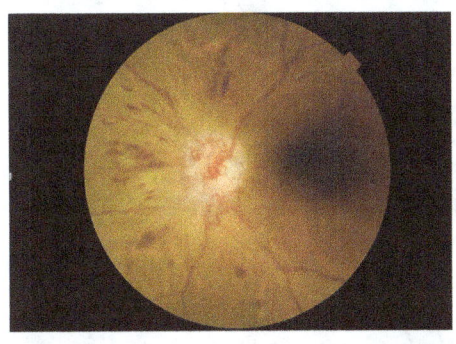

FIGURE S3.17 Papilloedema [L].

Source: (Courtesy of Dr. S. Basu, LV Prasad Eye Institute, Hyderabad, India)

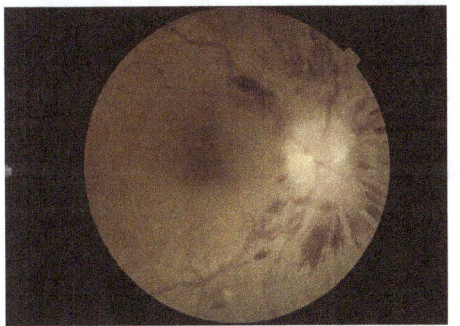

FIGURE S3.18 Papilloedema [R].

Source: (Courtesy of Dr. S. Basu, LV Prasad Eye Institute, Hyderabad, India)

OPTIC NEURITIS

The Swinging Flashlight Test (Figures S3.19–S3.22)

This is performed by shining a light in one eye (right) and observing the pupillary response; in section (A) earlier, the pupil of both eyes constricts demonstrating an intact afferent pathway. The light is then moved to the other (left) eye; both eyes remain dilated because the afferent pathway of the *left* eye is non-functioning (viz. optic neuritis) [1].

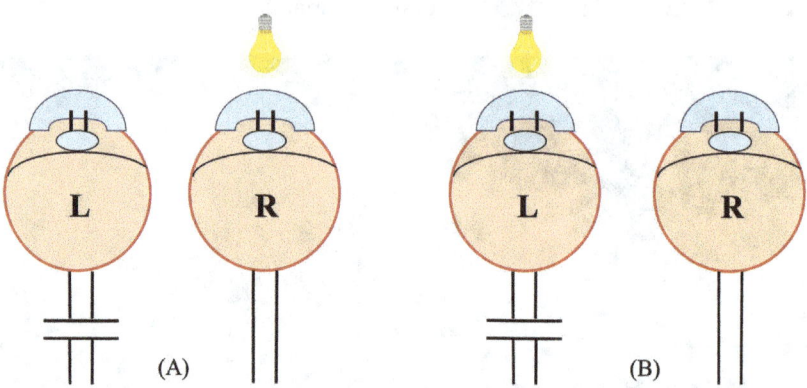

The Swinging Light Test for a RAPD (Relative Afferent Pupillary Defect).

FIGURE S3.19 Swinging flashlight test for a RAPD.

Source: (Courtesy of Mr. J.Z. Ong, RUMC, Penang, Malaysia)

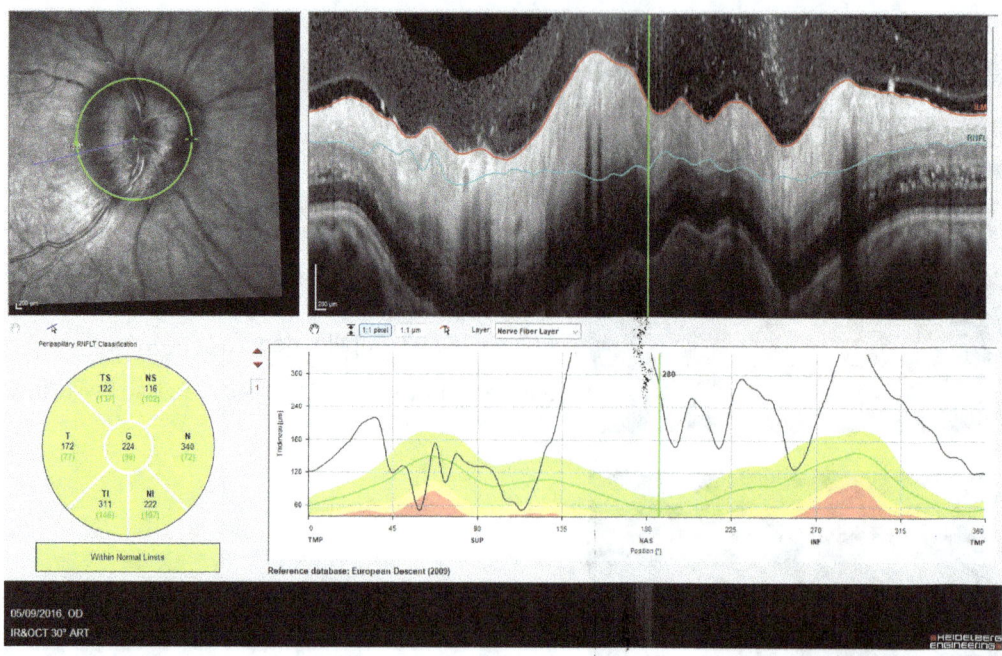

FIGURE S3.20 OCT image of early stage of optic neuritis shows swelling of disc (papillitis).

Source: (Courtesy of Drs. Marta Crespo-Rodriguez and Miguel Acosta-Darias, Hospital Universitario de Canarias, Spain)

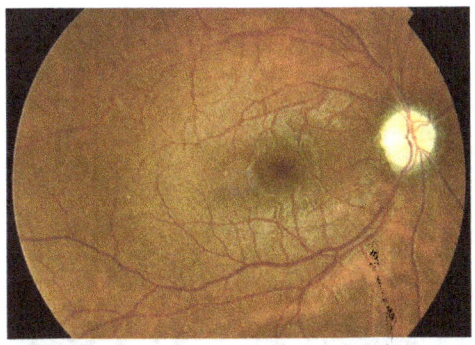

FIGURE S3.21 Final stage of optic neuritis shows complete atrophy of disc.

Source: (Courtesy of Drs. Marta Crespo-Rodriguez and Miguel Acosta-Darias, Hospital Universitario de Canarias, Spain)

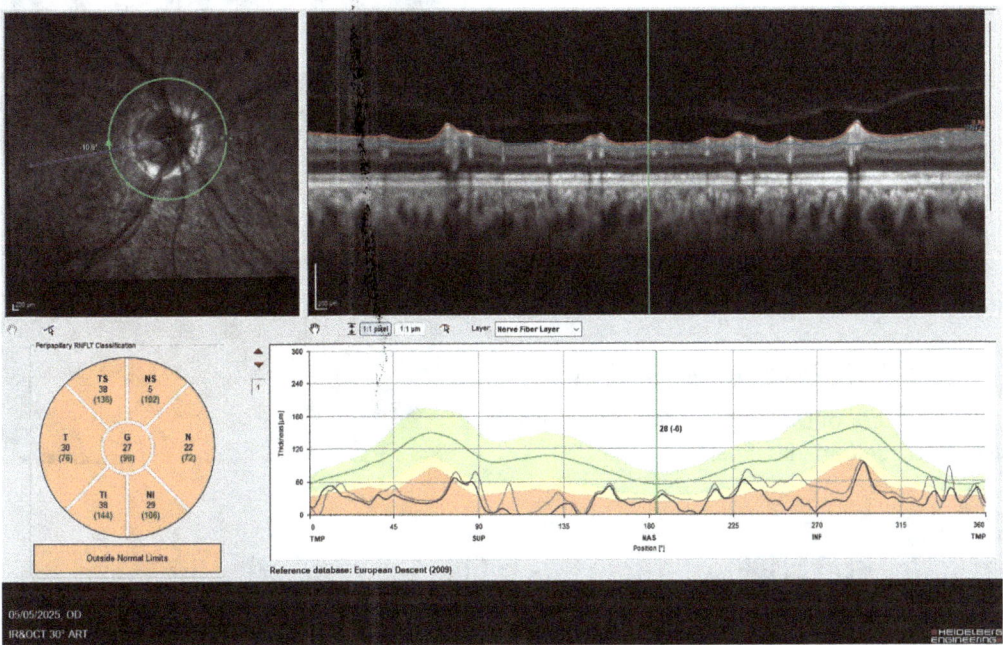

FIGURE S3.22 OCT of final stage of optic neuritis shows complete atrophy of disc.

Source: (Courtesy of Drs. Marta Crespo-Rodriguez and Miguel Acosta-Darias, Hospital Universitario de Canarias, Spain)

FLOATERS (FIGURE S3.23)

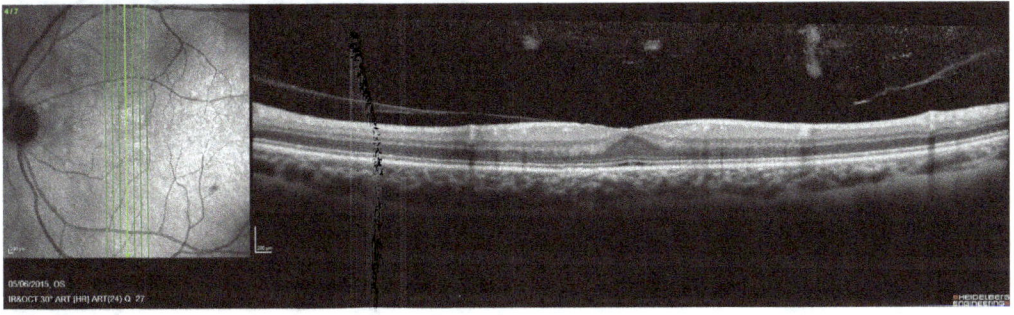

FIGURE S3.23 OCT of floaters with a normal macula.

Source: (Courtesy of Dr. Fatima Mesa-Lugo, Hospital Universitario de Canarias, Spain)

VEIN OCCLUSIONS (FIGURES S3.24 AND S3.25)

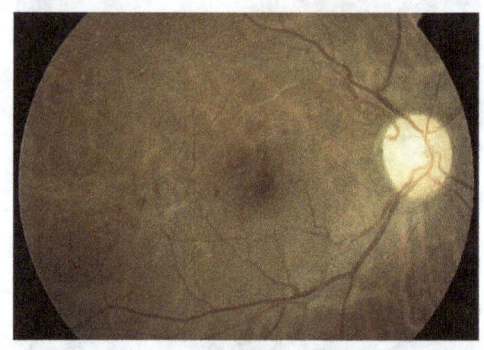

FIGURE S3.24 Branch retinal vein occlusion.

Source: (Courtesy of Dr. Fatima Mesa-Lugo, Hospital Universitario de Canarias, Spain)

FIGURE S3.25 Central retinal vein occlusion.

Source: (Courtesy of Dr. Fatima Mesa-Lugo, Hospital Universitario de Canarias, Spain)

MYELINATED NERVE FIBRES IN THE RETINA (FIGURES S3.26–S3.28)

Myelinated retinal nerve fibres (MRNF) are congenital anomalies that appear as grey-white opaque lesions on the retina with feathery edges that obscure details. These fibres are typically present at birth and are static lesions, occurring in about 1% of the population.

They may be located on the disc or elsewhere on the retina. MRNF can be associated with ocular findings, such as strabismus, high myopia and amblyopia.

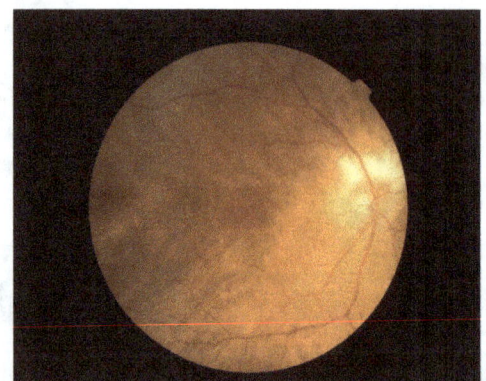

FIGURE S3.26 Myelinated nerve fibres.

Source: (Courtesy of Dr. Fatima Mesa-Lugo, Hospital Universitario de Canarias, Spain)

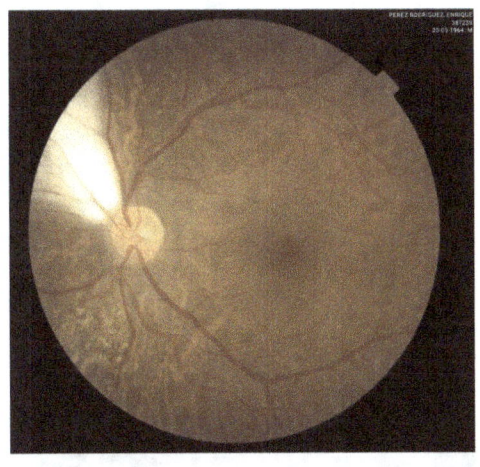

FIGURE S3.27 Myelinated nerve fibres.

Source: (Courtesy of Dr. Fatima Mesa-Lugo, Hospital Universitario de Canarias, Spain)

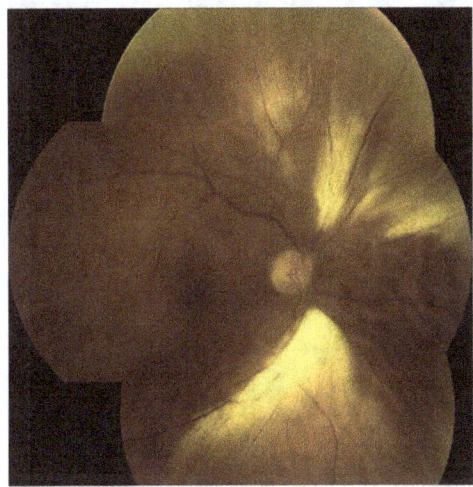

FIGURE S3.28 Optomap of myelinated nerve fibres.

Source: (Courtesy of Dr. Fatima Mesa-Lugo, Hospital Universitario de Canarias, Spain)

OPTIC NERVE HEAD PIT (FIGURE S3.29)

An optic nerve head pit is a rare congenital anomaly of the optic disc. It is typically a small, grayish-white excavation in the inferotemporal quadrant and typically unilateral, though 15% of cases are bilateral. While often asymptomatic and discovered during routine eye examinations, they can be associated with visual field defects, such as an enlarged blind spot or paracentral scotoma.

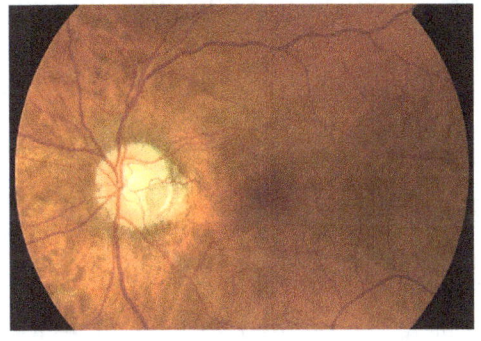

FIGURE S3.29 Optic nerve head pit.

Source: (Courtesy of Dr. Fatima Mesa-Lugo, Hospital Universitario de Canarias, Spain)

CHOROIDAL NAEVUS WITH DRUSEN (FIGURES S3.30 AND S3.31)

A choroidal naevus is a benign pigmented tumour in which drusen develop, indicating chronicity, since drusen take years to appear. It is an important differential diagnosis to a melanoma.

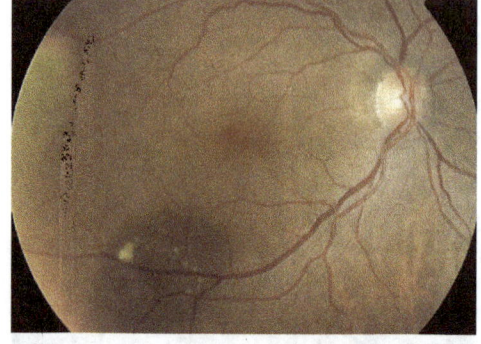

FIGURE S3.30 Choroidal naevus with drusen.

Source: (Courtesy of Dr. Fatima Mesa-Lugo, Hospital Universitario de Canarias, Spain)

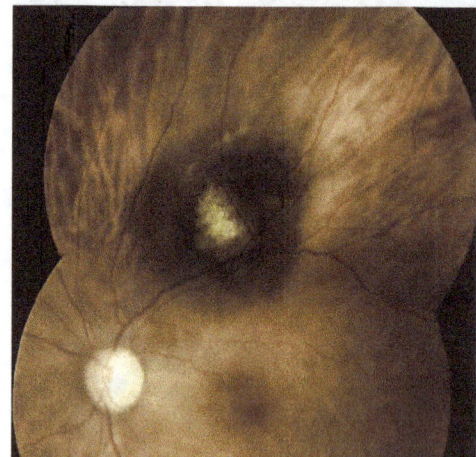

FIGURE S3.31 Choroidal naevus with drusen.

Source: (Courtesy of Dr. Fatima Mesa-Lugo, Hospital Universitario de Canarias, Spain)

NEURODEGENERATIVE CONDITIONS

The use of OCT for assessing changes in neuroinflammatory and neurodegenerative diseases, identified as imaging biomarkers, across the retina and optic nerve has allowed much greater understanding of the pathological processes as well as contributing to identifying early disease for better therapy [2]. In particular, it is possible to assess changes in the retinal nerve fibre layer, either thinning due to loss of ganglion and amacrine cells in the macula or optic disc areas, or an increase in the inner nuclear layer, reported as a sign of activation of Müller cells in patients with early diabetic retinopathy or multiple sclerosis.

Alzheimer's Disease (AD)

AD is associated with acquired cognitive decline with loss of past memory but retention of recent memory until that, too, is lost. This contrasts with age-related and vascular insufficiency (ischaemic) dementia when short-term memory is lost initially with retention of past memory. AD is now responsible for 60 to 80% of dementia cases. Refer to the following UK College of Optometrists Guidelines for conducting eye examinations in patients with dementia:

(https://www.college-optometrists.org/clinical-guidance/supplementary-guidance/dementia-and-the-eye-examination)

AD is characterised by the accumulation of extracellular amyloid-beta plaques and intracellular tau within the brain with a reduction in size of the cerebral cortex and expansion in size of the sinuses. These proteins cause inflammation with synaptic and neuronal loss that results in cerebral atrophy. Smaller amyloid-beta plaques are also found in the retina in the superior and inferior quadrants.

AD has three phases—a preclinical period that can extend to ten years or more, cognitive impairment and dementia. Biomarkers for the preclinical period include magnetic resonance imaging and cerebrospinal fluid analysis. OCT imaging has confirmed a reduction in the nerve fibre layer and ganglion cell number within the optic nerve. A UK study has shown that a thinner retinal nerve fibre layer is associated with lower cognitive test scoring, while a Dutch study has shown that it can be used as a biomarker of impending early dementia [2].

Parkinson's Disease (PD)

PD presents clinically with motor symptoms of tremor, bradykinesia, rigidity and dystonia, which are unilateral at onset but become bilateral later. Tremor occurs in about 70% of patients and is the most common initial symptom often described as shakiness or nervousness, usually beginning in one upper extremity. Non-motor symptoms include depression, anxiety, fatigue, constipation and sleep disorders.

Parkinson's disease is a progressive neurodegenerative disorder of the central nervous system. It is associated with depletion of dopaminergic neurons in the substantia nigra of the midbrain. A sub-population of amacrine cells in the retina are dopamine-releasing neurons, and a reduced concentration of retinal dopamine is found. Loss of the amacrine cells leads to thinning of the retinal ganglion cells. There is marked neuronal loss in the inferior disc quadrant with relative sparing of the nasal sector, similar to findings with primary open angle glaucoma (POAG); in addition, there is an increased incidence of PD in patients with POAG (16% versus 7% in controls) [2].

OCT shows a reduction in thickness of the nerve fibre layer, which can be measured. Early identification allows the start of medical and surgical therapy where possible. These patients should be referred for hospital care.

Schizophrenia

Schizophrenia is a progressive neurocognitive disorder also associated with a reduction in volume of the brain. OCT imaging of the retina shows significant thinning of the peripapillary nerve fibre layer and macular thinning and volume, compared to controls, with features correlating with duration of the disease [2].

Prions

Prions are known to exist in the cornea, causing a 'silent' infection in patients who later progress to Creutzfeldt-Jakob disease (CJD). The first recognised case of iatrogenic CJD occurred in 1974 in a 55-year-old woman given a corneal transplant 18 months earlier from a donor who had died unknowingly from the disease; the speed of transmission is notable. Homogenates from the brain of the deceased recipient were shown to transmit spongiform encephalopathy to chimpanzees. However, there is no test available for corneal or systemic infection by prions.

AGE-RELATED ISSUES

Cataract

The lens is derived from embryonic ectoderm and continues to grow throughout life, with new fibres being produced from the anterior epithelial stem cells after birth. The lens accommodative power decreases with age, while nuclear sclerosis increases the refractive index, causing a myopic shift.

The development of lens changes begins with the breakdown of proteins, common in older individuals, creating a cataract that reduces light transmission to give blurry vision. Cataracts also develop due to other factors, such as diabetes, where hyperglycemia causes changes in the refractive index of the lens, leading to formation of cortical fluid vacuoles and opacities. Additionally, trauma, chronic anterior uveitis and corticosteroid use can cause the development of secondary cataracts.

In early stages, a cataract may not significantly affect vision, but as it progresses, symptoms arise of glare, halos around lights, difficulty seeing at night and changes in refractive error. If these symptoms interfere with daily activities, cataract surgery is recommended to replace the opacified lens with an artificial monofocal or multifocal intraocular lens.

Varifocal or Bifocal Spectacles

These potentially attract a certain danger for the wearer, when climbing or descending steps, by blurring the inferior field of vision, resulting in slipping and falling. Older adults with health conditions that affect balance are particularly at risk. A typical injury is a trimalleolar fracture of the ankle climbing upstairs, or a transverse fracture falling downstairs, all due to loss of focus. Vulnerable individuals should be advised about this problem before fitting.

REFERENCES

1. Broadway GC. Comm Eye Health J 2012. PMID: 40151368 (https://pmc.ncbi.nlm.nih.gov/articles/PMC3588138/).
2. Vujosevic S et al. Eye 2023. PMID: 37944588 (https://doi.org/10.1038/s41433-022-02056-9).

S4: Application of Tear Osmolarity for a DED Grading Scheme and Conjunctival Scarring Disorders

Grading for dry eyes is given in Table 4.1.

TABLE S4.1 Grading for Dry Eyes

Severity Level	1	2	3	4
TYPE	Marginally Dry Eye	Questionably Dry Eye*	Dry Eye (sicca)	Keratoconjunctivitis sicca
SYMPTOMS				
Discomfort and severity	Mild and/or episodic under environmental stress	Moderate episodic or chronic, stress or no stress	Frequent or constant without stress, can be severe	Disabling and constant causing stress
Visual symptoms	None or episodic with fatigue	Annoying and/or activity-limiting episodic	Annoying, chronic and/or constant, limiting activity	Constant and/or possibly disabling
SIGNS				
Conjunctival injection	None to mild	None to mild	+/−	+/++
Conjunctival staining	None to mild	Variable	Moderate to marked	Marked
Corneal staining (severity/location)	None to mild	Variable	Marked central	Severe punctate erosions
Corneal/tear film signs	None to mild	Mild debris, ↓meniscus	Filamentary keratitis, mucus clumping, tear debris	Filamentary keratitis, mucus clumping, tear debris, ulceration
Lid/meibomian glands	MGD variably present	MGD variably present	MGD frequent	Trichiasis, keratinisation, symblepharon
TESTS				
TFBUT (sec) Normal = > 20	Variable	≤ 10	≤ 5	Immediate
Osmolarity mOsms/L Normal = 296+/−10	> 308	315 +/− 10	> 316	336 +/−22
Schirmer score (mm/5 min) Normal = > 15–20	Variable	≤ 10	≤ 5	≤ 2

Adapted from Shenton & Phewani 2014 (https://www.staffsloc.co.uk/uploads/lubricating-eye-drops.pdf).

* The Questionably Dry Eye (QDE) occurs in postmenopausal women. The primary cause is reduced function of the lacrimal gland, thought to be hormonal, which can be assessed by measuring the tear fluid lysozyme concentration when low levels are found [1,2]; lactoferrin concentrations can also be assayed to show dysfunction. There is aqueous deficiency and hyperosmolarity within the reduced tear film [2]. Patients complain of chronic discomfort, pain and dryness. Folliculitis is not found.

171

DOI: 10.1201/9781003606789-16

Patients with the QDE syndrome were followed up for eight years when they were *not* found to progress from a grade 2 to a grade 3 severity level. This finding distinguishes this patient group from those with Sjogren's disease (syndrome) (severity level 3 progressing to 4) who have an autoimmune aetiology. They can also be considered as aqueous-deficient dry eye (ADDE) syndrome (https://www. college-optometrists.org/clinical-guidance/clinical-management-guidelines/ dryeye_keratoconjunctivitissicca_kcs).

For DED caused by practolol toxicity, refer to *Section (D)*.

CONJUNCTIVAL SCARRING DISORDERS

Non-infectious conjunctival scarring disorders include a range of conditions that lead to fibrosis and damage to the conjunctiva.

a) *Ocular mucosal pemphigoid* is a rare, chronically progressive autoimmune disease characterised by recurrent inflammation and progressive fibrosis of the conjunctiva, which can lead to severe morphological and functional damage
b) *Stevens–Johnson syndrome* is a severe skin and mucous membrane reaction, often triggered by medications or infections, that can cause conjunctival scarring and ocular complications
c) *Rosacea*
d) *Practolol toxicity (drug withdrawn from market in 1975)*

All these disorders require early diagnosis and appropriate immune-modulatory therapy to prevent serious complications and preserve vision.

A) OCULAR MUCOSAL PEMPHIGOID

Ocular mucosal pemphigoid is a rare, chronically progressive autoimmune disease of the ocular surface. It belongs to a group of diseases whose common clinical correlate is the disruption of cohesion at the basement membrane. Recurrent inflammation with progressive fibrosis of the conjunctiva and damage to limbal stem cells are characteristic. If the course remains uncontrolled, severe morphological and functional damage can occur leading to blindness. Therefore, the *critical perception of initial subtle findings and early diagnosis are of great importance*. The aim of immunomodulatory therapy is to control the underlying inflammation and prevent the progression of fibrosis to avoid serious complications.

Clinical Details

Ocular mucous membrane pemphigoid (OMMP) predominantly affects both eyes. However, it can present itself asymmetrically, especially initially. *The suspicion of early manifestation is due to chronic recurrent conjunctivitis, which is also accompanied by a pronounced dry eye.* Since blepharitis with meibomian gland dysfunction is also present in both clinical pictures, this is often misinterpreted initially. Therefore, further clinical indications must be recorded. This applies to findings such as fibrotic changes in the plica region and nasal fornix.

The eyelids and conjunctiva should always be examined in order to detect symblephara and fornix shortening in the inferior and superior fornix at an early stage (Figures S4.1–S4.3). These findings are also the basis of the currently accepted staging classification (Table S4.2). Corneal epithelial defects can occur as early as stage I–II due to affection of the limbal corneal stem cells. Development of symblepharon is shown in Figure S4.4 (Stage III).

Pathogenesis and Diagnosis

Initially, the suspected diagnosis is made clinically. Pathogenesis is based on observations of immunopathological changes in the conjunctiva, the hallmark being binding of immunoglobulins and proteins of the complement system to the basement membrane of the mucosa. Since these patients have involvement of other mucosae in 50% of cases, other organ sites should be investigated [3].

The following tests are recommended for basic diagnosis.

1. Direct immunofluorescence from perilesional (mucous) skin for IgG, IgA, IgM and/or C3 at the basement membrane zone in direct IF and/or mucosal biopsy
2. Indirect immunofluorescence on human split skin
3. Serological examinations to identify the autoantigen, including ELISA and immunoblotting
4. Histology from mucous membrane lesions and clinical exclusion of differential diagnoses

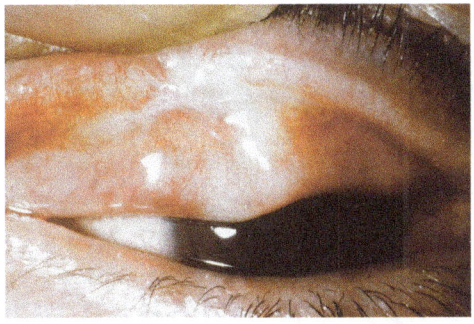

FIGURE S4.1 Ocular mucous membrane pemphigoid (Stage I).

Source: (Courtesy of Dr. D. Seal, London)

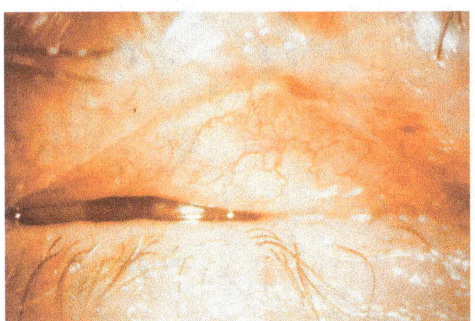

FIGURE S4.2 Mild conjunctival scarring due to pemphigoid (Stage I).

Source: (Courtesy of Dr. D. Seal, London)

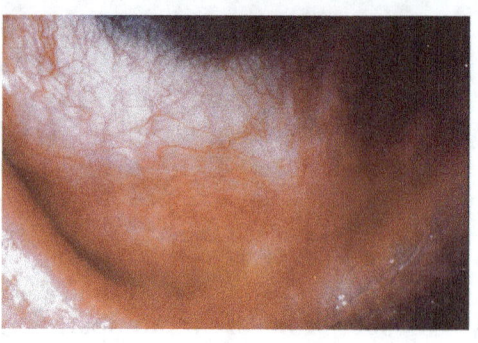

FIGURE S4.3 Conjunctival scarring due to ocular mucous membrane pemphigoid (Stage II).

Source: (Courtesy of Prof. U. Pleyer, Charité Hospital, Berlin, Germany)

TABLE S4.2 Classification of Ocular Mucous Membrane Pemphigoid into Four Stages

Stage	Clinical Signs	Loss of Fornix Depth (%)
I	Chronic conjunctivitis with subepithelial fibrosis	0–25%
II	Reduction of the inferior fornix	25–50%
III	Development of symblepharon	50–75%
IV	Ankyloblepharon and keratinisation of the ocular surface	75–100%

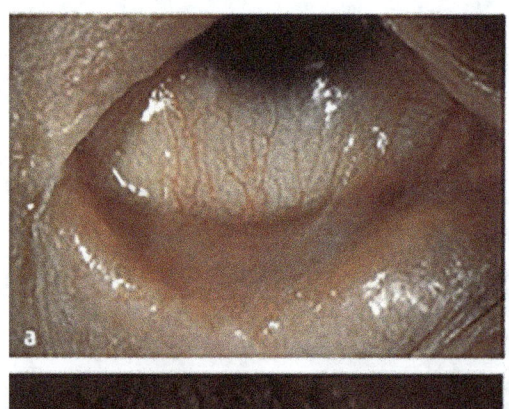
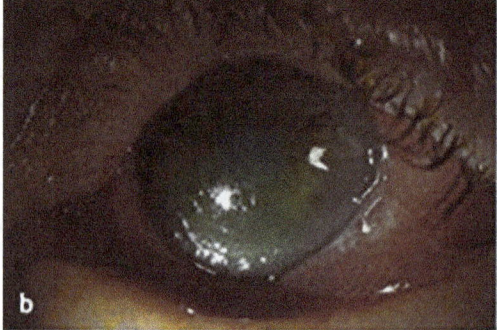
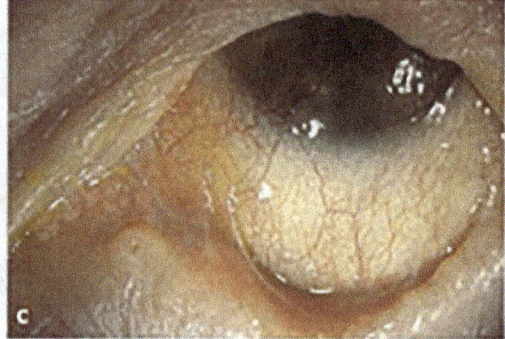

FIGURE S4.4 Severe conjunctival scarring due to ocular mucous membrane pemphigoid (Stage III).

Source: (Courtesy of Prof. U. Pleyer, Charité Hospital, Berlin, Germany)

TABLE S4.3 Extraocular Manifestations of Ocular Mucous Membrane Pemphigoid

Organ	Clinical Findings	Frequency (%)
Mouth	Desquamative gingivitis: erythematous plaques and maculae, blisters, erosions and erosions covered by pseudomembranes	> 85 %
Skin	Generalised involvement with recurrent, vesiculobullous, slightly scarring erosions	25–30%
	Localised involvement: erythematous plaques with recurrent vesicles, blisters on the scalp and face, healing with scarring	
Nose	Epistaxis, ulcerations, hoarseness, loss of voice	20–40%
Larynx	Sore throat, hoarseness, oedema, scarring	10–15%
Oesophagus	Ulcers, stricture, stenosis, dysphagia	10–15%
Anogenital	Skin lesions and spasms	10–20%

Key Points

1. Ocular mucous membrane pemphigoid (OMMP) is a rare autoimmune disease that is often problematic and needs to be treated systemically.
2. The care of these patients requires interdisciplinary cooperation.
3. Early clinical signs of ocular OMMP may present as fibrosis in the area of the nasal fornix and the semilunar plica (Table S4.3).
4. In the event of clinical suspicion, patients should be referred to a specialised centre for immuno-diagnostics and treatment at an early stage.
5. The diagnostic procedure should be based on the current guidelines, which includes several specific immunological procedures.
6. Even in the case of negative findings of immuno-diagnostics, adequate treatment measures must be initiated and clinically monitored.
7. The therapy of ocular OMMP is primarily based on systemically applied immunomodulatory substances that can be escalated/de-escalated in a step-by-step approach.
8. Adjuvant treatment measures must be given for disorders on the surface of the eye (keratoconjunctivitis sicca, trichiasis, possible infection and the need for frequent lubrication).

B) STEVENS–JOHNSON SYNDROME

Stevens–Johnson syndrome (SJS) is a rare condition that severely affects the skin and mucous membranes. It is mainly induced by drugs, less frequently by infections. SJS often presents with flu-like symptoms, painful red or purplish rash that spreads and blisters and mucosal involvement in the eyes, mouth and genitals. Depending on the extent of skin involvement, this is a life-threatening condition that requires intensive medical care.

In approximately 50% of these patients, ocular complications occur, which can lead to blindness without immediate ophthalmological treatment. The acute pattern, the unpredictable course and extreme variation in the manifestation of complications require an interdisciplinary treatment. *Early diagnosis and initiation of intensive lubrication and anti-inflammatory surface care are of utmost*

importance (https://www.aao.org/eyenet/article/management-of-stevensjohnson-syndrome-toxic-epider-2). Surgical reconstruction (amniotic membrane) is recommended in cases with recurrent non-healing.

Clinical Features

Due to the rarity of SJS, the initial phase of the reaction is not immediately recognised. The symptoms are like a banal infection, e.g. with sore throat, difficulty swallowing, fatigue, fever, redness, burning and watering of the eyes (Table S4.3). Clinical changes can range from unproblematic conjunctival hyperaemia to detachment of the surface epithelia of the conjunctiva and cornea. Acute, often purulent conjunctivitis exists in most patients and can precede the general symptoms (skin changes).

Timely ophthalmological inspection (within 48 hours) ensures a correct assessment of the severity and initiation of treatment in the sensitive initial phase of ocular involvement. Also, close follow-up is needed to prevent chronic consequences and to reduce ocular morbidity. The examination for corneal conjunctival defects is carried out with fluorescein dye staining with special attention to the eyelid margins. The conjunctiva, including fornix and tarsal portions, is examined for the development of epithelial defects and membranes (this always requires opening the eyelids). The precise documentation of all defects ensures the correct classification and initiation of therapy; use of a diagnostic/therapeutic algorithm is essential [4].

C) ROSACEA

Refer to Chapter 4 for full discussion (Figures S4.5 and S4.6).

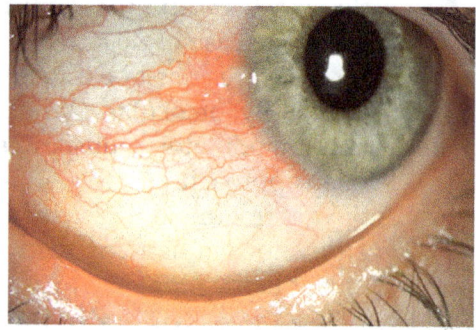

FIGURE S4.5 Rosacea blepharophyma with phlycten.

Source: (Courtesy of Dr. D. Seal, London)

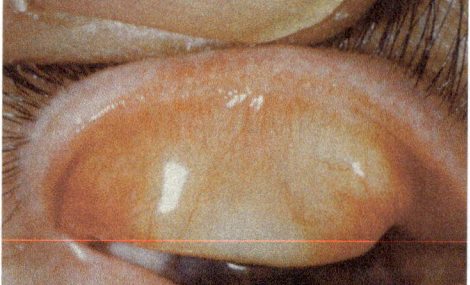

FIGURE S4.6 Rosacea disease showing upper lid thickening (scarring) in the absence of lid margin telangiectasia.

Source: (Courtesy of Dr. D. Seal, London)

D) PRACTOLOL TOXICITY

Drug-Induced Sclerosis of Mucosal Membranes and the Lacrimal Gland

Initially, patients presented with symptoms and signs of a dry eye (Chapter 4), which progressively worsened over six months from severity level 1 to levels 3 or 4 (Table S4.1, Figures S4.7 and S4.8) [5]; the mucosa of the mouth could also be involved. The external eye suffered from both aqueous deficiency and conjunctival sclerosis. In addition, there were symptoms and signs of sclerosis in other mucosal membranes, involving, in particular, the pleura and peritoneum, causing severe pain.

Historically, the lysozyme (or lactoferrin) test was used to assess the toxic effect of drugs on the lacrimal gland, viz. practolol [5]. This cardio-selective beta-blocking drug caused sclerosis of most mucosal membranes, as well as reducing lacrimal gland function; the tear lysozyme test was used to predict worsening drug effects, which were reversible in the early stage. In addition, patients with practolol 'toxicity' also developed antibodies to the intercellular cement substance (ICSA), found in the intercellular spaces between epithelial cells. This is similar to patients with pemphigus, demonstrating an autoimmune component to the adverse reaction.

Ocular symptoms and signs improved on withdrawal of the drug, but a reduction of tear secretion and tear lysozyme concentration persisted in most patients. The toxicity profile of practolol led to its withdrawal from the market in 1975.

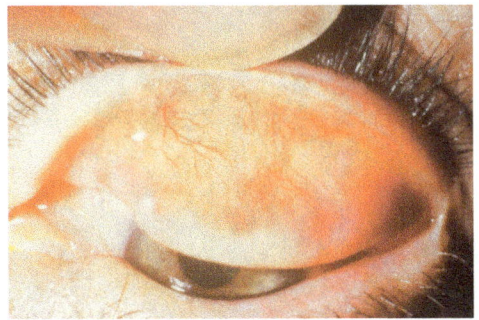

FIGURE S4.7 Conjunctival sclerosis from practolol toxicity (severity level 3).

Source: (Courtesy of Dr. D. Seal, London)

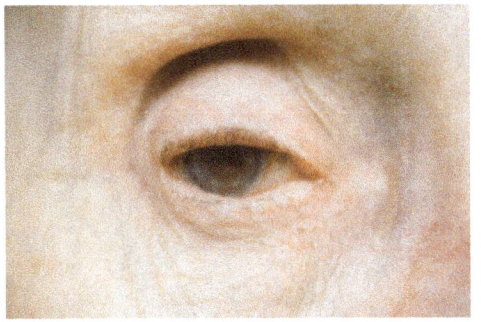

FIGURE S4.8 Dry eye (sicca, severity level 3) from practolol toxicity.

Source: (Courtesy of Dr. D. Seal, London)

REFERENCES

1. Mackie IA et al. Brit J Ophthalmol 1976. PMID: 1268164 (https://pmc.ncbi.nlm.nih.gov/articles/PMC1017470/).
2. Mackie IA et al. Brit J Ophthalmol 1981. PMID: 7448154 (https://pmc.ncbi.nlm.nih.gov/articles/PMC1039403/?page=8).
3. Hofman SC et al. J Dtsch Dermatol Ges 2022. PMID: 36383969 (http://doi.org/10.1111/ddg.14905).
4. Shanbhag SS et al. Am J Ophthalmol 2019. PMID: 31326519 (https://www.clinicalkey.com/#!/content/playContent/1-s2.0-S0002939419303290).
5. Mackie IA et al. Brit J Ophthalmol 1977. PMID: 17431 (https://pmc.ncbi.nlm.nih.gov/articles/PMC1042968/?page=6).

S5: Uveitis due to other causes

Syphilis, in its secondary stage, is a great mimic of other diseases that can present with retinochoroiditis and meningitis. Syphilitic neuroretinitis presents as papillitis, with peripapillary flame-shaped heamorrhages, periarteriolar sheathing and stellate macular exudates [1]. At this stage, there may be the characteristic macular-papular rash of secondary syphilis with "snail-track" mouth ulcers, or *the patient may be asymptomatic apart from a loss of visual acuity.*

Acute syphilitic posterior placoid chorioretinitis is an ocular manifestation of syphilis that has been characterised by spectral domain optical coherence tomography (SD OCT). In these cases, characteristic outer retinal abnormalities include disruption of the inner segment/outer segment band and nodular thickening of the RPE with loss of the linear outer segment/RPE junction. These findings may offer better prognostic evaluation since poor vision was seen in patients with disruption of outer retinal anatomy on SD OCT. Residual changes include optic atrophy. Necrotising retinitis may occur, associated with panuveitis and retinal vasculitis. Retinitis can become more extensive and bilateral in patients with AIDS.

Treatment for ocular syphilis should be similar to neurosyphilis. The patient requires high-dose intravenous penicillin G (3 MU, four-hourly with normal renal function), or high-dose intramuscular depository penicillin G with oral probenecid, given for two weeks. The patient's serology should be repeated to follow an expected reduction in titre of the nonspecific reagin test. If this reduction does not begin after six weeks, then the penicillin course must be repeated and the patient closely followed up in a specialist clinic. No reduction in titre is expected with the specific treponemal antigen serological tests.

Failure of the standard two-week course to treat the patient adequately is common when progression to the tertiary stage of neurosyphilis can occur. Together with the classical presentation of tabes dorsalis (shooting pains in the legs with a "shuffle" type of walking), this can present as pseudo-retinitis pigmentosa with a progressive decrease in visual acuity and nyctalopia (night blindness), when the rod cells in the retina gradually lose their ability to respond to light. Findings include a diffuse, granular appearance of the retinal pigment epithelium throughout both fundi with choroidal atrophy.

Systemic findings include Argyll-Robertson pupils (small, irregular and reactive to accommodation but not to light) and reduced or absent reflexes. Other AR-like pupils can occur in the setting of diabetes mellitus, neurosarcoidosis, chronic alcoholism, encephalitis, multiple sclerosis, Lyme disease and herpes zoster.

Patients may also present with abstruse signs of meningovascular disease, with cranial nerve palsies, or generalised vascular disease with peri- and endarteritis, while a gumma (syphilitic granuloma) can occur anywhere.

179

DOI: 10.1201/9781003606789-17

Congenital syphilitic chorioretinopathy persists for life with poor vision, narrowing of retinal vessels, optic disc pallor and peripheral pseudo-retinitis pigmentosa; iritis and interstitial neuritis may also be present.

BORRELIOSIS (LYME DISEASE)

Although ocular manifestations are a rare feature of this tick-borne disease, the spirochete (*Borrelia burgdorferi*) invades the eye early and may remain dormant, accounting for both early and late ocular manifestations. A nonspecific follicular conjunctivitis occurs in approximately 10% of patients with early Lyme disease, while keratitis occurs within a few months of onset and is characterised by nummular *interstitial* opacities. Inflammatory events include orbital myositis, episcleritis, uveitis, vitritis and retinal vasculitis.

Lyme disease presents as bilateral keratitis with indistinct infiltrates scattered throughout the corneal stroma. It resolves with corticosteroid treatment without sequelae, suggesting an immunopathological basis. Cogan-1 syndrome is an important differential diagnosis presenting with interstitial keratitis, hearing loss and other neurological symptoms. If not treated with immunomodulatory agents, permanent hearing loss will result.

In some cases, when serology is negative, a vitreous tap is required for diagnosis by PCR. Neuro-ophthalmic manifestations include bilateral mydriasis, neuroretinitis, pigmentary retinopathy, involvement of multiple cranial nerves, optic atrophy and disc oedema. Seventh cranial nerve paresis can lead to neuroparalytic keratitis. In endemic areas, Lyme disease may be responsible for approximately 25% of new-onset Bell's palsy.

The diagnosis can be difficult and is usually based on a history of exposure within an endemic area and positive serology. Erythema migrans has been considered an important clinical sign of Lyme disease, but it is present in only about 30% of patients.

Response to treatment has been considered as a diagnostic sign. Serology in Lyme disease is difficult, and the diagnosis should never be solely based on it. In contrast, there are patients described where the organism has been cultured from the eye in the presence of negative serology so that seronegativity cannot exclude vitritis due to borreliosis. PCR has been used successfully to confirm borreliosis within the vitreous and cerebrospinal fluid. Interestingly, the bladder has been identified as a reservoir of the organisms, and urine PCR has been found positive in patients with ocular borreliosis.

The use of oral beta-lactam antibacterials (phenoxymethylpenicillin [penicillin V], amoxicillin, cefuroxime axetil) and oral tetracyclines have been recommended as effective first-line treatment for between 10 to 21 days. Oral macrolides are considered second-line agents, as their clinical efficacy has been less effective.

TOXOCARIASIS

Toxocara canis and *T. catis* are worms whose natural hosts are the dog or cat. Humans are an accidental host, infected from ingesting the ova (Figure S5.1) from contaminated soil, in whom the larval stage develops, causing visceral and ocular "larva migrans," but adult worms are not found.

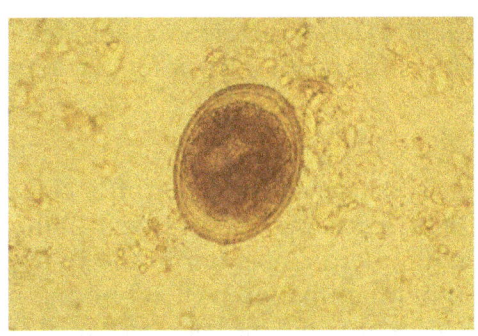

FIGURE S5.1 Egg of *Toxocara canis* from contaminated soil with dog faeces.

Source: (Courtesy of Dr. D. Seal, London)

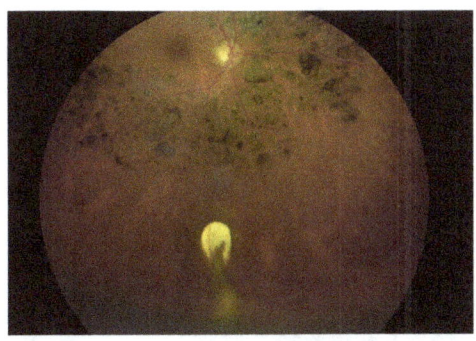

FIGURE S5.2 Retinochoroiditis due to *Toxocara canis* larva.

Source: (Courtesy of Dr. Fatima Mesa-Lugo, Hospital Universitario de Canarias, Spain)

The parasite is widespread, and in some tropical countries, seroconversion may be found in up to 90%, whereas in Europe, the infection level is between 3% and 30%. It has been reported as a cause for posterior uveitis in 3% to 18% of children.

These larvae migrate around the body and occasionally deposit themselves in the central nervous system, including the retina (as the second stage larva) (Figure S5.2). Here, they can present as a retinochoroiditis or as a granulomatous reaction resembling a possible tumour, for which eyes have been eviscerated in the past (https://www.ncbi.nlm.nih.gov/books/NBK576384/).

Clinical Presentation

Three major clinical presentations have been described:

1) Peripheral granuloma may occur bilaterally, presenting as "pars planitis." Secondary complications may result from traction at the posterior pole.
2) Posterior pole granuloma is a large white granuloma, often with traction bands to the mid-periphery of the retina, usually accompanied by some cellular vitreous infiltration.
3) Endophthalmitis: mainly unilateral presentation with all signs of panuveitis, including hypopyon and severe vitreous infiltration; retinal detachment can be a presenting sign.

Diagnosis

Serological diagnosis only confirms previous exposure and does not imply whether the retinal lesion is that of toxocariasis or not. Furthermore, *the serological*

test may be negative when a choroidal lesion is present, so it is unreliable and should not be used. Intraocular diagnosis is required with a fine needle biopsy for cytology and PCR for *Toxocara* DNA.

Treatment

If the retinal lesion is peripheral, treatment is conservative, but if it is close to the macula, treatment is warranted. Diethylcarbamazine is given orally for three weeks at 3 mg/kg. There may be an allergic reaction to the dying larva, requiring prednisolone to suppress the inflammation. When blindness results, it is usually unilateral, but bilateral cases are known. Therapy can also be given with albendazole or with a single dose of ivermectin (Appendix 6).

TOXOPLASMOSIS

Refer to Chapter 5. For the latest information on management of the infection, refer to the new guidelines by the International Ocular Toxoplasmosis Study Group set up in 2020 [2].

NON-INFECTIOUS CAUSES OF POSTERIOR UVEITIS

Acute Posterior Multifocal Placoid Pigment Epitheliopathy (APMPPE)

APMPPE presents with a short history of progressive blurring of vision. There are multiple, discrete, cream-coloured lesions with ill-defined margins deep within the macular area and retina in the posterior pole. Mild to severe vision loss occurs early (especially if it involves the optic nerve with later scarring) *but is normally transient.* It is usually, but not always, bilateral and self-limiting. The lesions leave some pigmentation, but visual acuity improves even without treatment, provided the optic nerve is spared.

APMPPE occurs between ages 16 to 40 with a mean of 27 years. It usually occurs during a systemic infection, such as tuberculosis (Figures S5.3 & S5.4) (reflecting current experience), brucellosis or late-stage syphilis [1] but can be associated with other disorders, including Lyme disease. It is considered an immune reaction in the choroid rather than direct invasion by the microbe. When due to tuberculosis (Figures S5.3 and S5.4), it may be synonymous with multifocal choroiditis. APMPPE may occur with a closed tuberculous pulmonary lesion as opposed to miliary tuberculosis (TB) disease; refer to Appendix 5 for TB testing.

Refer for investigation and specific therapy, including anti-tuberculous antibiotics and corticosteroids. Recurrence of APMPPE is unusual.

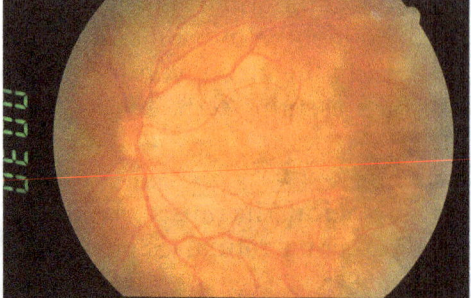

FIGURE S5.3 Ampiginous choroiditis (APMPPE) due to tuberculosis. Pre-treatment.

Source: (Seal & Pleyer, Ocular Infection, 2007)

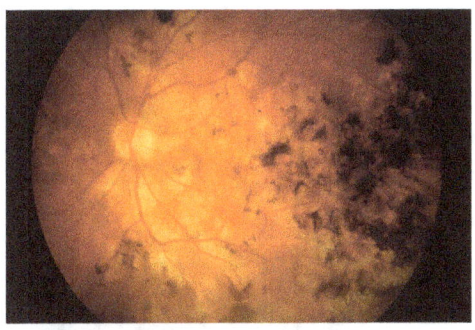

FIGURE S5.4 Ampiginous choroiditis (APMPPE) due to tuberculosis. Post-treatment showing considerable scarring within the retina.

Source: (Seal & Pleyer, Ocular Infection, 2007)

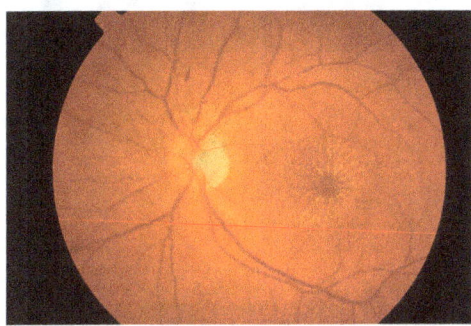

FIGURE S5.5 Leber's idiopathic stellate neuroretinitis.

Source: (Seal & Pleyer, Ocular Infection, 2007)

Leber's Idiopathic Stellate Neuroretinitis

This condition presents with *sudden loss of vision following a viral-type illness*, such as hepatitis A, cat-scratch fever (Tey MS *et al*. The clinical spectrum of ocular bartonellosis: a retrospective study at a tertiary centre in Malaysia. J Ophthalmic Inflam 2020 PMID: 33191467) or leptospirosis, and occasionally after other systemic infections, including *Toxocara*. It may also occur in the early stage of asymptomatic neurosyphilis, and appropriate tests for syphilis should always be performed.

During the first week after onset of decreased visual acuity, the only finding is swelling of the optic disc, but one week later, a typical macular star (Figure S5.5) is present. This is not a maculopathy but is caused by vascular leakage from the optic nerve head with reabsorption of serum when lipid precipitates in a stellate pattern. The swelling of the optic disc may be mild, segmental or massive; it is not related to demyelinating disease. A differential diagnosis includes leakage from the parafoveal capillaries with diabetes mellitus and hypertension.

There is no specific therapy. The disc swelling begins to decrease after two weeks and resolves within ten weeks. The macular star begins to decrease after one month but requires up to one year for complete resolution. The prognosis for vision is good, but there are exceptions.

Multiple Evanescent White Dot Syndrome

Viral-induced chorioretinitis has been postulated as a cause for some of the transient white dot syndromes. *The patient has usually suffered a flu-like illness in the week before presentation.* A multifocal primary inflammatory choriocapillaritis is seen as multiple white dots in the paramacular area that can be documented by fluorescein angiography at the retinal pigment epithelial layer. The disease is usually unilateral in young adults who *present with a sudden loss of vision*, decreasing to between 20/20 (6/6) and 20/300 (6/90), sometimes with a temporal scotoma. There can be vitreal cells and a blurring of the disc margin. Symptomatic macular lesions have responded to oral corticosteroid therapy. Recovery to normal vision usually occurs after six weeks.

INTERSTITIAL KERATITIS (REFER TO CHAPTER 5) (SEE FIGURES S5.6 AND S5.7)

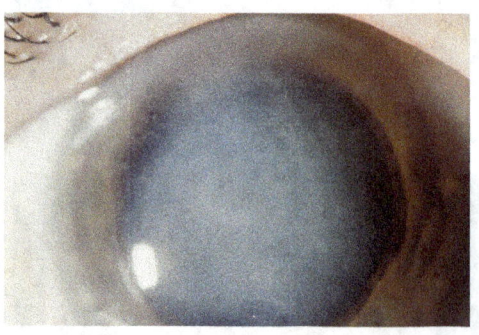

FIGURE S5.6 Interstitial keratitis due to congenital syphilis.

Source: (Seal & Pleyer, Ocular Infection, 2007)

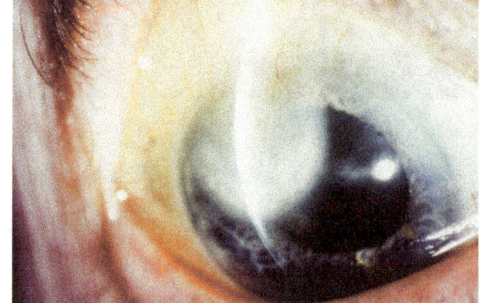

FIGURE S5.7 Interstitial keratitis of unknown cause with neovascularization.

Source: (Courtesy of Dr. D. Seal, London)

REFERENCES

1. Neri P et al. J Ophthalmic Inflamm Infect 2022. PMID: 35192047 (https://https://doi.org/10.1186/s12348-022-00286).
2. Yougeswaran K et al. Brit J Ophthalmol 2023. PMID: 35197262 (https://doi.org/10.1136/bjophthalmol-2022-321091).

S6: Infections

The following atopic patient (female, age 25) suffered *Staphylococcus aureus* folliculitis on her eyelids (Figure S6.1), with inflammatory conjunctivitis and limbitis (Figure S6.2). She showed type IV (delayed-type) hypersensitivity, due to cell-mediated immunity (Chapter 10), following intradermal challenge of *St. aureus* protein A, resulting in a 20 cm wide zone of induration after 48 hours (Figure S6.3), which subsided after 3 days [1]. Killed *St. aureus* cells also gave an indurated reaction, but smaller at 5 cm, while in a patient with seborrhoeic blepharitis (Figure S6.4), the reaction was negative (Figure S6.5).

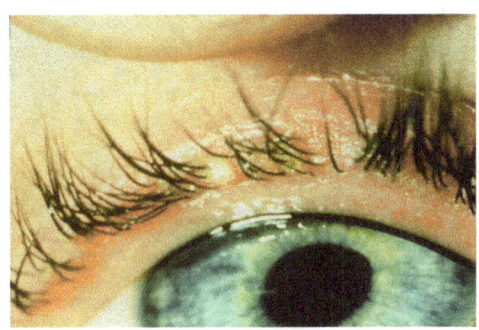

FIGURE S6.1 Folliculitis due to *St. aureus* (Gram-positive cocci) [patient Ch].

Source: (Courtesy of Dr. D. Seal, London)

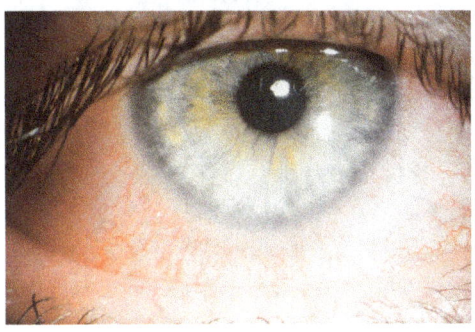

FIGURE S6.2 Inflammatory conjunctivitis and limbitis due to *St. aureus* on lids [patient Ch].

Source: (Courtesy of Dr. D. Seal, London)

DOI: 10.1201/9781003606789-18

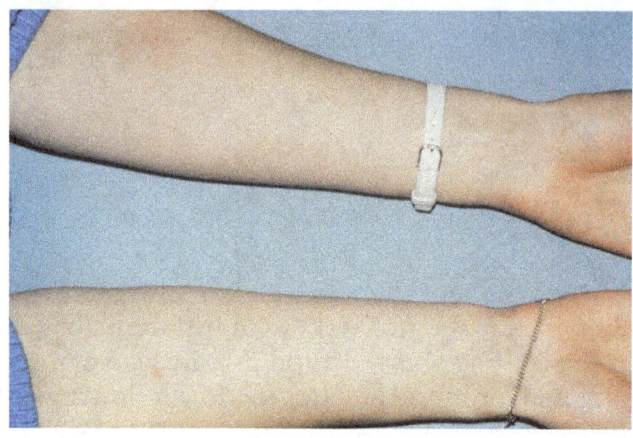

FIGURE S6.3 [L] arm—enhanced reaction to intradermal challenge of *St. aureus* protein A. [R] arm—enhanced reaction to intradermal challenge of *St. aureus* killed cells [L]; saline subcutaneous injection [central] and coagulase-negative staphylococcus [CNS] (*St. epidermidis*) killed cells [R] which gave a negative reaction [patient Ch].

Source: (Courtesy of Dr. D. Seal, London)

SEBORRHOEIC BLEPHARITIS (FIGURES S6.4 AND S6.5)

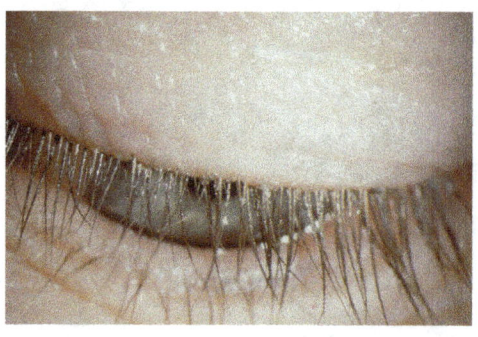

FIGURE S6.4 Seborrhoeic blepharitis [patient F].

Source: (Courtesy of Dr. D. Seal, London)

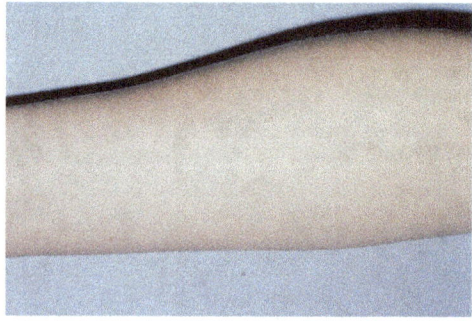

FIGURE S6.5 CNS killed cells [L], saline [central] and *St. aureus* killed cells [R] gave a *negative* intradermal reaction in seborrheic blepharitis [patient F].

Source: (Courtesy of Dr. D. Seal, London)

ERYSIPELAS DUE TO *STREPTOCOCCUS PYOGENES*

This infection (Figure S6.6) is due to intradermal penetration of *Streptococcus pyogenes*. It commonly affects the face but can occur at any site. Treatment is with systemic penicillin or cephalosporin, or a quinolone if not available, for two weeks; other therapy is palliative.

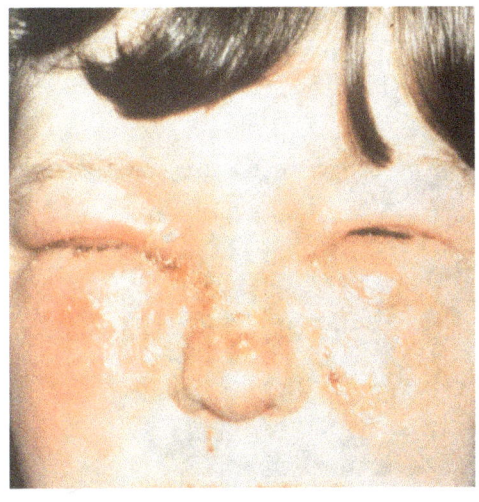

FIGURE S6.6 Erysipelas due to *Streptococcus pyogenes* (Gram-positive cocci).

Source: (Courtesy of Dr. D. Seal, London)

BACTERIAL KERATITIS (FIGURES S6.7–S6.9)

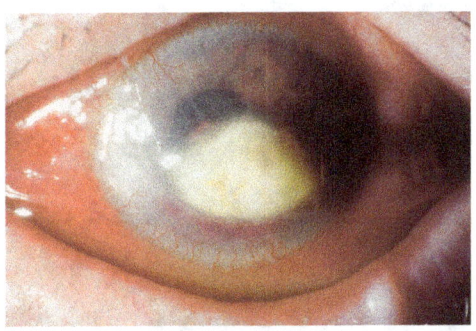

FIGURE S6.7 Exposure keratitis with secondary infection by *Moraxella sp.* (Gram-negative rods).

Source: (Seal & Pleyer, Ocular Infection, 2007)

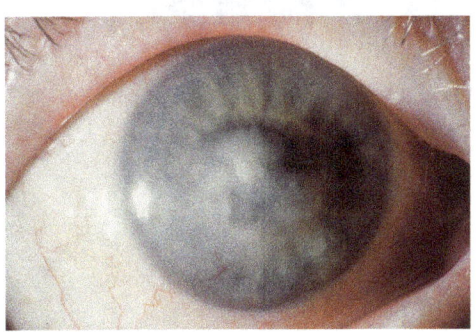

FIGURE S6.8 Keratitis due to *Acintobacter sp.* (Gram-negative rods) in lipid keratopathy on FML.

Source: (Seal & Pleyer, Ocular Infection, 2007)

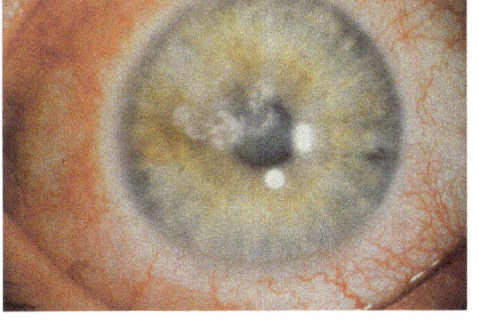

FIGURE S6.9 Keratitis due to *Nocardia sp.* (acid fast bacillus) in a patient with a delayed, unrecognised infection (Appendix 5).

Source: (Seal & Pleyer, Ocular Infection, 2007)

Acanthamoeba **Keratitis**

Early presentation of three contact lens wearers (CLWs) at two weeks; each complained of a sore, watering eye with photophobia (Figures S6.10–S6.12)

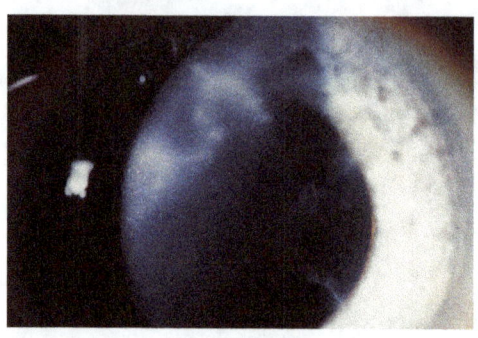

FIGURE S6.10 Typical keratoneuritis of *Acanthamoeba* infection.

Source: (Seal & Pleyer, Ocular Infection, 2007)

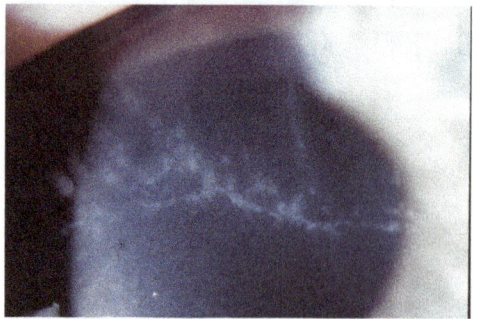

FIGURE S6.11 High power slit lamp view of *Acanthamoeba* pseudo-dendrite and corneal nerve above.

Source: (Seal & Pleyer, Ocular Infection, 2007)

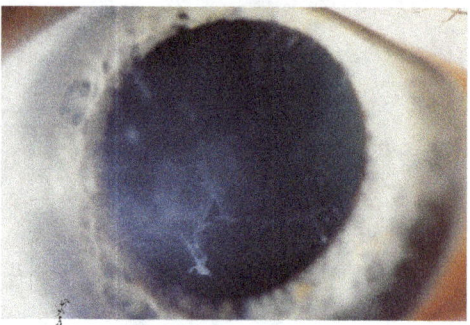

FIGURE S6.12 Epithelial oedema, early infiltration and radial keratoneuritis.

Source: (Seal & Pleyer, Ocular Infection, 2007)

Early presentation of a CLW at three weeks (Figure S6.13):

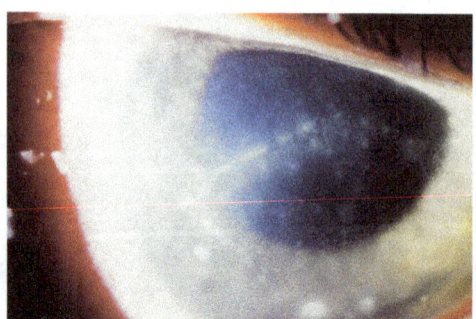

FIGURE S6.13 Typical keratoneuritis of *Acanthamoeba* infection and early ring abscess formation (high power view).

Source: (Seal & Pleyer, Ocular Infection, 2007)

Dual infection of *Acanthamoeba* and secondary microaerophilic streptococci (Figure S6.14):

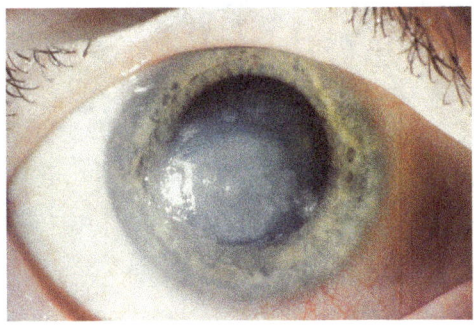

FIGURE S6.14 *Acanthamoeba* infection with secondary microaerophilic streptococcal infection causing a 'crystalline' keratopathy.

Source: (Seal & Pleyer, Ocular Infection, 2007)

Dual infection of *Acanthamoeba* and *Pseudomonas aeruginosa* in a tropical climate (refer to Chapter 7, see Figure S6.15):

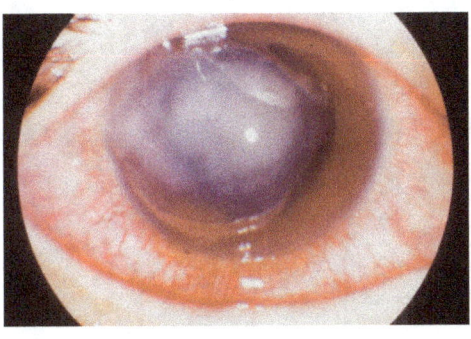

FIGURE S6.15 Combined *Acanthamoeba* and *Pseudomonas aeruginosa* infection in Malaysia.

Source: (Courtesy of Dr. D. Seal, London)

HERPETIC EYE DISEASE

Herpes Simplex

Herpes simplex infection of lid and face (Figure S6.16):

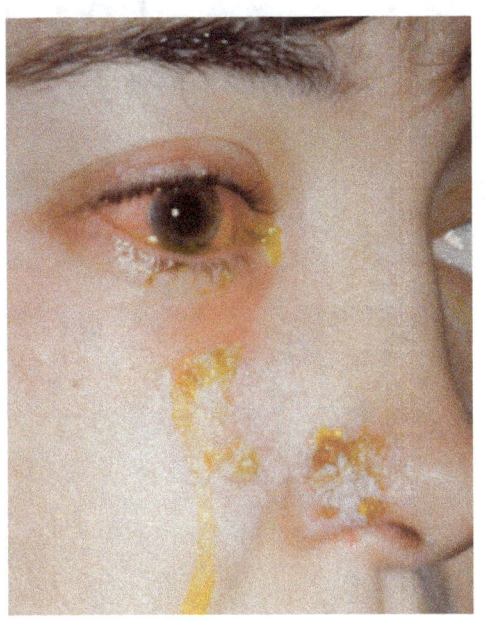

FIGURE S6.16 Herpes simplex infection of lid and face.

Source: (Courtesy of Dr. D. Seal, London)

Primary infection—dendritic ulcer (Figure S6.17):

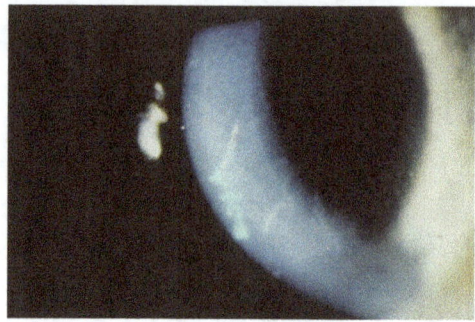

FIGURE S6.17 Dendritic ulcer due to herpes simplex (fluorescein stain and blue light).

Source: (Courtesy of Dr. D. Seal, London)

Stromal Herpetic Keratitis (Figure S6.18)

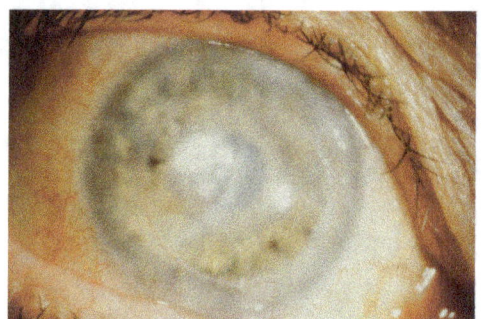

FIGURE S6.18 Stromal herpetic keratitis under a protective contact lens.

Source: (Courtesy of Dr. D. Seal, London)

Progressive Herpetic Disease (Figures S6.19–S6.24)

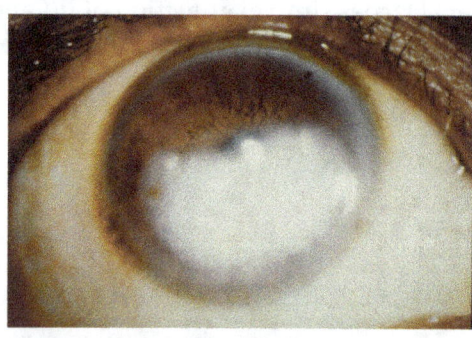

FIGURE S6.19 Herpes simplex keratopathy.

Source: (Courtesy of Dr. D. Seal, London)

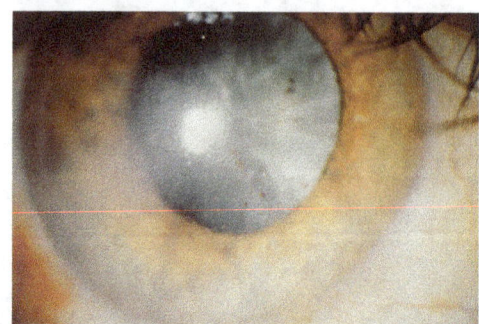

FIGURE S6.20 Recurrence of herpes simplex infection in a graft.

Source: (Courtesy of Dr. D. Seal, London)

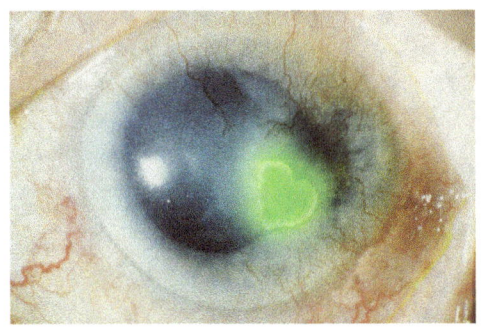

FIGURE S6.21 Herpetic keratitis and uveitis.

Source: (Seal & Pleyer, Ocular Infection, 2007)

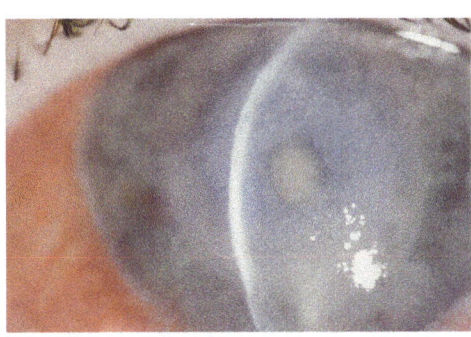

FIGURE S6.22 Herpetic keratitis with secondary *Staphylococcus aureus* infection.

Source: (Seal & Pleyer, Ocular Infection, 2007)

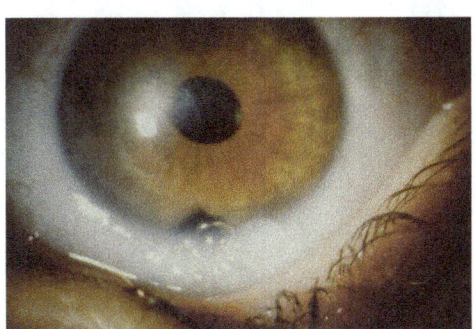

FIGURE S6.23 Herpes simplex infection with high ocular pressure managed with trabeculectomy.

Source: (Courtesy of Dr. D. Seal, London)

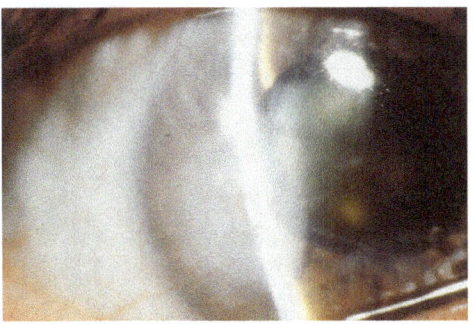

FIGURE S6.24 Herpetic eye perforated.

Source: (Courtesy of Dr. D. Seal, London)

Drug-Induced Epithelial Toxicity From F3T and Idoxuridine

Trifluorothymidine, also known as F3T, is a topical antiviral agent used in the treatment of herpes keratitis, effective for dendritic and geographic ulcers, but can cause epithelial toxicity (Figures S6.25 and S6.26).

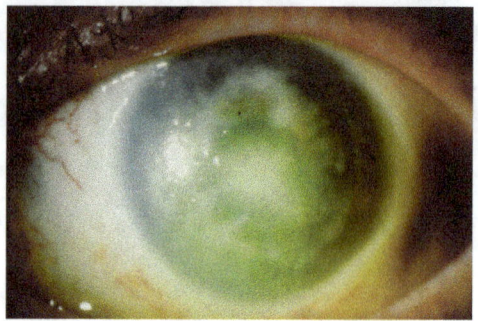

FIGURE S6.25 Corneal epithelial toxicity from F3T in a herpetic eye (lissamine green stain).

Source: (Courtesy of Dr. D. Seal, London)

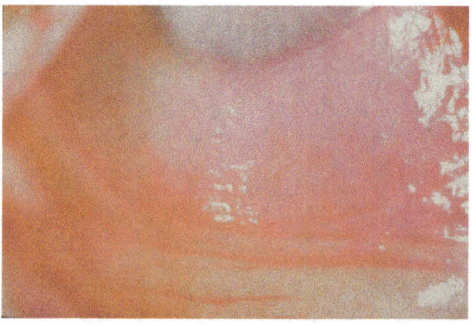

FIGURE S6.26 Conjunctival epithelial toxicity from idoxuridine (rose bengal) stain.

Source: (Courtesy of Dr. D. Seal, London)

REFERENCE

1. Ficker L et al. Role of Cell-Mediated Immunity to Staphylococci in Blepharitis. Am J Ophthalmol 1991. PMID: 2012150 (https://doi.org/10.1016/s0002-9394(14)72383-9).

S7: Tropical and Global Eye Conditions

Progressive corneal opacity due to trichiasis (Figures S7.1 and S7.2):

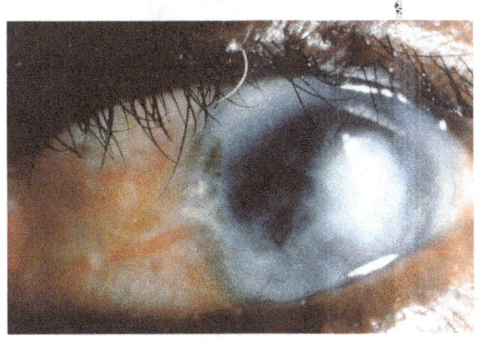

FIGURE S7.1 Corneal opacity—visible corneal opacity over the pupil that spreads to cause blindness.

Source: (Seal & Pleyer, Ocular Infection, 2007)

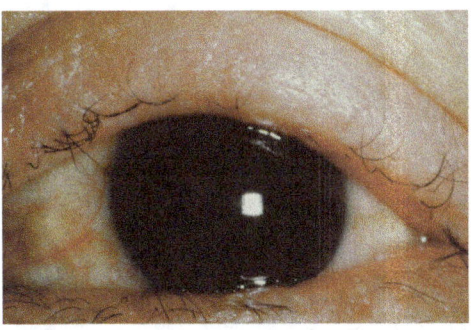

FIGURE S7.2 The typical 'scaphoid' lid of trachoma.

Source: (Courtesy of Dr. D. Seal, London)

TRIC—trachoma inclusion conjunctivitis (Figure S7.3)

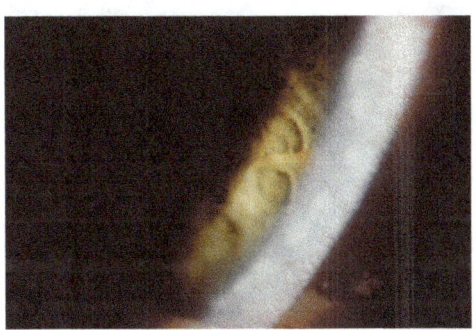

FIGURE S7.3 Marginal infiltrates at the limbus due to TRIC.

Source: (Courtesy of Dr. D. Seal, London)

193

DOI: 10.1201/9781003606789-19

This milder syndrome is covered in Chapter 6.

ONCHOCERCIASIS—LIFE CYCLE (FIGURE S7.4)

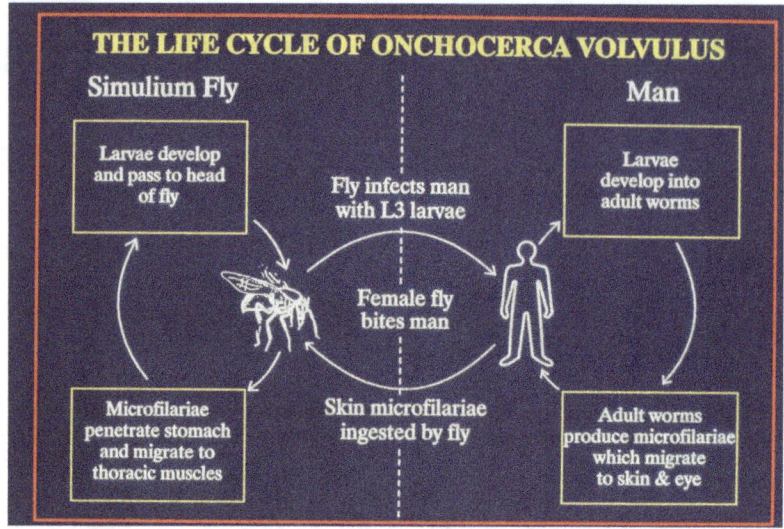

FIGURE S7.4 The life cycle of *Onchocerca volvulus*.

Source: (Seal & Pleyer, Ocular Infection, 2007)

FUNGAL KERATITIS (FIGURES S7.5 AND S7.6)

The corneal injury came from a 'cheese' plant (*Monstera deliciosa*) native to the tropical forests of southern Mexico.

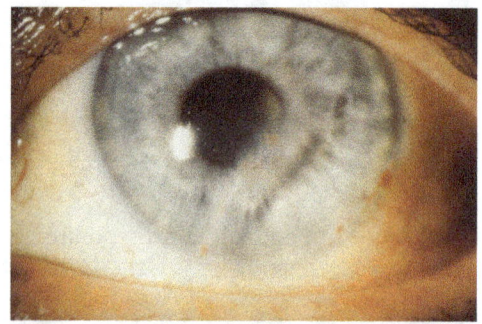

FIGURE S7.5 Cheese plant (*Monstera deliciosa*) injury causing fungal keratitis (dry infiltration with no hypopyon).

Source: (Courtesy of Dr. D. Seal, London)

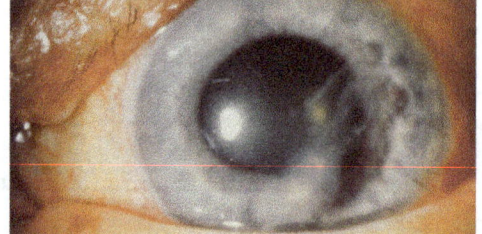

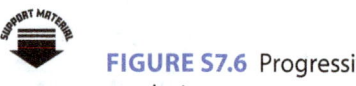
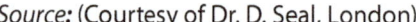

FIGURE S7.6 Progressive invasion of stroma before resolution.

Source: (Courtesy of Dr. D. Seal, London)

The keratitis became progressively worse but then resolved with antifungal antibiotics.

PREVENTION OF INFECTION IN CATARACT SURGERY AND MANAGEMENT OF SACCULAR ENDOPHTHALMITIS (REFER TO CHAPTER 7)

The global prevalence of cataract, as a cause of blindness, was published as a meta-analysis in 2024 [1]. In 2020, among all ages, 43.3 million were assessed to be blind from cataract, and 295 million suffered with moderate severe vision impairment (MSVI). The number of people with severe cataract has risen over the past 30 years, despite a decrease in the age-standardised prevalence of cataract, due to population growth and longer survival. This indicates that cataract treatment programs have been beneficial, but population growth and aging have outpaced their impact, requiring increased global capacity for cataract surgery.

Prophylaxis of Postoperative Endophthalmitis Following Cataract Surgery

The European Society of Cataract and Refractive Surgeons (ESCRS) set up a large prospective, randomised, double-blind, placebo-controlled study for use of *'intracameral (IC) cefuroxime antibiotic to prevent postoperative endophthalmitis following cataract surgery'* within nine European countries in 2002, that took five years to complete and involved 16,603 operations [2]. The prospective study confirmed previous retrospective studies with an infection rate of 0.05% (2/4,052, both due to coagulase-negative staphylococci) in those receiving IC cefuroxime (1 mg in 0.1 mL normal saline injected into the anterior chamber at the end of surgery) and of 0.35% (12/4,054) [nearly seven times higher] in those without IC cefuroxime; five out of the ten culture-positive cases were due to streptococci, three due to coagulase-negative staphylococci, one due to *P. acnes* and one mixed due to *Staphylococcus aureus* and *P. acnes* [3].

The study was based on a 2 × 2 factorial design, with intracameral cefuroxime and topical perioperative levofloxacin factors resulting in four treatment groups. The comparison of case and non-case data was performed using multivariable logistic regression analyses. Odds ratios (ORs) associated with treatment effects and other risk factors were estimated (refer to Chapter S8).

While moxifloxacin (Appendix 6), with a broader antibacterial spectrum, was not available for the ESCRS study, the principle established—of a large reduction in postoperative endophthalmitis following use of an intracameral antibiotic *at the time of cataract surgery*—holds true and relevant for the future; use of an intracameral antibiotic at the end of cataract surgery is now adopted worldwide (https://eyewiki.org/Intracameral_Medications_Following_Cataract_Surgery).

In 2017, a large retrospective study was concluded involving 600,000 patients given moxifloxacin by the intracameral route at the time of cataract surgery [4]. While interesting, it suffers from the problems of retrospective studies but does show that the technique can be performed satisfactorily with a different antibiotic (moxifloxacin) to cefuroxime to achieve a similarly good result. However, the study depended on historical controls and included changes of surgeons and intraocular lenses.

The Aravind Hospital Group (India), where the 2017 study was conducted, now sells small volume ampoules of moxifloxacin for intracameral use*, available worldwide; their production facilities are FDA and CE approved. Alcon

Laboratories (Fort Worth, Texas, USA) produces a single-use vial of moxifloxacin at 5 mg/ml (use 0.1 mL containing 0.5 mg [500 micrograms]); it is available from Imprimis Pharmaceuticals, San Diego, USA.

Auromox* Moxifloxacin 0.5% w/v (Aurolab, India)	For routine intracameral injection of 0.1 mL (0.5 mg) at the time of cataract surgery to prevent postoperative endophthalmitis

* Each ampoule contains 1.0 mL and is sufficient for eight (nine) patients.

Intracameral 'ready-to-use' cefuroxime is only available in the UK and European Union (refer to Chapter 7). It is produced by Thea Pharmaceuticals (Clermont-Ferrand, France) as a single-use product (Aprokam) being a powder dissolved in 0.9% sterile saline available in Europe (not the USA); the diluent contains 1 mg cefuroxime in 0.1 mL normal saline. The cefuroxime is supplied in vials containing 50 mg, to which 5 mL of 0.9% sterile saline is added, to give a solution at 10 mg/ml (use 0.1 mL containing 1 mg).

Acute Endophthalmitis Post-Cataract Surgery

This is an emergency that requires vitrectomy and intravitreal antibiotics in hospital.

Chronic Endophthalmitis Post-Cataract Surgery

Macrophages within the anterior chamber (AC) are not always able to kill bacteria, such as *Propionibacterium acnes* and coagulase-negative staphylococci (CNS). This is well illustrated in chronic 'saccular' or granulomatous endophthalmitis due to *P. acnes* (Figure S7.7) and, less frequently, CNS.

Macrophages phagocytose *P. acnes* and CNS within the capsule fragment but are unable to kill the bacteria due to the lack of a functioning cell-mediated immune system with cytokine expression so that these bacteria are able to multiply within them (Figure S7.8). Macrophages within the AC function as tolerogenic APCs rather than as scavenger cells. There is a chronic inflammatory reaction recognised clinically as 'saccular', plaque or granulomatous endophthalmitis with white plaque in the capsular bag. The AC tap is often culture-negative because the bacteria are intracellular only, but a PCR test can be positive (Appendix 5). The bacteria may be killed when released from the macrophages by the antibacterial effect within the aqueous humour.

Our hypothesis suggests that the continued intracellular replication of the bacteria may allow the macrophage to express MHC class II molecules and to give a limited Th1 response (Chapter 10) that is susceptible to suppression with

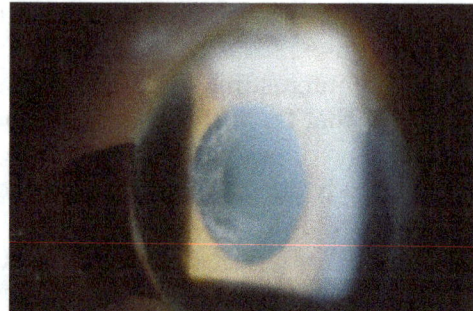

FIGURE S7.7 Saccular postoperative endophthalmitis due to *P. acnes* pre-treatment; responded well to azithromycin.

Source: (Courtesy of Dr. D. Seal, London)

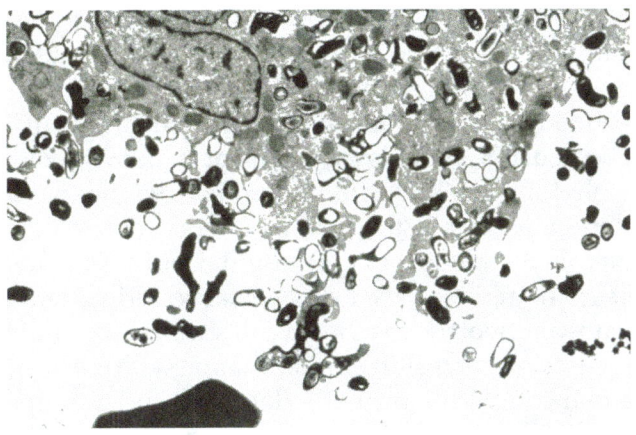

FIGURE S7.8 Electron microscopy of intracellular *P. acnes* (lens epithelium).

Source: (Courtesy of Dr. D. Seal, London)

corticosteroids. This explains why the inflammation returns when corticosteroid therapy is withdrawn and why the capsule fragment may need to be removed surgically, after which there is no recurrence of chronic inflammation.

The most appropriate antibiotic to use is clarithromycin or azithromycin, by the oral or intravitreal route, which penetrates into the AC and is concentrated up to 200 times intracellularly within macrophages to kill intracellular bacteria; therapeutic success has been reported with oral therapy at 500 mg bd without the need for surgical removal of the capsule and intraocular lens. Clarithromycin can be injected intravitreally with a nontoxic dose of up to, but not more than, 1.0 mg in 0.1 mL. A trial of antibiotic therapy is warranted.

EMERGING VIRUS DISEASES

Emergent and resurgent infectious diseases are major worldwide causes of systemic morbidity and death. Among them, viral and bacterial agents—including West Nile virus, dengue fever, chikungunya, Rift Valley fever, Zika virus, Ebola virus and rickettsioses—have been associated with an array of ocular manifestations [5]. These include anterior uveitis, retinitis, chorioretinitis, retinal vasculitis and optic nerve involvement. Proper clinical diagnosis of any of these infectious diseases is based on epidemiological data, history, systemic symptoms and signs and the pattern of ocular involvement. The diagnosis is confirmed by detection of specific antibody in serum or by PCR. Ocular involvement associated with emergent infections usually has a self-limited course, but it can result in persistent visual impairment. There is currently no proven specific treatment for arboviral diseases, and therapy is mostly supportive. Vaccination for humans against these viruses is still in the research phase but is now available for chikungunya virus. VIMKUNYA, developed by Bavarian Nordic, is a non-replicating VLP vaccine approved for use in individuals aged 12 years and older in the United States, European Union and the United Kingdom. Doxycycline is the treatment of choice for rickettsial diseases. Prevention, including public health measures to reduce the number of mosquitoes and personal protection measures, remains the mainstay for arthropod vector and zoonotic disease control.

West Nile Fever Virus

Ocular infection with West Nile virus (WNV) is a rare but significant manifestation of the virus, which is primarily transmitted through mosquito bites. The infection can lead to various ocular complications, including uveitis, retinitis, choroiditis and optic neuritis. Patients may present with symptoms, such as blurred vision, floaters, photophobia and ocular pain. The diagnosis is typically based on clinical examination, patient history and laboratory tests to detect WNV antibodies or viral RNA in the blood or cerebrospinal fluid. Imaging technology, like OCT and fluorescein angiography, helps visualise retinal and choroidal lesions. Treatment is mainly supportive, as there is no specific antiviral therapy for WNV. Management focuses on controlling inflammation with corticosteroids and monitoring for potential complications. Early detection and appropriate management are crucial to prevent long-term visual impairment.

Dengue Fever Virus

Ocular infection with dengue fever is a notable complication of this mosquito-borne viral disease. Dengue fever can lead to various ocular manifestations, including dengue-related maculopathy, uveitis, retinal heamorrhages and optic neuropathy (Figures S7.9 and S7.10). Symptoms are nonspecific, including blurred vision, floaters and photophobia. The diagnosis of ocular involvement is based on clinical findings and patient history. Imaging studies, like optical coherence tomography (OCT) and fluorescein angiography, can help visualise retinal and choroidal involvement. Laboratory tests are used to detect dengue virus antibodies or viral RNA in the blood. The most common general symptom of the disease is a high fever, often reaching up to 104°F (40°C). Also, severe headache, muscle and joint pain, nausea, vomiting and swollen glands are suggestive symptoms. A rash may appear, typically a few days after the onset of fever. In more severe cases, known as dengue haemorrhagic fever, bleeding from the nose and blood in the stool, accompanied by abdominal pain and vomiting, occur. These severe manifestations can lead to shock and even death.

Treatment is mainly supportive, as there is no specific antiviral therapy for dengue fever. Management focuses on controlling inflammation with corticosteroids and monitoring for potential complications. Early detection and appropriate management are crucial to prevent long-term visual impairment. A vaccine has

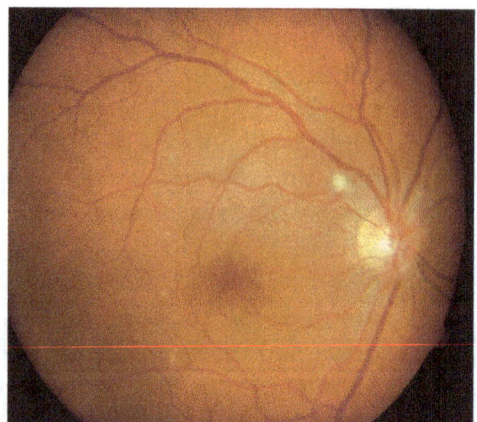

FIGURE S7.9 Dengue fever fundus photograph showing pale-yellow dots being foci of inflammation around live virus.

Source: (Courtesy of Prof. U. Pleyer, Charité Hospital, Berlin, Germany)

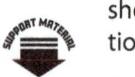

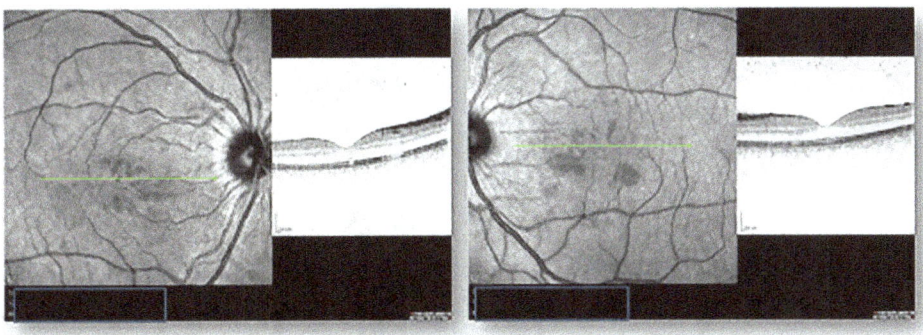

FIGURE S7.10 Dengue fever showing areas of virus-induced inflammation.

Source: (Courtesy of Prof. U. Pleyer, Charité Hospital, Berlin, Germany)

recently been approved. Qdenga, developed by Takeda Pharmaceuticals, is a live attenuated vaccine. It is approved for use in USA, UK and the European Union for those aged 4 years and older regardless of prior dengue infection status, making it suitable for both endemic populations and travellers. WHO recommends Qdenga for children aged 6–16 years in areas with high dengue transmission.

Chikungunya virus

Infection with the chikungunya virus can lead to various ocular complications, including anterior uveitis, posterior uveitis and panuveitis (Figures S7.11 and S7.12). The virus is transmitted primarily by Aedes mosquitoes. Patients may present with nonspecific signs and symptoms, such as eye pain, redness, blurred vision, photophobia and floaters. The diagnosis is based on clinical examination, patient history and laboratory tests to detect chikungunya virus antibodies or serological viral RNA. More recently, imaging techniques, like OCT and fluorescein angiography, can help to visualise retinal and choroidal lesions. Current treatment is only supportive, as there is no specific antiviral therapy for this virus. Management focuses on controlling inflammation with corticosteroids and monitoring for potential complications.

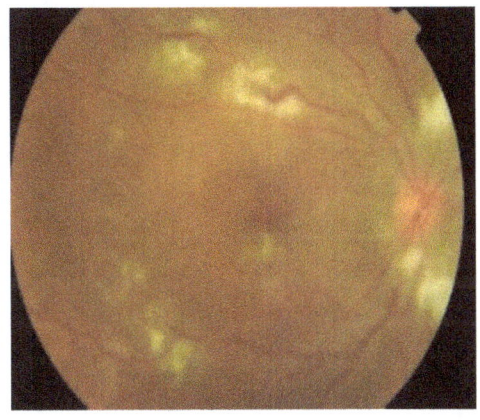

FIGURE S7.11 Right eye. Chikungunya virus showing hyperaemic papillitis, cotton wool spots and vasculitis.

Source: (Courtesy of Prof. U. Pleyer, Charité Hospital, Berlin, Germany)

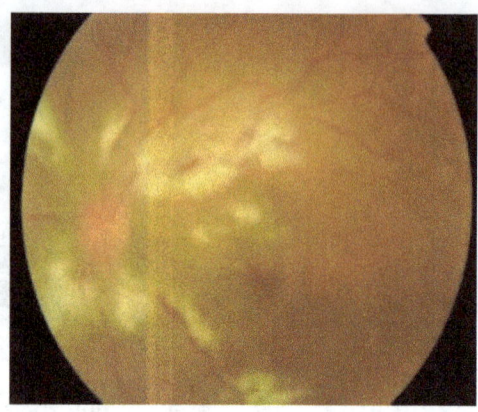

FIGURE S7.12 Left eye. Chikungunya virus photograph with similar findings.

REFERENCES

1. Vision Loss Expert Group. Eye 2024. PMID: 38461217 (https://doi.org/10.1038/s41433-024-02961-1).
2. ESCRS Endophthalmitis Study Group. J Cataract Refract Surg 2007. PMID: 17531690 (https://doi.org/10.1016/j.jcrs.2007.02.032).
3. Montan PG et al. J Cataract Refract Surg 2002. PMID: 12036639 (http://doi.org/10.1016/s0886-3350(01)01269-x).
4. Haripriya A et al. Ophthalmol 2017. PMID: 28214101 (http://doi.org/10.1016/j.ophtha.2017.01.026).
5. Venkatesh A et al. Eye 2021. PMID: 33514902 (https://doi.org/10.1038/s41433-020-01376-y).

S8: Assessment of Risk of Exposure between Diseases and Non-Diseased Controls

In epidemiology, an analytical prospective study is a type of observational study that follows a group of individuals, known as a *cohort*, over a specified time period, to examine the relationship between an exposure (risk factor) and the subsequent development of a health outcome or disease.

Refer to Chapter 8 for examples.

QUESTIONNAIRE REPORTING STUDY

A questionnaire in a survey study typically involves a set of systematically written questions to gather data from respondents. They provide information that is not directly available from other sources. It can be a self-administered format or an interview. Questions can be open-ended or close-ended. They are essential in epidemiology, as they allow assessment of the distribution of health-related conditions, lifestyle factors, habitual factors and risk factors. It enables the investigator to conduct further analytical and descriptive research.

Refer to Chapter 8 for examples.

ASSESSMENT OF RISK EXPOSURE BETWEEN DISEASED AND NON-DISEASED CONTROLS

Odds Ratio (OR)

The odds ratio is the ratio of the odds of exposure among diseased persons to non-diseased controls.

It is calculated as follows:

	Diseased (Cases)	Non-Diseased (Controls)
With history of exposure	a	b
Without history of exposure	c	d

$$\text{Odds ratio} = \frac{odds\ of\ exposure\ in\ disease}{odds\ of\ exposure\ in\ non-disease} = \frac{a/c}{b/d} \ or \ \frac{a \times d}{b \times c}$$

Population Attributable Risk (PAR)

The population attributable risk is the proportion of a disease incidence in a population that can be attributed to an exposure or risk factor. It shows the difference

DOI: 10.1201/9781003606789-20

between exposed disease incidence and non-exposed disease incidence. It is a significant measure in public health, as it informs us how much of the disease burden in a population can be potentially prevented if the exposure risk factor was removed (refer to Supplementary Chapter S7).

Confounding Factors

A third variable that is linked to the independent variable (exposure) and the dependent variable (outcome) can create a false association between them.

For a variable to be known as a confounding factor, it must satisfy three criteria:

1. It is associated with the independent variable (exposure).
2. It is a risk factor for the dependent variable (outcome).
3. It is not a consequential effect of the exposure (i.e. is not in the causal pathway).

S9: Peripapillary Atrophy and Myopic Crescent

Peripapillary atrophy (PPA) describes atrophy or thinning in the layers of the retina and retinal pigment epithelium around the optic nerve head. It is often detected during a regular eye examination and is usually not a cause for concern, as it can be present in healthy individuals. However, PPA can be associated with glaucoma, where it may indicate a higher risk or progression of the disease.

PPA can be divided into two zones: the alpha zone and the beta zone. The beta zone, which is closer to the inner part of the optic nerve, is present in about 15% to 20% of normal eyes; it is more strongly associated with glaucoma and may enlarge as the disease progresses. The alpha zone is further out from the optic nerve.

There is no treatment for PPA, and it typically does not cause any symptoms or vision loss. However, there is significant association between PPA, glaucomatous optic nerve damage and visual field loss. PPA is commonly observed together with high myopia, estimated to be present in about 20% of cases.

The prominent broad markings (tigroid fundus), further from the disc—from 5 to 10 o'clock in the L eye (Figure S9.1) and approximately symmetrical in the R eye (Figure S9.2)—are choroidal vessels visible through the RPE (retinal pigment epithelium) layer lying deep to the retina.

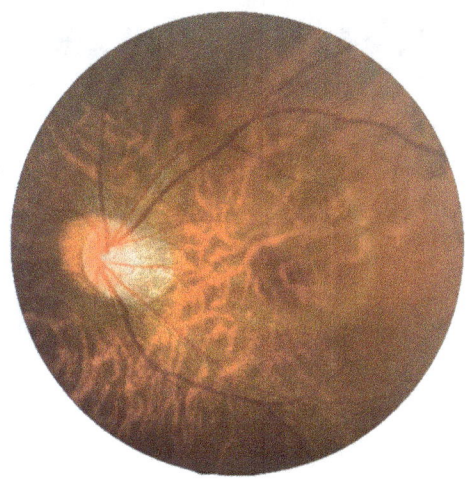

FIGURE S9.1 Myopic (L) eye in 21-year-old male (axial length 27.34), power—7D, showing PPA and a myopic crescent with no symptoms.

Source: (Courtesy of Mr. J.Z. Ong)

203

DOI: 10.1201/9781003606789-21

The crescent on the temporal edge of the retina is common in myopes and longstanding; the globe curvature may be slightly more concave medial to that demarcation.

MYOPIC CRESCENT

Myopia can lead to changes in the retina, including the development of a myopic maculopathy, which may involve a ring-like structure associated with macular degeneration. This condition is caused by thinning of the peripheral retina and stretching of the macula.

A myopic crescent (Figure S9.2) is a white or grayish-white crescentic area located on the temporal side of the optic disc in the retina of a myope. The crescent is caused by atrophy of the choroid, allowing the sclera to become visible. It is more commonly seen in pathological axial myopia. In highly myopic eyes, the crescent can be divided into two zones with fluorescent angiography: an inner zone that is consistently hypofluorescent and an outer zone with delayed choroidal filling. Enlargement of the myopic crescent may occur.

The presence of a myopic crescent may indicate an increased risk of morbidity, including myopic progression, development of myopic maculopathy and open-angle glaucoma. The size of the crescent tends to increase with age and can grow as myopia progresses.

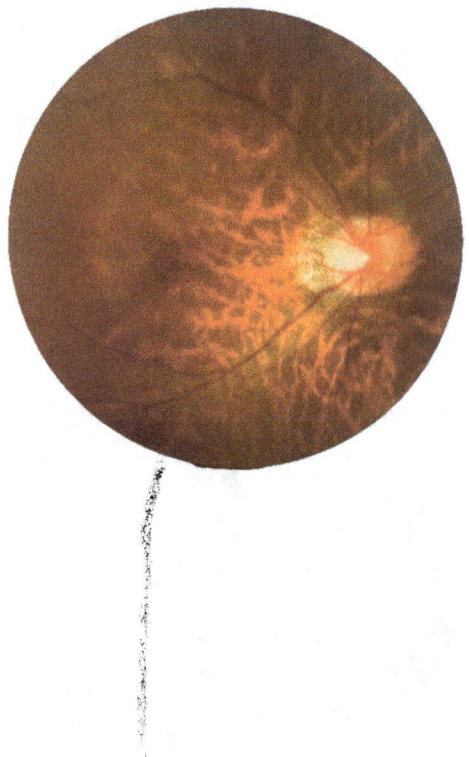

FIGURE S9.2 Myopic (R) eye in 21-year-old male (axial length 27.36), power—7D, showing PPA and a myopic crescent with no symptoms.

Source: (Courtesy of Mr. J.Z. Ong)

S10: Localised Immune Complex Disease, Immune Deposition in the Cornea and Mucosal-Associated Lymphoid Tissue

Localised immune complex disease occurs in the peripheral cornea by the activation of the C1 component of complement and the formation of C5a, which is chemotactic for polymorphonuclear cells (PMNs). This also causes release of IL–8. The marginal ulceration that occurs in the autoimmune connective tissue diseases, such as rheumatoid arthritis, is thought to be immune complex–mediated, involving rheumatoid factor (IgM) directed against self-IgG. The integrin ICAM-1-b2 is involved in neutrophil invasion as part of this inflammatory process.

A similar mechanism has been proposed for marginal ulceration associated with blepharitis due to *Staphylococcus aureus*, as an alternative explanation to the DTH theory by Mondino, although both mechanisms may interact. It is suggested that toxins of *St. aureus* cause punctate epithelial breakdown that allows staphylococcal antigens, especially protein A, to penetrate the epithelium and complex with IgM found in the peripheral cornea. This is conceived to activate the C1 complement and its cascade to C5a, causing tissue damage. It is also a possibility that the marginal ulceration that occasionally occurs in chlamydial infection is due to immune complex disease.

IMMUNE DEPOSITION IN THE CORNEA

The cornea is unique in that insoluble complexes, formed by soluble antigens and antibodies when each is at equal concentration, can be visualised as localised rings in the corneal stroma (Figure S10.1); the cornea acts like a 'gel plate' for immunoprecipitation. When either the antigen or the antibody is present in excess concentration, the complexes remain soluble. The reaction occurs between a microbial antigen in the central cornea and an antibody (IgG) that diffuses across the cornea from the limbal vessels. Centripetally migrating PMNs degranulate within the ring. Such an example is illustrated in Figure S10.1, when there was an *Acanthamoeba* infection under partial host control at three months. The depositions produced are called Wessley rings, which appear as double circles, and while they have often been associated with herpetic keratitis, they have also been recognised with bacterial, fungal and viral infections.

MUCOSA-ASSOCIATED LYMPHOID TISSUE

The immune protection at mucosal surfaces, including the ocular surface, is maintained in part by mucosa-associated lymphoid tissue (MALT). One of the

DOI: 10.1201/9781003606789-22

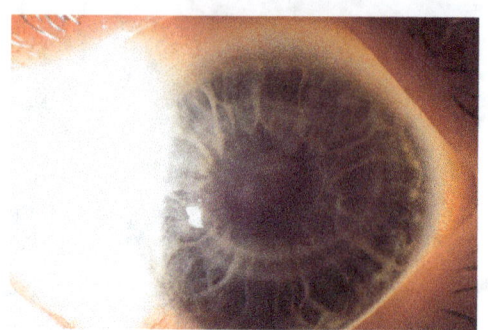

FIGURE S10.1 Wessley rings around a healed scar from *Acanthamoeba* infection.

Source: (Seal & Pleyer, Ocular Infection, 2007)

main functions of MALT is to establish a balance between immunity and tolerance in order to prevent destruction of the delicate mucosal tissues by constant inflammatory reactions, which applies in particular to the eye. This is maintained by an anti-inflammatory cytokine milieu in mucosal tissues and is most likely regulated by antigen-presenting dendritic cells as key regulators of the immune system. They normally favour anti-inflammatory T- or B-cell responses in mucosal locations. A major defense mechanism of MALT is the production of secretory immunoglobulins, mainly of the IgA and partly of the IgM isotype, by differentiated B cells (plasma cells). In contrast to the IgG isotype that prevails in the blood, IgA has very little complement-binding activity and, therefore, does not initiate inflammatory reactions during host defense. IgA attaches to bacteria to 'coat' them, reducing their adhesion to epithelial cells.

The lymphoid cells of MALT migrate in a regulated fashion, guided by specialized vessels, adhesion molecules and soluble chemotactic factors. They migrate between the different mucosal organs, which are hence assumed to constitute a functionally interrelated mucosal immune system. By these migration pathways, MALT is also connected to the central immune system. MALT is a regular component of the normal human ocular surface and termed eye-associated lymphoid tissue (EALT) [1].

MALT consists of a diffuse lymphoid tissue (A) and of an organised follicular tissue (B) (Figure S10.2). Mucosal tissues in general are composed of two sheets—the surface epithelium (e), with its basement membrane (bm), and an underlying lamina propria (lp)—that both contain lymphocytes. The lamina propria is composed of loose connective tissue with small blood vessels (b), afferent lymph vessels (l) and numerous cells, including lymphoid cells (T lymphocytes [black], B-lymphocytes [blue], plasma cells [p]).

Accessory cells occur, including fibroblasts (f), macrophages (m), mast cells (mc) or dendritic cells (dc). Intraepithelial lymphocytes are mainly CD8þ suppressor/cytotoxic T cells, whereas in the lamina propria of the diffuse tissue (A), they occur in roughly equal numbers together with CD4 T helper cells. Follicular lymphoid tissue (B) is formed by accumulations of B lymphocytes with parafollicular T-cell zones, vessels and an overlying specialised follicle-associated epithelium for antigen transport towards the follicle. Naive lymphocytes enter follicular regions via blood vessels (b) and make contact with antigens; antigen-specific lymphocytes

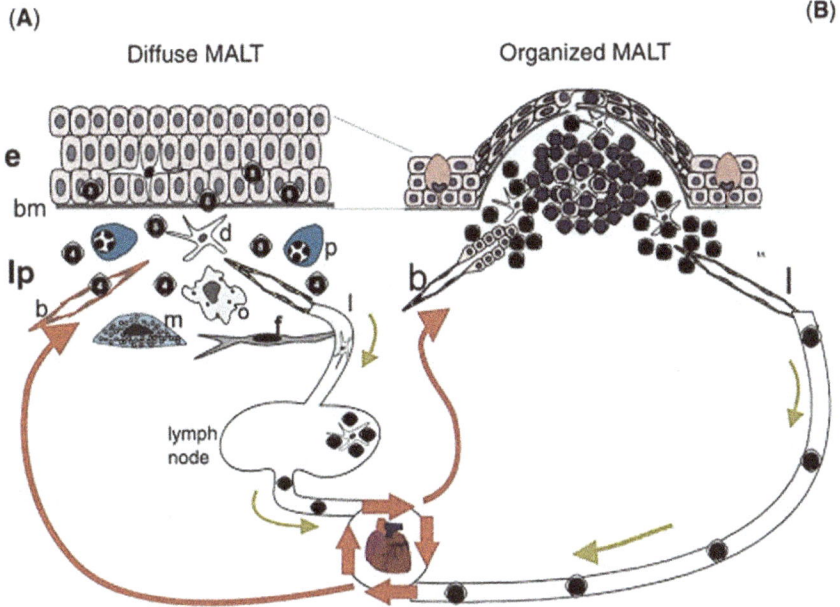

FIGURE S10.2 Schematic diagram of mucosa-associated lymphoid tissue (MALT).

proliferate, differentiate and leave via lymphatics (l). They finally reach the blood circulation and may later emigrate to populate the same or other mucosal tissues as effector cells (T cells and plasma cells).

EYE-ASSOCIATED LYMPHOID TISSUE

Lymphoid cells are a normal tissue constituent and form continuous mucosa-associated lymphoid tissue in the lacrimal gland, conjunctiva and lacrimal drainage system.

The ocular surface is an integral part of the mucosal immune system of the body. The diffuse lymphoid tissue, with an effector function by lymphocytes and plasma cells, is continuous from the lacrimal gland along the excretory ducts into the conjunctiva as conjunctiva-associated lymphoid tissue (CALT) and continues through the lacrimal canaliculi inside the lacrimal drainage system as lacrimal drainage-associated lymphoid tissue (LDALT). The lymphoid tissue of these three organs together constitutes EALT (Figure S10.3). Similar ocular antigens are detected in the follicular tissue of CALT and LDALT.

Effector cells that are primed in follicular tissue against ocular surface antigens can migrate in a regulated fashion via specialised vessels between the organs of EALT and the other parts of the mucosal immune system and can hence provide them with effector cells that are specifically directed against antigens that occur at the ocular surface.

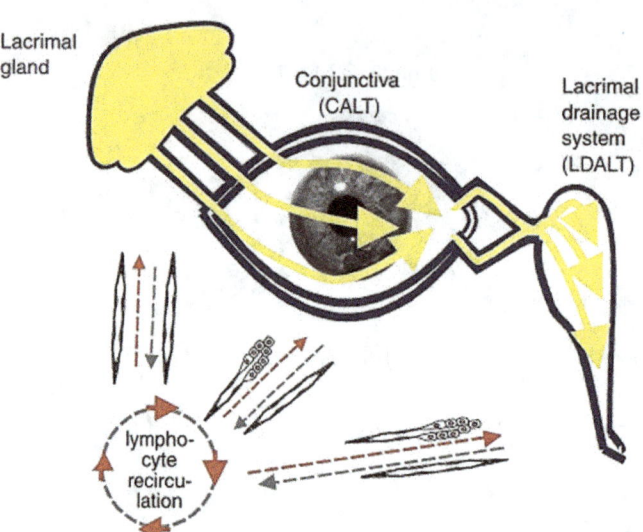

Lacrimal gland

Conjunctiva (CALT)

Lacrimal drainage system (LDALT)

lympho-cyte recircu-lation

FIGURE S10.3 Schematic diagram of eye-associated lymphoid tissue (EALT).

REFERENCE

[1] Knop E et al. Clinical Aspects of MALT. In: U Pleyer, BJ Mondino (eds), Essentials in Ophthalmology. Uveitis and Immunological Disorders. Berlin, Heidelberg: Springer 2004/2005, pp 65–89.

S11: Pharmacokinetics and Pharmacodynamics

INTRODUCTION

Drug penetration into the eye is influenced by many factors, including characteristics of the drug administered (e.g. lipophilicity versus hydrophilicity), route of drug administration, frequency of dosing, degree of ocular inflammation, and surgical status of the eye. Types of drug formulations include drops, ointments, and injections, both commercial and produced "in-house" in the pharmacy department. All these factors are reviewed for their influence on drug penetration into the eye and also on their removal out of the eye.

Appendices 1 and 6 give drug formularies for ophthalmic drugs most commonly used in primary eye care, with mechanisms of action and target effects, for therapeutic use. For mechanisms by which drugs give immune suppression (cyclosporine, corticosteroids, and nonsteroidal anti-inflammatory drugs [NSAIDs]), refer to Chapter 10.

LIPOPHILICITY/HYDROPHILICITY

Drugs (including antibiotics) are chemical compounds that can be characterised as to their solubility in water. A coefficient named the lipid/water solubility coefficient (or ether/water solubility coefficient) describes to what extent the compound is freely soluble in either kind of solvent. It is this solubility ratio that determines how well the drug will penetrate cell membranes and be retained within compartments, how easily it can be dissolved in nontoxic solvents for human use, how safely it can be administered, and what the pharmacokinetic characteristics will be in regard to a specific targeted tissue.

The greater the lipophilicity of the compound, the greater the penetration through the lipid-containing membranes of cell walls. However, to administer a drug with a very high lipid/water solubility ratio requires dissolution in a solvent that is not aqueous, and these solvents themselves are usually toxic to cell membranes and would also be noxious when administered via the bloodstream. Therefore, dissolution of highly lipophilic compounds in specific solvents is feasible in the laboratory but not feasible for administration in clinical medicine without specially developed delivery systems.

Familiar examples of a relatively lipophilic antibiotic are chloramphenicol, levofloxacin, and clarithromycin. Highly lipophilic antibiotics are fewer in number than the relatively hydrophilic antibiotics used extensively in clinical medicine. The penicillins, cephalosporins, and aminoglycosides are relatively water-soluble, and these comprise the majority of antibiotics used. The quinolone

DOI: 10.1201/9781003606789-23

group of antibiotics (moxifloxacin, ciprofloxacin, ofloxacin, levofloxacin, and gatifloxacin) is relatively more lipophilic than cephalosporins, but data specific to each antibiotic should guide the clinical use and expectations; moxifloxacin gives the highest levels within ocular tissues.

DIFFUSION

Simple diffusion is the most common method of drug transfer from one space or tissue of the body to another or from one compartment to another. It involves the movement of solute particles from an area of higher concentration to one of lower concentration by transfer through tissues and interfaces. Once diffusion has occurred, drug concentrations within adjacent compartments become stabilised according to the drug's partition coefficient (Figure S11.1).

Diffusion is affected by factors such as the concentration of drug presented at a tissue interface (concentration gradient), molecular weight of the drug, membrane permeability (inflamed or non-inflamed), tissue binding, active transport mechanisms, surgical status of the eye, and others, including formulation of the drug itself.

EPITHELIAL BARRIER

The epithelia of the bulbar conjunctiva and cornea are relatively impermeable to even water-soluble agents of small molecular size applied topically. Proprietary ophthalmic preparations, such as gentamicin sulphate, are available as drops (0.3%) or ointments at high concentration (e.g. 0.3–1.0%) relative to their effective antimicrobial concentration and are thus active in the treatment of surface ocular

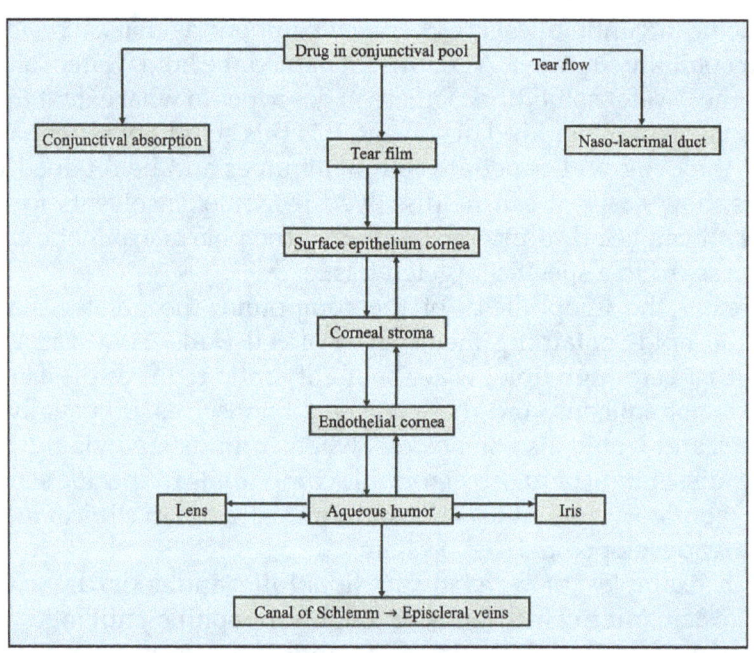

FIGURE S11.1 Partition flow for drug transfer from topical drops to aqueous humour.

Source: (Courtesy of Mr. J.Z. Ong, RUMC, Penang, Malaysia)

infection (e.g. conjunctivitis). Antibiotics with a relatively high lipid-water solubility coefficient (such as chloramphenicol, moxifloxacin, and levofloxacin) can penetrate the conjunctiva and cornea much better to enter deeper tissues at more effective concentrations. For a topically applied antibiotic to penetrate to the aqueous humour, it has to pass through the various layers of the cornea, as illustrated in Figure S11.1.

If the surface epithelium is breached, as with corneal ulceration, water-soluble drugs can diffuse into the anterior segment of the eye in high concentration. This can be enhanced by the use of fortified eye drops, whose concentrations exceed those of commercial preparations. However, this route is ineffective in providing useful concentrations in the posterior segment of the eye because there is a diffusion barrier across the lens-zonule compartment and across the anterior vitreous.

The barrier offered by the epithelium of the ocular surface can be circumvented therapeutically by delivering a bolus of drug under the conjunctiva (subconjunctival injection) or more deeply into the orbit (sub-Tenon's injection). These periocular routes will deliver effective antimicrobial concentrations into the anterior segment of the eye (cornea and anterior chamber) and, to some extent, into the posterior segment (the vitreous) but should not be relied upon to deliver a sufficiently high concentration of antibiotic to satisfactorily treat bacterial endophthalmitis.

Penetration of the different quinolone antibiotics—moxifloxacin, ciprofloxacin, ofloxacin, levofloxacin, and gatifloxacin—into the anterior chamber from the topical drop route, or by oral therapy, vary widely between the different compounds, with moxifloxacin and levofloxacin achieving the highest levels in the aqueous humour due to their relative lipophilicity.

BLOOD-OCULAR BARRIERS

There are two main barrier systems in the eye (Figures S11.2 & S11.3). The first regulates exchange between blood and aqueous humour in which inward movement predominates—the blood-aqueous barrier. Aqueous humour is secreted into the posterior chamber by the ciliary processes and flows through the pupil into the anterior chamber to leave via the trabecular meshwork. Important diffusional solute exchange takes place between the aqueous and not only the surrounding tissues but also with the vitreous.

The blood aqueous barrier is formed by two layers of cells: the endothelium of the iris blood vessels and the non-pigmented inner layer of the ciliary epithelium. These cell layers impair transport of blood proteins to maintain an osmotic and chemical equilibrium. However, the ciliary vascular endothelium is permeable to blood-borne solutes that give a concentration of 1% of proteins found in the plasma. The ciliary body has a pivotal role in regulating all inner ocular fluids via its large surface covered by the ciliary processes. There is active secretory transport of sodium, chloride, and bicarbonate providing the osmotic force for the production of the aqueous, as well as maintaining ascorbic acid at a higher level than in plasma. The ciliary body is also responsible for a free continuous flow of ions, amino acids, and vitamins from the aqueous into the vitreous.

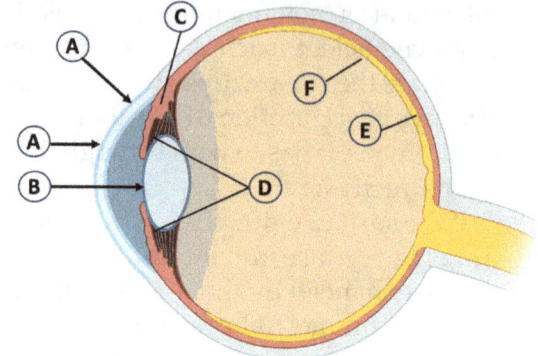

FIGURE S11.2 Barriers of penetration of drugs, including antibiotics, into the eye.

Source: Courtesy of Dr. D. Seal, London (drawn by Mr. J.Z. Ong, RUMC, Penang Malaysia) [1]

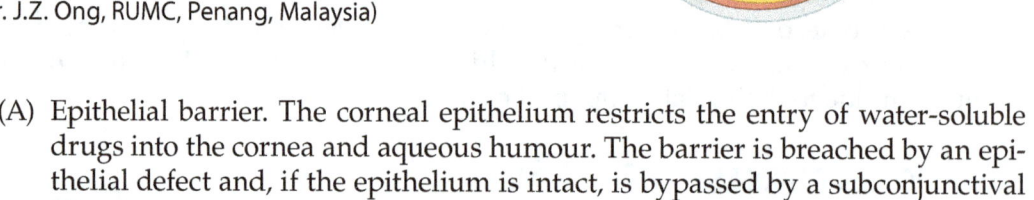

FIGURE S11.3 *Active transfer* (cefazolin and penicillins) and *passive transfer* (gentamicin and aminoglycosides) routes out of the eye. Quinolone antibiotics are removed by both the active and passive transport routes.

Source: Courtesy of Dr. D. Seal, London (drawn by Mr. J.Z. Ong, RUMC, Penang, Malaysia)

(A) Epithelial barrier. The corneal epithelium restricts the entry of water-soluble drugs into the cornea and aqueous humour. The barrier is breached by an epithelial defect and, if the epithelium is intact, is bypassed by a subconjunctival injection.

(B) Bulk flow of aqueous humour out of the eye, and the presence of an intact lens and zonule, retard the diffusion of drugs from the anterior chamber into the vitreous humour.

(C) Blood-aqueous barrier: limits the entry of drugs from the blood into the aqueous.

(D) The epithelia of the iris and ciliary body pump anionic drugs out of the aqueous.

(E) Blood-retinal barrier: Limits the entry of drugs into the vitreous from the systemic circulation. Externally is the pigment epithelial barrier.

(F) Internally is the retinal capillary endothelial barrier. There is an outward pumping of anions across the retina by the retinal pigment epithelium and the endothelial cells of the retinal vessels.

In contrast, the second barrier in the posterior segment affects outward movement from the retina into the blood—the blood-retinal barrier. It is responsible for the homeostasis and microenvironment of the retina. It also serves to remove waste products of metabolic activity from within the eye. There are no diffusional barriers between the extracellular fluid of the retina and the adjacent vitreous nor with the posterior chamber of the anterior segment so that the functions of both anterior and posterior segments work together. The blood-retinal barrier is formed by a combination of the endothelium of retinal blood vessels, the retinal pigment epithelium, and retinal glial cells. The endothelial cells of the retina have functional and morphological differences compared with those of other organs. They have narrow tight junctional structures composed of a complex called the zonulae occludentes. They impair cellular transport of hydrophilic compounds. The retinal pigment epithelium is in the outer blood-retinal barrier and is also sealed with extensive zonulae occludentes. High activities of barrier selective enzymes contribute to a protective function, but essential nutrients are transported into the vitreous by carrier-selective mechanisms.

Equally important are the active transport mechanisms that remove ions from the vitreous. The microenvironment of the retina resembles the extracellular fluid of the brain. It is regulated by active transport processes located within the barrier cells. There are three main sites of transport out of the eye: the endothelial cells of the retinal vessels, the retinal pigment epithelium, and the ciliary epithelium. Within the retinal barrier, there is active transport of potassium to blood with a net magnesium flux in the opposite direction. *Organic anions, such as prostaglandins and related compounds,* that are produced but not metabolised within the eye, and *anionic drugs, such as penicillins, cephalosporins, and zwitterions, such as ciprofloxacin (quinolones), are removed from the extracellular fluid of the retina by active transport across the blood-retinal barrier cells* similarly to the renal tubular clearance mechanism.

This active transport system is inhibited by probenecid, which can be used to maintain higher levels of anionic drugs in the eye; *however, this may interfere with outward transport of prostaglandins.* Use of oral probenecid (500 mg every 12 hours) retards outward transport of penicillins, cephalosporins, and ciprofloxacin (quinolones) across the retinal capillary endothelial cells, thus extending the half-life of the drug within the vitreous. Probenecid also raises the plasma level by blocking secretion of these drugs by the proximal renal tubule.

Cationic compounds and drugs, such as the aminoglycosides (gentamicin, tobramycin), vancomycin, erythromycin, and rifampicin, are not actively transported out of the eye by the blood-retinal barrier and *have to leave the posterior compartment by diffusing forward into the anterior chamber and aqueous humour.*

Ciprofloxacin and the other quinolones are removed by both the active and passive transport routes.

The barriers referred to the globe do not exist for other orbital structures. Thus, infections within the orbit or ocular adnexae (the eyelids, lacrimal gland, and nasolacrimal system) are readily treatable with systemic antibiotics.

The result of the blood-retinal barrier described earlier is an active transport system for the anionic drugs (penicillin, cephalosporins) out of the eye, giving a half-life of approximately eight hours when given intravitreally, as opposed to the passive diffusion forward of the cationic drugs (gentamicin and other aminoglycosides, vancomycin, rifampicin, and erythromycin), giving a half-life of approximately 24 hours. This means that a combination injection given intravitreally of a cephalosporin, viz. ceftazidime, and an aminoglycoside or vancomycin, have different half-lives, which must be considered in the management of the clinical infection. However, for reasons given later, in the presence of inflammation removal of the actively absorbed drug, viz. cephazolin is delayed, resulting in a longer half-life than without inflammation. In contrast, the passively transported drug eliminated by forward diffusion, e.g. aminoglycosides (gentamicin, tobramycin), has enhanced removal. The combination of a cephalosporin and an aminoglycoside given intravitreally thus becomes acceptable in practice for treatment of the acutely infected and inflamed eye.

EFFECTS OF INFLAMMATION

These barriers affect the ocular distribution of drugs, the potential of systemically administered drugs to enter the vitreous, as well as the retention of drugs after direct delivery by vitreous tap.

In the uninflamed eye, the highest aqueous concentration using the systemic route will be achieved by lipid-soluble drugs, such as chloramphenicol or the quinolones. Negligible concentrations will be achieved using water-soluble drugs, particularly those in anionic form (such as the penicillins and cephalosporins), which are actively transported out of the eye.

In the inflamed eye, after systemic antibiotic administration, the concentrations achieved in the ocular compartments are increased, owing to partial breakdown of the blood-aqueous barrier, so that effective antimicrobial concentrations may be reached in the aqueous. However, concentrations reached in the vitreous with parenteral therapy are always much lower than those achieved in the aqueous, even in the inflamed eye with endophthalmitis. Vitreous concentrations after high-dose systemic therapy in such situations will be sub-therapeutic after initial doses and lower than those achievable by subconjunctival injection.

The highest antibiotic levels are gained by direct injection into the vitreous, which is always favoured in the treatment of serious endophthalmitis. However, giving the same antibiotic by the intravenous route as that given by an intravitreal tap will prolong effective levels in the vitreous and should be practiced in the treatment of acute bacterial endophthalmitis.

Infectious endophthalmitis creates sufficient intraocular inflammation to compromise the function of the retinal pump mechanism that helps to eliminate antibiotics, such as cephazolin, thereby prolonging their half-life in the vitreous of the normal eye from approximately 6.5 to 10.4 hours. At the same time, surgical alteration of the eye, such as lensectomy and/or vitrectomy, changes the inner anatomy of the eye, affecting overall elimination characteristics.

In contrast, gentamicin, which is not removed by the retinal pump mechanism, does not show any prolongation of half-life in the vitreous of the inflamed or infected eye but instead has a reduction of 50% from 20 to 10 hours because of its elimination by the anterior route. A similar reduction is given with aphakia, but this is not further increased with inflammation or infection. For vancomycin, aphakia and vitrectomy reduce vitreous vancomycin levels, compared with phakic non-vitrectomised eyes, so that only 25 mg/mL remains out of a dose of 2 mg given 48 hours earlier.

INTRAVITREAL INJECTION OF ANTIBIOTICS, VITRECTOMY, AND TOXICITY

Direct intravitreal antibiotic injection is now the "standard of practice" for treatment of infectious endophthalmitis. Direct intravitreal injection of an antibiotic in the highest nontoxic dose delivers high, instantaneous antibiotic levels where they are needed—at the focus of infection inside the vitreous space. "Debulking" of the vitreous with surgery (partial or full vitrectomy) will also remove part of the infectious load and allow the antibiotic to diffuse easily within the cavity. The goal of intravitreal antibiotic injection is to sterilise the vitreous cavity as early as possible to reduce the destructive effect of the bacteria on the retina.

With intravitreal injection, antibiotic levels are delivered that are bactericidal, at least for a period of time. These high antibiotic levels are needed for eradication of bacteria in this closed avascular space. The purpose of injecting the highest dose that is nontoxic to the retina is to ensure that antibiotic levels destructive to bacteria are delivered in a single injection and that they are maintained above a sub-therapeutic level for as long as possible, while the intravitreal level of antibiotic is declining. Bacteria kill rates are a function not only of drug concentration but also of contact time with the bacterium, as well as the numbers involved.

When diagnosed early, there will be a smaller number of actively replicating bacterial cells than with a late diagnosis when there is a large number of static bacterial cells present. Antibiotics, such as cephalosporins, that act against the bacterial cell wall require replicating cells for their bactericidal effect. The same situation applies to aminoglycosides that act on the cell ribosome but to a lesser extent. Treatment at a late stage involves a changed environment with pH change, hypoxia, nutrient shortage, and non-replicating bacteria, which additionally reduces the effectiveness of the antibiotic. This is when vitrectomy is needed to "evacuate the pus."

The concentration of antibiotic in the vitreous cavity after an intravitreal injection is generally calculated by dividing the dose injected by the average volume of the vitreous, in humans 4.5 mL (refer to end of chapter). However, the presence of infection/inflammation, aphakia, and vitrectomy affect the immediate and early antibiotic levels distributed throughout the vitreous space after intravitreal injection.

After instantaneous antibiotic levels are established by intravitreal injection, the drug half-life then determines the rate of decline or reduction of drug levels within the vitreous space. Drug elimination is affected by factors including the degree of inflammation, the elimination route for the antibiotic in question (anterior or posterior), tissue binding of drug, and the surgical status of the eye, such as aphakia or vitrectomy.

Inflammation prolongs the half-life of cefazolin after intravitreal injection in the non-surgical eye. In this instance, as described earlier, damage to the retinal pump mechanism actually serves to prolong the retention of those drugs within the vitreous cavity that are eliminated via the posterior route. However, drugs eliminated via the anterior route, viz. gentamicin, are not subject to this effect, and inflammation will decrease their half-life or retention after an intravitreal injection, as will removal of the cataractous lens.

In aphakic, vitrectomised eyes, the rate of antibiotic decline in the vitreous space can still be faster. The vitreous gel that sequesters the injected bolus of drug, and promotes gradual diffusion throughout the vitreous cavity, has been removed.

The increasing use of vitrectomy demands that the toxicity of the injected dose and the method of intravitreal injection be reconsidered. When injected into the vitreous gel, gradual diffusion of antibiotic occurs. However, where vitrectomy has been performed, the injection should be given slowly so that these relatively high concentrations of antibiotic, or their vehicles, are not "squirted" with force onto the retina itself. This is especially important with gentamicin. The dose of 0.4 mg in 0.1 mL has been reduced to 0.2 mg because of suspected macular infarction due to toxicity, as has the dose of amikacin (0.2 mg), although it is not equipotent, and amikacin is less effective per mg as a bactericidal drug than gentamicin. Gentamicin and other antibiotics should be reduced in concentration by a further 50% (for gentamicin to 0.1 mg) if given intravitreally when a full vitrectomy is performed.

Most cases of gentamicin toxicity occur after a 0.4 mg dose in eyes that have undergone a vitrectomy. The retinal toxicity of gentamicin may have been exacerbated due to the methods used to prepare the intraocular injection in some places. By irregular means of creating the intraocular injection (drawing up concentrated commercial products within one tuberculin syringe in "series"— in poor order) in the syringe and not going through the more cumbersome serial dilutions first in separate vials that also dilute out the toxins in the vehicle, clinicians have deviated in the past from standard clinical procedures and recommendations.

INTRACELLULAR AND EXTRACELLULAR LEVELS OF ANTIBIOTICS

Once an antibiotic or another drug reaches a particular tissue within the eye, its concentration will be partitioned between the cellular and extracellular (EC) space. There is a big difference in cellular penetration between the various antibiotics that, surprisingly, is not related to their ionic charge. Polymorphonuclear (PMN) cells are used in laboratory experiments and are representative of levels expected within macrophages.

Antibiotics can be classified according to whether their PMN/EC ratio is less than or greater than 1. Those antibiotics with a ratio of < 1 have a lower concentration within the PMN cell than within the extracellular tissue. In contrast, those antibiotics with a ratio > 1 become concentrated within the cell. The penicillins, cephalosporins, and all the aminoglycosides have a ratio of < 1. The ratio is highest for azithromycin (also representative of clarithromycin) at 226, clindamycin at 43, erythromycin at 14, and the various quinolones at between 10.9 and 3.7. Chloramphenicol, which has been much used in the past due to its lipophilicity, and therefore, cell membrane penetration, only has a ratio of 2.2.

Chronic low-grade infection, often presenting as a "hypopyon uveitis" that develops six weeks or more after phacoemulsification cataract surgery and lasts for months, can be due to "saccular" plaque or capsular bag endophthalmitis (refer to Supplementary Chapter S7). The bacteria causing this type of infection are usually *P. acnes,* diphtheroids, or coagulase-negative staphylococci. They are found within macrophages lining the capsule fragment. To eradicate these intracellular bacteria (Figure S7.8), there is need to use antibiotics that penetrate well into macrophages, such as the erythromycin derivatives *azithromycin and clarithromycin.*

Clarithromycin was first used for this purpose in an individual case of "saccular" (plaque) endophthalmitis (Figure S7.7), confirmed by PCR, which responded well to treatment and resulted in a quiet eye without the need for any surgical removal of the lens. Since then, clarithromycin has been used similarly by others and in a randomised trial of therapy for chronic subacute endophthalmitis, when patients responded much better to this therapy than those who did not receive clarithromycin.

Clarithromycin is given orally as 500 mg every 12 hours and is well absorbed. It penetrates well into both the anterior and posterior segments and is then concentrated into macrophages at up to 200-fold [1]. The expected concentrations in vitreous 3, 6, 8, 11, and 24 hours after administration are as follows: 0.11, 0.257, 0.27, 0.307, and 0.108 mg/mL [1]. The expected concentration of clarithromycin in the iris is 6.2 mg/g, demonstrating its concentration into cells [1].

Quinolones are given by the topical route for treating bacterial conjunctivitis and prophylaxis of endophthalmitis following phacoemulsification cataract surgery. Levofloxacin is a quinolone that is both lipophilic (fat soluble) and hydrophilic (water soluble). This allows it to penetrate through the corneal epithelial barrier into the stroma and anterior chamber in good levels reaching 4.4 mg/mL (mean value) in the aqueous humour at 60 minutes after the third postoperative dose (3); two doses of 0.5% drops were given half-hourly in the one hour before cataract surgery, and three doses of 0.5% drops were given every five minutes immediately after surgery.

Studies have consistently shown that levofloxacin is better absorbed into the anterior chamber by the topical or oral route than ofloxacin by a two- to eightfold factor greater than ciprofloxacin. Moxifloxacin has given equally good penetration to levofloxacin. Moxifloxacin is the most active quinolone effective against methicillin-resistant *Staphylococcus aureus* (MRSA) that is not susceptible to levofloxacin and has better activity against streptococci.

Antibiotics have an inhibitory (bacteriostatic) and killing (bactericidal) effect on the bacterial cell. Bacteriostatic antibiotics, such as chloramphenicol, tetracycline, low-dose erythromycin, and sulphonamides bind to ribosomes to inhibit messenger RNA translation and, therefore, protein production. The bacterial cell cannot divide but remains viable, the killing effect depending on PMN cells and macrophages. Other antibiotics, such as penicillins and cephalosporins, which attach to penicillin-binding proteins, prevent cell wall formation, resulting in cell death. The aminoglycosides (gentamicin, tobramycin, and amikacin) bind to ribosomes irreversibly with a bactericidal effect not requiring PMNs. Laboratory testing involves assessing the minimum inhibitory concentration and minimum bactericidal concentration and usually refers to the MIC90 and the MBC90, when the values quoted reflect those likely to be found effective against 90% of the isolates.

GLOBE SIZE AND INTRAVITREAL INJECTIONS

Teichmann [2] and Fechner and Teichmann [3] have considered the variation in the volume of vitreous, from 1.7 to 16.5 mL, for globe sizes of axial lengths from 16 mm to 34 mm, respectively (2, 3). For the 90% of eyes that have an axial length between 21 mm and 26 mm, the expected volume of the whole globe varies from 4.2 to 9.2 mL, respectively, of which the vitreous constitutes 75% to 85%, giving an average value for the vitreous from 4.0 mL to 7.5 mL. For the average eye with an axial length of 23.5 mm, the globe volume would be 6.5 mL (vitreous volume of 5.2 mL). The effect of injecting an antibiotic would be to dilute the expected concentration (26 mm, 7 diopters [D]) in the myopic, long eye by approximately 38%.

OVERUSE OF TOPICAL DROPS

Excessive topical therapy with single or multiple drugs can result in toxic epitheliopathy, as shown in Figure S11.4.

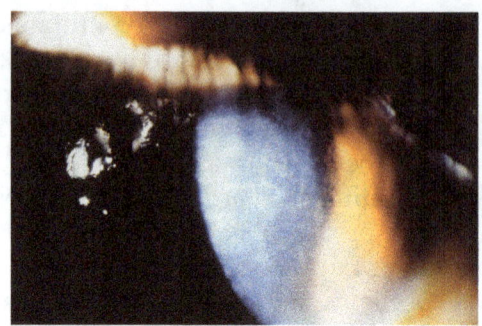

FIGURE S11.4 Toxic epitheliopathy induced by medication with drops.

Source: (Courtesy of Dr. D. Seal, London)

REFERENCES

1. Seal D, Pleyer U. Ocular Infection. 2nd ed. Informa Healthcare USA Inc. 2007. ISBN-10: 0-8493-9093-1.
2. Teichmann KD. J Cat Refract Surg 2002. PMID: 12388051 (https://doi.org/10.1016/s0886-3350(02)01671-1).
3. Fechner PU, Teichmann KD. Ocular Therapeutics—Pharmacology and Clinical Application. Thorofare, NJ, USA: Slack Inc. 1998: 11, pp 451–470.

PART 3
Appendices

Appendix 1: Drug Prescribing and Formularies

A variety of healthcare professionals are involved in the delivery of primary eye care, including family medical practitioners, medical practitioners with an ophthalmic qualification, optometrists, ophthalmic nurses and ophthalmologists. The role and scope of practice of these professionals varies considerably (Arnould et al. Eye 2024 PMID: 38472379 [https://doi.org/10.1038/s41433-024-03010-7]) (https://ecoo.info/).

Regarding therapeutic agents, medical practitioners use and prescribe medication in all jurisdictions within their scope of their professional practice. Access to diagnostic and therapeutic drugs by optometrists varies with geographical location. In Europe, the UK is the only country to allow optometrists to use and supply therapeutic agents. Under current medicines legislation, all UK optometrists are able to use diagnostic ophthalmic drugs, including mydriatics, cycloplegics and topical anaesthetics; they also use and supply topical antibiotics, chloramphenicol and fusidic acid and 'over-the-counter' ophthalmic formulations, such as lubricants, antihistamines and mast cell stabilisers.

In 2008, statutory legislation was introduced to enable UK optometrists who had undergone further training to prescribe any licensed medicine (except for controlled drugs or medicines for parenteral administration) for conditions affecting the eye and the surrounding tissues, within their recognised area of expertise and competence. The scope of optometrist-independent prescribing is informed by the College of Optometrists' Clinical Management Guidelines (CMGs), which provide evidence-based information on the diagnosis and management of eye conditions that present with varying frequency in primary and first-contact care (https://www.college-optometrists.org/clinical-guidance/clinical-management-guidelines). UK optometrists with an independent prescribing qualification need additional accreditation to manage glaucoma (Designing glaucoma care pathways using GLAUC-STRAT-FAST—College of Optometrists).

Evidence-based clinical guidelines for the management of ocular hypertension, open-angle glaucoma and angle closure glaucoma are available [1–3].

In other European countries, viz. Ireland, Switzerland, Finland, Norway, Sweden and the Netherlands, optometrists are permitted only to use diagnostic drugs; however, this is practiced in a limited number of other EU countries outside a legal framework [4]. In addition, there is no harmonisation for test standards for contact lens disinfecting solutions within the EU [5].

Optometrists in the USA can prescribe topical medication for ocular diseases, including glaucoma, while use of oral medication varies between different states. Australia and New Zealand allow optometrists to prescribe a range of topical and oral medications for eye conditions.

The following tables present commonly used drugs in ophthalmic primary care, grouped by their classification and use.

DIAGNOSTIC OPHTHALMIC DRUGS

By dilating the pupil, mydriatics facilitate ophthalmoscopic examination of the fundus. Short-acting antimuscarinic mydriatics, such as tropicamide, usually

DOI: 10.1201/9781003606789-25

achieve mydriasis within 20 minutes and last up to six hours. Since antimuscarinics bind to pigment, they may take longer to act on darker irises. Combining an antimuscarinic with the sympathomimetic phenylephrine produces more effective pupil dilation. Longer-acting mydriatics, including cyclopentolate hydrochloride and atropine, are used therapeutically to alleviate ciliary spasm or prevent posterior synechiae in anterior uveitis.

Cyclopentolate is mostly used to perform cycloplegic refraction in children to obtain an accurate assessment of refractive error. In this context, atropine is useful for very dark-eyed children, where the level of pigment prevents sufficient cycloplegia.

Topical ocular anaesthetics are used for diagnostic procedures involving contact between ophthalmic instruments and the eye—e.g. tonometry, pachymetry or gonioscopy. They are also used for corneal foreign body removal and minor surgical procedures.

Commonly used vital stains are fluorescein and lissamine green. Fluorescein is an orange-red powder that when dissolved in water becomes an intense, bright-yellow-green fluorescent dye that penetrates damaged corneal epithelial cells and can highlight areas of epithelial disruption or damage. It is also used topically in diagnostic procedures such as Goldman applanation tonometry. Lissamine green stains devitalised or dead cells and is preferred for conjunctival staining to diagnose and grade dry eye disease (DED).

Group	Drug (Formulation)	Action	Indication
MYDRIATIC	Tropicamide (0.5%, 1% eye drops)	Antimuscarinic	Mydriasis for fundoscopy
	Phenylephrine (2.5%, 10% eye drops)	Sympathomimetic	Mydriatic for fundoscopy
CYCLOPLEGIC	Atropine (1% eye drops)	Antimuscarinic	Cycloplegic refraction*
	Cyclopentolate (0.5%, 1% eye drops)	Antimuscarinic	Cycloplegic refraction
ANAESTHETIC	Tetracaine (0.5%, 1% eye drops)**	Ester-type topical anaesthesia	Applanation tonometry**
	Proxymetacaine 0.5% eye drops (proparacaine)	Ester-type topical anaesthesia	Applanation tonometry
	Oxybuprocaine (0.4% eye drops)	Ester-type topical anaesthetic	Applanation tonometry
	Lidocaine (4% eye drops)	Amide-type topical anaesthetic	Applanation tonometry

* Cycloplegics are also be used therapeutically to alleviate ciliary spasm or prevent posterior synechiae in anterior uveitis.

** Topical anaesthetics are also used for corneal foreign body and minor surgical procedures.

THERAPEUTIC OPHTHALMIC DRUGS

Anti-Infectives

There is a wide range of antibacterial ophthalmic drugs available that exert their effect by a variety of mechanisms, including acting on the bacterial cell wall, disrupting the plasma membrane or inhibiting bacterial protein or DNA synthesis. Broad-spectrum antibiotics—e.g. chloramphenicol and gentamicin—are typically used for treating superficial bacterial infections such as conjunctivitis. Topical fluoroquinolones—e.g. ofloxacin, ciprofloxacin and levofloxacin—are an established empirical treatment for suspected microbial keratitis. However, newer generation fluoroquinolone moxifloxacin has been shown to have superior activity against quinolone-resistant strains.

Antivirals are used in ophthalmology for the treatment of herpes simplex, varicella zoster and cytomegalovirus infections.

Group	Drug (Formulation)	Action	Indication
ANTIBIOTIC	Azithromycin (1.5% eye drops)	Macrolide antibiotic	Treatment of superficial bacterial infections
	Chloramphenicol (0.5% eye drops, 1% eye ointment)	Bacteriostatic antibiotic	Treatment of superficial bacterial infections
	Ciprofloxacin (0.3% eye drops, 0.3% eye ointment)	Fluoroquinolone antibiotic	Treatment of more serious eye infections, e.g. microbial keratitis
	Fusidic acid (1% viscous eye drop)	Bacteriostatic steroid antibiotic	Treatment of superficial bacterial infections (particularly *St. aureus*)
	Gentamicin (0.3% eye drops)	Aminoglycoside	Treatment of superficial infections of the eye and adnexa caused by susceptible bacteria
	Levofloxacin (0.5% eye drops)	Fluoroquinolone antibiotic	Treatment of more serious eye infections, e.g. microbial keratitis
	Moxifloxacin (0.5% eye drops)	Fluoroquinolone antibiotic	Treatment of more serious eye infections, e.g. microbial keratitis
	Ofloxacin (0.3% eye drops)	Fluoroquinolone antibiotic	Treatment of more serious eye infections, e.g. microbial keratitis
ANTISEPTIC	Povidone-iodine (5% eye drops)	Antiseptic	Post-procedural infection control
	Propamidine (0.1% eye drops)	Aromatic diamidine disinfectant	Treatment of minor bacterial infections (also has antifungal and anti-amoebic properties)
ANTIVIRAL	Aciclovir (30 mg/g eye ointment)	Synthetic nucleoside analogue	Topical treatment of herpes simplex keratitis
	Ganciclovir (0.15% eye gel)	Synthetic nucleoside analogue	Topical treatment of herpes simplex keratitis

CORTICOSTEROIDS AND OTHER ANTI-INFLAMMATORY PREPARATIONS

Topical corticosteroids are used for the treatment of inflammatory eye conditions such as uveitis or to reduce postoperative inflammation following surgery. Whilst there is no official potency hierarchy for topical ocular steroids, it is generally accepted that prednisolone acetate and dexamethasone are used when inflammation is severe and that prednisolone sodium phosphate, fluorometholone or loteprednol are used for mild inflammation. It is important to be aware of steroid-related ocular hypertension and glaucoma when using topical steroids [6] (refer to College of Optometrists' CMGs for—Steroid-related ocular hypertension and glaucoma).

Topical non-steroidal anti-inflammatory drugs (NSAIDs) are often used before surgery to prevent prostaglandin-mediated miosis and, postoperatively, as an alternative to steroid eye drops to avoid steroidal adverse effects. Topical NSAIDs are also used therapeutically in the treatment of inflammatory conditions of the anterior eye—e.g. episcleritis.

Topical mast cell stabilisers (MCS) and antihistamines, which reduce inflammatory mediator release or counteract their effects, are used as anti-allergy treatments in common allergic conditions, such as seasonal allergic conjunctivitis. Newer generation topical antihistamines—e.g. olopatadine—have dual-acting antihistamine and mast cell stabilising properties and require fewer applications to achieve symptomatic relief. Mast cell stabilisers—e.g. sodium cromoglicate—inhibit degranulation of mast cells by limiting the release of histamine and the other vasoactive mediators. Mast cell stabilisers are most effective when administered prior to the triggering of the allergic reaction and should, therefore, be used prophylactically.

Ciclosporin is an immunomodulatory drug that is used topically in the treatment of severe DED and sight-threatening allergic eye disease—e.g. atopic keratoconjunctivitis and vernal keratoconjunctivitis—when alternative treatments have failed to treat the underlying condition.

Group	Drug (Formulation)	Action	Indication
STEROIDS*	Betamethasone (0.1% eye drops)	Corticosteroid	To prevent or treat non-infectious inflammation of the eye
	Dexamethasone (0.1% eye drops	Corticosteroid	To prevent or treat non-infectious inflammation of the eye
	Fluorometholone (0.1% eye drops)	Corticosteroid	To prevent or treat non-infectious inflammation of the eye
	Loteprednol (0.5% eye drops)	Corticosteroid	To prevent or treat non-infectious inflammation of the eye
	Prednisolone (0.5%, 1% eye drops)	Corticosteroid	To prevent or treat non-infectious inflammation of the eye
NSAIDs	Diclofenac (0.1% eye drops)	Inhibition of cyclooxygenase (COX)-1 and-2	Reduction of perioperative miosis and postoperative inflammation, control of ocular pain and discomfort associated with corneal epithelial defects, relief of the ocular signs and symptoms of seasonal allergic conjunctivitis
	Bromfenac (900 µg/ml eye drops)	Inhibition of cyclooxygenase (COX)-1 and-2	Reduction of perioperative miosis and postoperative inflammation
	Flurbiprofen (0.03% eye drops)	Inhibition of cyclooxygenase (COX)-1 and-2	Reduction of perioperative miosis and postoperative inflammation
	Kerorolac (0.5% eye drops)	Inhibition of cyclooxygenase (COX)-1 and-2	Reduction of perioperative miosis and postoperative inflammation
ANTIHISTAMINES	Antazoline (0.5% eye drops)	Antihistamine	Treatment of seasonal and perennial allergic conditions
	Azelastine (0.05% eye drops)	Dual-acting antihistamine and MCS	Treatment of seasonal and perennial allergic conditions
	Ketotifen (0.025% eye drops)	Dual-acting antihistamine and MCS	Treatment of seasonal and perennial allergic conditions

(Continued)

(*Continued*)

Group	Drug (Formulation)	Action	Indication
	Olopatadine (0.1% eye drops)	Dual-acting antihistamine and MCS	Treatment of seasonal and perennial allergic conditions
MAST CELL STABILISERS	Sodium cromoglicate (2% eye drops)	MCS	Prophylaxis and symptomatic treatment of acute and chronic allergic conjunctivitis
	Lodoxamide (0.1% eye drops)	MCS	Prophylaxis and symptomatic treatment of acute and chronic allergic conjunctivitis
CICLOSPORIN	Ciclosporin (1mg/ml, eye drops)	Calcineurin inhibitor	Treatment of severe keratitis in dry eye disease and severe allergic eye disease

* *Corticosteroids are also available in fixed combinations with antibiotics—e.g. neomycin, tobramycin, polymyxin B.*

GLAUCOMA MEDICATIONS

Published clinical guidelines for primary open-angle glaucoma suggest that medical treatment (i.e. topical eye drops) is a reasonable first-line therapy for the majority of glaucoma patients. Clinicians usually initially prescribe a single intraocular pressure (IOP)-lowering medication (monotherapy), chosen from one of the following drug classes: prostaglandin analogues, beta-blockers, carbonic anhydrase inhibitors or alpha-2 adrenergic agonists. The highest reduction in IOP is obtained with prostaglandin analogues, e.g. Latanoprost, followed by non-selective beta-blockers, e.g. Timolol. If the initial therapy is ineffective or not tolerated, switching to another monotherapy is recommended, rather than adding a second drug. However, if the target IOP is not reached, then combination therapy, using drugs of different classes, can be considered. A number of fixed combinations are available, which typically combine a beta-blocker with a drug from one of the other therapeutic classes.

Oral acetazolamide is widely used in the emergency treatment of raised IOP following acute angle closure, in conjunction with other ocular hypotensive medications.

Group	Drug (Formulation)	Action	Indication
PROSTAGLANDIN AND PROSTAMIDE ANALOGUES	Latanoprost (50 µg/ml eye drops)	Increased uveoscleral aqueous outflow	Reduction of elevated intraocular pressure in patients with open-angle glaucoma and ocular hypertension
	Travoprost (10 µg/ml eye drops)	Increased uveoscleral aqueous outflow	Reduction of elevated intraocular pressure in patients with open-angle glaucoma and ocular hypertension
	Tafluprost (15 µg/ml eye drops)	Increased uveoscleral aqueous outflow	Reduction of elevated intraocular pressure in patients with open-angle glaucoma and ocular hypertension
	Bimatoprost (prostamide analogue) (100 µg/ml eye drops)	Increased uveoscleral aqueous outflow	Reduction of elevated intraocular pressure in patients with open-angle glaucoma and ocular hypertension

Group	Drug (Formulation)	Action	Indication
BETA-BLOCKERS	Timolol (0.5%, 0.1% eye drops)	Decreased aqueous humour production	Reduction of elevated intraocular pressure in patients with open-angle glaucoma and ocular hypertension
	Betaxolol (0.25% eye drops)*	Decreased aqueous humour production	Reduction of elevated intraocular pressure in patients with open-angle glaucoma and ocular hypertension
	Levobunolol (0.5% eye drops)	Decreased aqueous humour production	Reduction of elevated intraocular pressure in patients with open-angle glaucoma and ocular hypertension
CARBONIC ACID INHIBITORS	Dorzolomide (2% eye drops)	Decreased aqueous humour production	Reduction of elevated intraocular pressure in patients with open-angle glaucoma and ocular hypertension
	Brinzolomide (1% eye drops)	Decreased aqueous humour production	Reduction of elevated intraocular pressure in patients with open-angle glaucoma and ocular hypertension
	Acetazolamide (250 mg tablets)	Decreased aqueous humour production	Reduction of elevated intraocular pressure in patients with acute angle closure prior to referral for specialist treatment
MIOTICS	Pilocarpine (1%, 2% eye drops)	Increases aqueous outflow by contraction of the ciliary muscle and traction on the trabecular meshwork	Miotic, for reversing the action of weaker mydriatics and in the emergency treatment of glaucoma
RHO KINASE INHIBITORS	Netarsudil (50 µg/ml eye drops)	Increased trabecular outflow of aqueous and reduced episcleral venous pressure	Reduction of elevated intraocular pressure in patients with open-angle glaucoma and ocular hypertension
	Ripasudil (0.4% eye drops)	Increased trabecular outflow of aqueous	Reduction of elevated intraocular pressure in patients with open-angle glaucoma and ocular hypertension
ALPHA AGONISTS	Brimonidine (0.2% eye drops)	Decreased aqueous humour production	Reduction of elevated intraocular pressure in patients with open-angle glaucoma and ocular hypertension
	Apraclonidine (0.5% eye drops)	Decreased aqueous humour production and increased uveoscleral outflow	Control or prevention of post-surgical elevations in intraocular pressure that occur in patients after anterior segment laser surgery

* Non-selective beta-blocker

OCULAR LUBRICANTS AND OTHER DRY EYE PREPARATIONS

Ocular lubricants, available as eye drops, gels and ointments, are used to alleviate discomfort from conditions where the tear film is reduced or unstable, particularly DED. They are also used to prevent exposure keratitis in patients with eyelid abnormalities, such as ectropion. Lubricating eye ointments may be applied at night or used to lubricate the ocular surface in cases of recurrent corneal epithelial erosion.

Acetylcysteine is a mucolytic agent that is used in the treatment of filamentary keratitis and other ocular conditions characterised by abnormal mucus production.

Preservative-free eye drops are recommended for patients with conditions that require frequent use of lubricating drops due to the risk of preservative toxicity. Similarly, contact lenses should not be worn when preserved eye drops are used.

Group	Drug (Formulation)	Action	Indication
LUBRICANTS*	Hypromellose (0.3%, 0.5% eye drops)	Inert, viscoelastic polymer	Low-viscosity lubricant for the treatment of mild tear deficiency or unstable tear film
	Polyvinyl alcohol (1.4% eye drops)	Water-soluble synthetic polymer	Low-viscosity lubricant for the treatment of mild tear deficiency or unstable tear film
	Carbomers (0.2% eye gel)	Hydrophilic, high molecular weight polymer of acrylic acid	Medium-viscosity lubricant for the treatment of mild tear deficiency or unstable tear film
	Sodium hyaluronate (0.1%, 0.2%, 0.4% eye drops)	Sodium salt of hyaluronic acid	Medium-viscosity lubricant for the treatment of mild tear deficiency or unstable tear film
	Carmellose (0.5%, 1% eye drops)	Inert, viscoelastic polymer	Medium-viscosity lubricant for the treatment of mild tear deficiency or unstable tear film
	Macrogols (eye gel)	Polyethylene glycol 400 (PEG 400) and propylene glycol, hydroxypropyl guar	Medium-viscosity lubricant for the treatment of mild tear deficiency or unstable tear film
	Liquid paraffin (eye ointment)	Mineral oil and lanolin alcohol	Lubrication and protection of the eye in conditions such as exposure keratitis, recurrent corneal erosions and keratoconjunctivitis sicca
MUCOLYTIC	Acetylcysteine (5% eye drops)	Synthetic acetylated derivative of the amino acid L-cysteine	Relief of dry-eye diseaseassociated with deficient tear secretion and impaired or abnormal mucus production

* Preservative-free formulations are widely available.

SYSTEMIC MEDICATION USED IN OPHTHALMOLOGY

Although most pharmacological interventions used in ophthalmology involve the use of topical preparations, there are several ophthalmic indications for systemic medication. The following table includes a selection of drugs that are commonly used in the treatment of ocular conditions.

Group	Drug (Formulation)	Action	Indication
SYSTEMIC ANTIBIOTICS	Doxycycline (50 mg, 100 mg capsules)	Broad-spectrum antibiotic belonging to the tetracycline class. Its primary action is to inhibit bacterial protein synthesis. It can also inhibit the production of pro-inflammatory mediators, which makes it useful in treating inflammatory conditions such as ocular rosacea.	Doxycycline has been found to be clinically effective in the treatment of a variety of infections caused by susceptible strains of Gram-positive and Gram-negative bacteria. Most used in ophthalmology for the treatment of posterior blepharitis and ocular rosacea.
	Minocycline (50 mg, 100 mg tablets)	As previously mentioned	Minocycline has been found to be clinically effective in the treatment of a variety of infections caused by susceptible strains of Gram-positive and Gram-negative bacteria. It has a spectrum of activity similar to other tetracyclines but is more active against *Staphylococcus aureus*.
	Azithromycin (250 mg, 500 mg tablets)	Macrolide antibiotic that works by inhibiting bacterial protein synthesis	Used in the treatment of skin and soft tissue infections in adults and children
	Erythromycin (250 mg, 500 mg tablets)	As previously mentioned	As previously mentioned
	Amoxicillin (250 mg, 500 mg capsules)	Broad-spectrum antibiotic belonging to the penicillin class. Its primary action is to inhibit the synthesis of bacterial cell walls.	For the treatment of bacterial infections by susceptible organisms NOT effective against *St. aureus* (susceptible to penicillinase)
SYSTEMIC ANTIHISTAMINES	Cetirizine (10 mg tablet)	Non-sedating antihistamine	For the control of the symptoms of hay fever including ocular symptoms
	Cholorphenamine (4 mg tablet)	Antihistamine	For the control of the symptoms of hay fever including ocular symptoms
CARBONIC ACID INHIBITOR	Acetazolomide (250 mg tablet)	Reduction of aqueous secretion	Emergency treatment of acute-angle closure

REFERENCES

1. NICE. Glaucoma: Diagnosis and Management. NICE Guideline NG81 2022. Accessed 18/08/25 (https://www.nice.org.uk/guidance/ng81/).
2. European Glaucoma Society. Terminology and Guidelines for Glaucoma. 5th ed. 2020. Accessed 18/08/25 (https://www.eugs.org/).
3. Royal College of Ophthalmologists. Management of Angle Closure Glaucoma Guideline 2022. Accessed 18/8/25 (https://www.rcophth.ac.uk/resources-listing/management-of-angle-closure-glaucoma-guideline/).

4. European Council of Optometry and Optics. Blue Book 2020. Accessed 18/08/25 (https://ecoo.info/wp-content/uploads/2022/02/ECOO_BlueBook_2020-compressed_png.pdf).
5. Bradley CS et al. Clin Optom (Auckl). 2021. PMID: 34522149 (https://doi.org/10.2147/OPTO.S235679. eCollection 2021).
6. College of Optometrists. Clinical Management Guidelines. Steroid-Related Ocular Hypertension and Glaucoma 2025. Accessed 03/09/25.

Appendix 2: Infection Control in Clinical Settings

Patients receiving treatment within a clinic environment are at risk of contracting an infection from another patient or from a healthcare worker. Such an unexpected outcome can arise from contact with the practitioner's hands or from ophthalmic equipment in contact with the eye. Courteous handshakes should be avoided.

Adenovirus is a highly contagious virus that can rapidly cross-infect others. Patients with acutely infected eyes, particularly with haemorrhagic conjunctivitis (due to enterovirus 70 or coxsackie A24v), should always be segregated. They should be examined, *wearing disposable gloves,* in a separate room where equipment can be carefully disinfected between patients.

Hand-washing: perform before and after handling the lids of any infected eye using an antiseptic impregnated liquid soap preparation from an elbow- or floor-operated container. Such hand-wash preparations include 10% povidone-iodine (Betadine scrub), which is bactericidal and virucidal, or 4% chlorhexidine (Hibiscrub), which is only bactericidal and ineffective against adenovirus. Hand-washing should be practised with both soap and an alcoholic hand rub, which is virucidal (Figures A2.1, A2.2, A2.3).

Slit lamp microscope and other equipment: the head rim and chin rest should be wiped with a disposable alcoholic rub.

Eye drops: only single-use should be used in clinics.

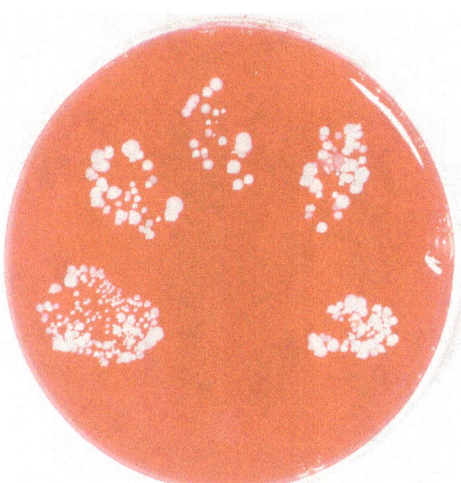

FIGURE A2.1 Bacterial culture of fingertips that have NOT been washed.

DOI: 10.1201/9781003606789-26

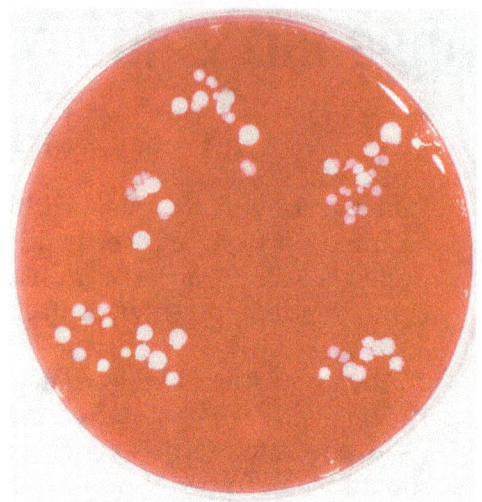

FIGURE A2.2 Bacterial culture of fingertips washed with soap.

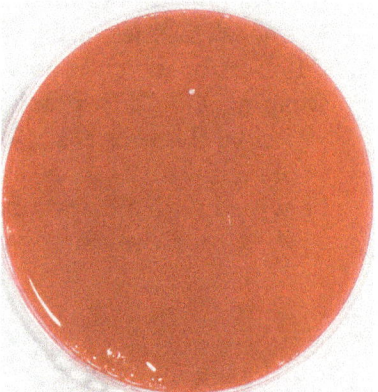

FIGURE A2.3 Culture of fingertips washed with soap *followed by an alcoholic rub.*

Appendix 3: Detailed Diagram of Immunity against Infection in the Cornea

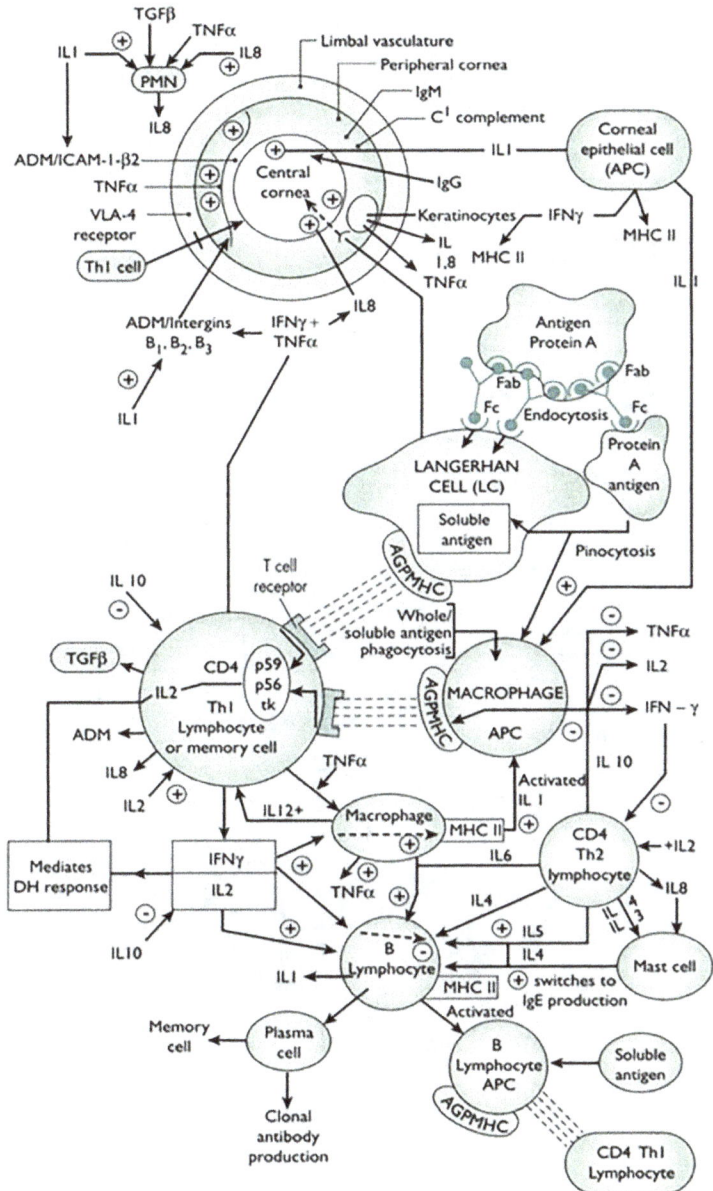

FIGURE A3.1 Immunity against infection in the cornea with *St. aureus* as the example antigen. ADM: adhesion molecules. IL: interleukin. AGPMHC: antigenic oligopeptide MHC (major histocompatibility complex) group. APC: antigen-presenting cells. CD: cluster-determinant antigen. IFN: interferon. PMN: polymorphonuclear cell. Th: T helper lymphocyte. TNF: tumour necrosis factor. VLA: very late antigen (super IgG receptor). Tk: tyrosine kinase p59 and p56.

Source: (Seal D, Pleyer U. Ocular Infection, 2nd Edition 2007)

DOI: 10.1201/9781003606789-27

Appendix 4: Classic and Alternative Complement Pathways

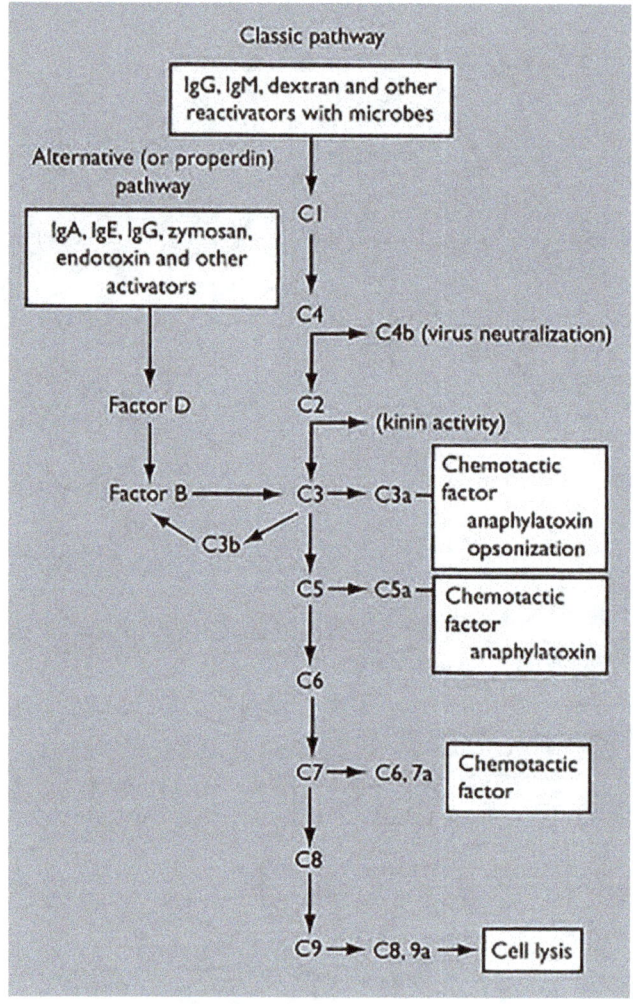

FIGURE A4.1 Classic and alternative complement pathways.

Source: (Seal D, Pleyer U. Ocular Infection, 2nd Edition 2007)

DOI: 10.1201/9781003606789-28

Appendix 5: Corneal Scrape and Laboratory Testing

HOW TO PERFORM A CORNEAL SCRAPE AND CULTURE FOR MICROBIAL KERATITIS

A blade is best for a corneal scrape, but calcium alginate swabs can be used instead except for deep stromal infection, when a biopsy may be needed. Scrapes are best obtained following one drop of unpreserved proparacaine, which has the least inhibitory effect on bacterial growth. Preservatives will inhibit bacterial replication, while some anaesthetics have intrinsic antimicrobial properties. In children under 5 years, sedation is useful.

The surface material from the ulcer should be debrided using a swab. This material may be plated onto culture medium but is less helpful since it contains mostly cellular debris and mucus. The second scrape should be taken for microscopy and the third for culture. Using a Kimura spatula, a large-gauge sterile needle or a disposable surgical blade, the base and edge of the ulcer is firmly scraped as most likely to yield organisms. A freshly sterile instrument is used for each sample. In the presence of deep ulceration, a small trephine may be used to obtain an adequate specimen; another method is to pass a 6–0 silk suture through the affected area.

Some bacteria are found at the edge of an active ulcer (*Streptococcus pneumoniae, Pseudomonas aeruginosa*), while others are often found within the corneal ulcer (*Moraxella sp.*). The material gathered should be firmly spread on to a clean glass slide, to create a thin film, which is air dried; refer to stains later. The second scrape should be similarly used, but emulsified in a drop of saline, or lactophenol blue, to make a wet preparation under a coverslip for *Acanthamoeba*, if suspected. The third scrape should be spread on to blood and 'chocolate' agar for bacteria and Sabouraud's agar for fungi. Fluid media (preferably brain-heart infusion or thioglycollate broth) should be inoculated with the same blade to allow microaerophilic culture. Thioglycollate broth can be used as both a transport and growth medium for actinomycetes of lacrimal canaliculitis and other microbes requiring microaerophilic growth conditions.

In addition, specialised media should be inoculated for mycobacteria if the keratitis is chronic, although the atypical *Mycobacterium chelonae* will grow on blood agar incubated for one week at 37°C. Culture media for bacteria are incubated at 37°C for 48 hours, ideally in 5% CO_2, and for fungi at 30°C for three weeks.

When *Acanthamoeba* keratitis is suspected, a specimen should also be collected for culture on appropriate media (non-nutrient agar seeded with live or killed *E. coli*) incubated at 30°C for one week.

For a chronic ulcer, blood agar should be incubated for one week in 4% CO_2 to facilitate growth of *Nocardia sp.* Anaerobic cultures should be considered when there is an unsatisfactory response to therapy; *Propionibacterium acnes* requires up to 14 days for growth.

Gram Stain for an Air-Dried Slide From a Corneal Scrape

The Gram stain is used to differentiate bacteria into two groups: Gram-positive and Gram-negative, based on the structure of their cell walls. The procedure

DOI: 10.1201/9781003606789-29

involves a series of staining steps that allow for the visualization of bacterial morphology and cell wall characteristics under a microscope.

Step 1: The air-dried slide from the corneal scrape is flooded with crystal violet, a basic dye that stains all bacteria purple. The stain is left on for one minute, after which the slide is rinsed gently with water to remove excess dye.

Step 2: Iodine is added to the slide, acting as a mordant that forms a complex with the crystal violet, making it more insoluble and enhancing its retention in the bacterial cell wall. The iodine is left on the slide for one minute, followed by another rinse with water.

Step 3: A decolourizing agent, often a mixture of ethanol and acetone, is applied drop by drop until the purple colour stops running out. This step is critical, as it differentiates between Gram-positive and Gram-negative bacteria. Gram-positive bacteria retain the crystal violet-iodine complex due to their thick peptidoglycan layer, while Gram-negative bacteria lose the stain because of their thinner peptidoglycan layer and outer membrane.

Step 4: After decolourization, the slide is stained with neutral red or safranin, a red counterstain. This step ensures that Gram-negative bacteria, which have lost the primary blue stain, appear pink or red, while Gram-positive bacteria remain purple.

Step 5: The slide is rinsed with water to remove any excess counterstain and then examined under a microscope with a × 100 lens and oil immersion. The bacteria visualised are classified as cocci or rods and Gram-positive (blue) (see Figures A5.1–A5.3) or Gram-negative (red) (see Figure A5.4); their morphology allows provisional identification, especially for the Gram-positive cocci (GPC), clusters being staphylococci and chains being streptococci. The Gram stain also stains fungi, including yeasts (*Candida sp.*) and hyphae. Sunlight makes an excellent light source for the microscope mirror.

The Gram stain of a corneal scrape is an invaluable and cheap tool for making an early diagnosis of microbial keratitis and establishing the type of infection, particularly if it is mixed between bacteria and fungi in the tropics. It can also be performed without electricity!

Modified Ziehl–Neelsen Stain for *Nocardia sp.* on a Corneal Scrape

The modified Ziehl–Neelsen stain is used to identify *Nocardia sp.* because these bacteria are partially acid-fast only and are decolourised with the strong (20%) acid/alcohol used in the full-strength stain. This technique differentiates nocardia from other bacteria and is a critical step in diagnosing it as an opportunistic infection in the cornea (see Figure S6.9).

Method:

Primary stain: add carbol fuchsin for five minutes to stain the bacteria bright red (heating the slide is not necessary as for mycobacteria). Rinse gently with water.

Decolourize: add a weak acid (1% sulfuric acid) to decolourize the corneal scrape (as opposed to 20% for mycobateria) for five *seconds*. Rinse gently with water.

Counterstain: add methylene blue for three minutes, which stains the non-acid-fast background and other bacteria blue. Rinse gently with water and allow to air dry before viewing.

Examine: place the slide under a microscope with an oil immersion lens at × 100. The nocardia bacteria are seen as pink, filamentous, branching rods against a blue background (see Figure A5.5).

ACRIDINE ORANGE STAIN FOR BACTERIA ON A CORNEAL SCRAPE

Acridine orange is a fluorescent stain used in microscopy to detect bacteria by intercalating into their nucleic acids, causing bacteria to appear as bright, orange-red bodies. It is a sensitive and rapid method that can be more effective than the Gram stain for screening when bacterial loads are low. The staining requires a fluorescent microscope and works best at an acidic pH, where it differentiates bacteria from host cells and debris (see Figure A5.6).

Examples of stained bacteria are shown below

Bacteria

Staphylococcus aureus (GPC) (laboratory culture; Figure A5.1).

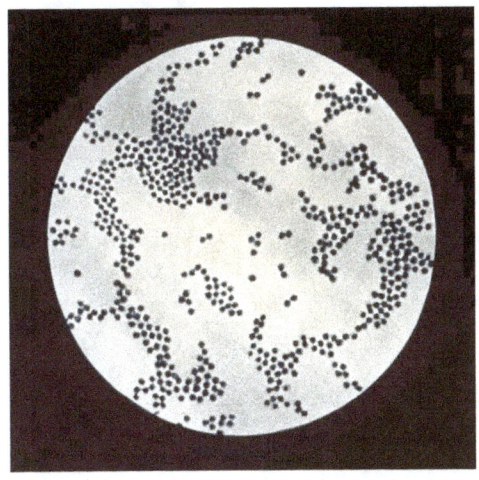

FIGURE A5.1 Gram stain showing GPC in clusters.

Source: (Courtesy of Dr. D. Seal, London)

- *Streptococcus pyogenes* (GPC) (laboratory culture; Figures A5.2 and A5.3).

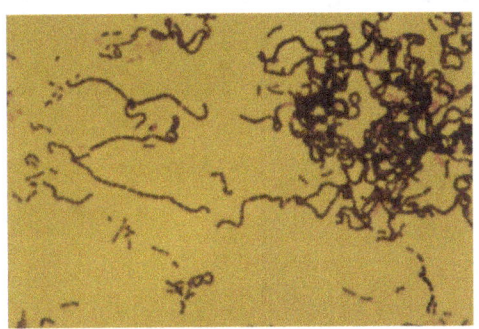

FIGURE A5.2 Gram stain showing GPC in chains.

Source: (Courtesy of Dr. D. Seal, London)

Arachnia propionica (GPR) (pus from the lacrimal canaliculus).

FIGURE A5.3 Elongated characteristic Gram-positive rods (GPR) of *Arachnia propionica* from dacrocystitis.

Source: (Courtesy of Dr. D. Seal, London)

- *Moraxella sp.* (corneal scrape; Figure A5.4).

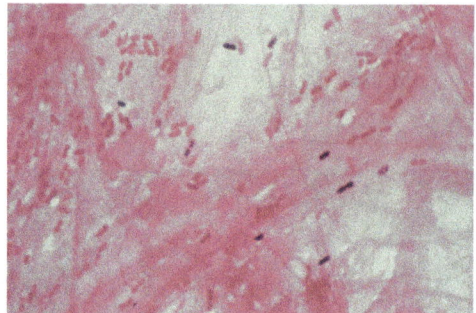

FIGURE A5.4 Short Gram-negative rods (GNR) from keratitis.

Source: (Courtesy of Dr. D. Seal, London)

- *Nocardia sp.* (corneal scrape; Figure A5.5).

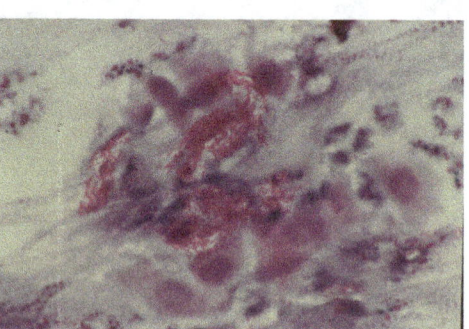

FIGURE A5.5 Carbol-fuchsin staining red bacteria of *Nocardia sp.* against corneal scrape material.

Source: (Courtesy of Dr. D. Seal, London)

- Modified Ziehl–Neelsen stain [L] and acridene orange stain [R] of a corneal scrape (Figure A5.6).

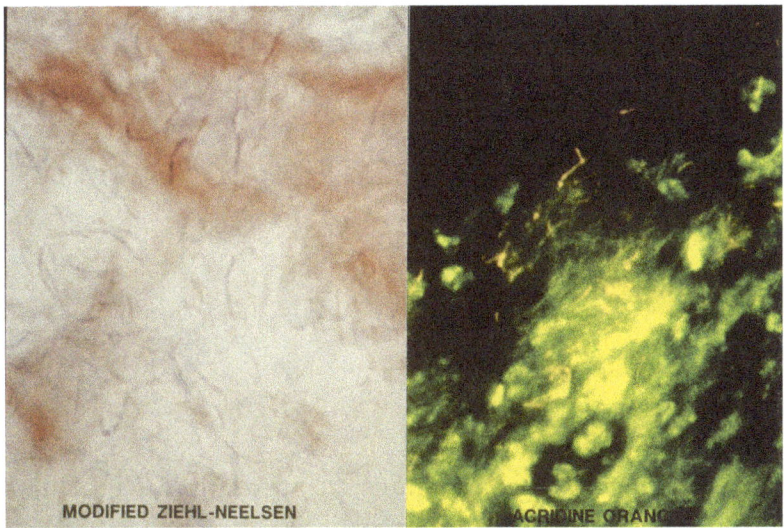

FIGURE A5.6 *Nocarida sp.* staining red [L], staining yellow [R].

Source: (Courtesy of Dr. D. Seal, London)

Wet Preparation for a Corneal Scrape

Use a clean slide with one drop of lactophenol blue for fungal hyphae (Figures A5.7 and A5.8) or saline (for *Acanthamoeba*) (Figure A5.9). The blade or needle can be agitated into a drop of saline in a sterile tube or rubbed into the saline drop on the slide if an adequate specimen. Place a clean cover slip on top of the drop and examine under the microscope. Amoebae and fungi are larger than bacteria and can be seen under the ×40 objective lens.

- Lactophenol blue stain for fungi (wet preparation) of a corneal scrape.

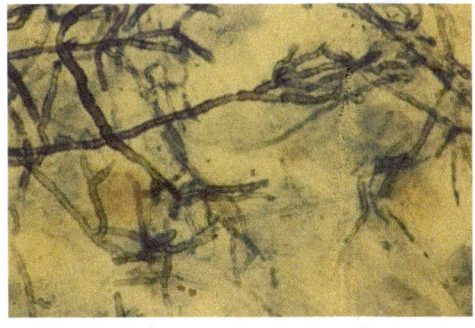

FIGURE A5.7 Lactophenol blue stain showing branching septate hyphae of *Curvularia sp.*

Source: (Seal & Pleyer, Ocular Infection, 2007)

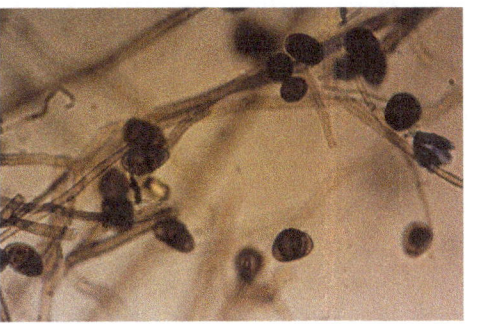

FIGURE A5.8 High-power view of *Curvularia sp.* showing brown conidia with transverse septa.

Source: (Seal & Pleyer, Ocular Infection, 2007)

Acanthamoeba seen in a wet preparation.

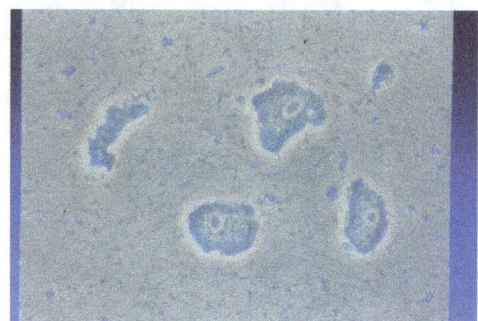

FIGURE A5.9 *Acanthamoeba* trophozoites stained with wet lactophenol blue.

Source: (Courtesy of Dr. D. Seal, London)

Thioglycollate broth:
   This broth can be used both as a transport medium and as a culture medium for micro-aerophilic bacteria (Figure A5.10).

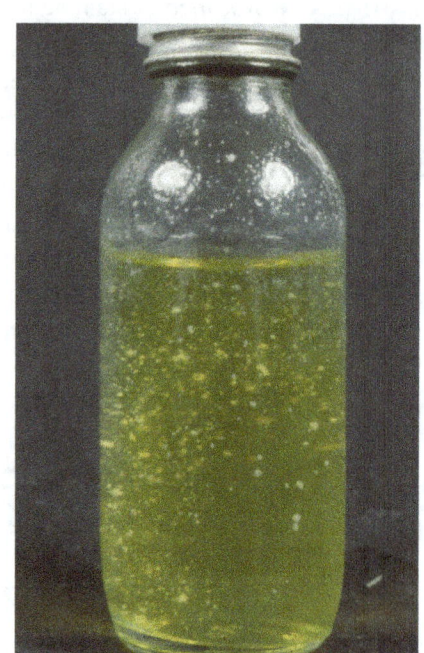

FIGURE A5.10 Bread-crumb colonies of *Arachnia propionica* in thioglycollate broth.

Source: (Seal & Pleyer, Ocular Infection, 2007)

RAPID TESTS USING DNA TECHNOLOGY

   PCR (polymerase chain reaction) test kits are available for field work for bacteria, viruses, chlamydia, protozoan and filarial infections, as well as rapid diagnosis of difficult-to-culture bacteria, viz. *Mycobacterium tuberculosis*

   (*https://www.gov.uk/government/news/new-study-shows-mhra-collaboration-with-hospital-dna-sequencing-service-cuts-time-to-diagnose-infections*).

QUANTIFERON TUBERCULOSIS TEST

The QuantiFERON-TB Gold test, also known as the IGRA (interferon-gamma release assay) test, is a blood test used to detect immune responses to tuberculosis (TB) infection. It is more advanced and faster than the traditional skin test and is not affected by previous BCG vaccinations, making its results more reliable. The test involves taking a blood sample and mixing it with substances that simulate bacteria. If the immune cells in the blood react, it indicates a *Mycobacterium tuberculosis* infection.

The QuantiFERON-TB Gold Plus (QFT-Plus) assay is an *in vitro* diagnostic test that uses a peptide cocktail to stimulate cells in heparinised whole blood. Detection of interferon-gamma by ELISA is used to identify responses to these peptide antigens associated with infection by *Mycobacterium tuberculosis*. Samples for the test must be kept at room temperature and reach the laboratory within 16 hours of collection to ensure accurate results. The QuantiFERON-TB Gold test is particularly suitable for screening large numbers of healthy people in contact tracing or health screening programs (https://www.qiagen.com/kr/products/diagnostics-and-clinical-research/infectious-disease/quantiferon-tb-gold-test).

Appendix 6: Formulary of Drugs for Ocular Use in Specialist Care

Drugs for use in ocular conditions [specialist use for licensed prescribers worldwide]

ANTI-INFECTIVES

a) Antibiotics (effectivity against specific bacteria)

GROUP	DRUG	ACTION	USE
G+veC: Gram-positive cocci	G-veR: Gram-negative rods	TRIC: Trachoma and Inclusion Conjunctivitis	
ANTIBIOTIC (anti-bacterial)	Amoxicillin oral	Bactericidal on cell wall	Streptococci, Haemophilus, G-veR (NOT for *St. aureus, Ps. aeruginosa*)
	Amoxicillin/clavulanic acid (co-amoxiclav)	Bactericidal on cell wall	As for amoxicillin but including *St. aureus*
	Flucloxacillin oral	Bactericidal on cell wall	*St. aureus*, Streptococci (NOT for G-veR and *Ps. aeruginosa*)
	Fusidic acid 1% w/w viscous eye drop	Bacteriostatic inhibits protein synthesis Has anti-inflammatory cyclosporin-like activity	*St. aureus* ONLY. Used to treat rosacea blepharitis (associated with *St. aureus*)
	Erythromycin 0.5% eye ointment, oral	Bacteriostatic macrolide inhibits protein synthesis	*St. aureus*, Streptococci, *P. acnes*, Haemophilus, Neisseria, Chlamydia, Mycoplasma, *Treponema pallidum*. (NOT for G-veR including *Ps. aeruginosa*)
	Azithromycin eye drops 1.5% UK, 1.0% USA, oral	Bacteriostatic macrolide inhibits protein synthesis	More active and broader spectrum than erythromycin. Used for TRIC treatment and eradication (NOT for G-veR and *Ps. aeruginosa*)
	Doxycycline oral	Bacteriostatic (tetracycline) inhibits protein synthesis	Broad spectrum G+veC and G-veR (NOT for *Ps. aeruginosa*)
	Minocycline oral	Bacteriostatic (tetracycline) inhibits protein synthesis	*P. acnes* (use only for meibomianitis and acne treatment)

DOI: 10.1201/9781003606789-30

GROUP	DRUG	ACTION	USE
	Chloramphenicol 0.5% eye drops, 1% eye ointment	Bacteriostatic inhibits protein synthesis	Broad spectrum G+veC and G-veR (NOT for *Ps. aeruginosa*)
	Gentamicin 0.3% eye drops	Bactericidal aminoglycoside	*St. aureus,* G-veR and *Ps. aeruginosa* (NOT for streptococci)
	Cipro/Ofloxacin 0.3% eye drops, oral for sight-threatening conditions only	Bactericidal fluoroquinolone	*St. aureus,* Streptococci, Neisseria, G-veR and *Ps. aeruginosa*
	Levofloxacin 0.5% eye drops, oral for sight-threatening conditions only	Bactericidal fluoroquinolone	*St. aureus,* Streptococci, Neisseria and G-veR (NOT for *Ps. aeruginosa*)
	Moxifloxacin 0.5% eye drops, oral for sight-threatening conditions only	Bactericidal fluoroquinolone	Enhanced activity against *St. aureus,* Streptococci, G+veC, Neisseria, G-veR inc. *Ps. aeruginosa* and *Mycobacterium chelonae.* Broad spectrum. Use as first line treatment until bacterial type known
	Auromox Moxifloxacin 0.5 mg (Aurolabs, Madurai—625 020, Tamil Nadu, India.)		For routine intracameral injection of 0.5 mg in 0.1 ml at the time of cataract surgery to prevent postoperative endophthalmitis
	Aprocam Cefuroxime 1 mg (Théa Pharmaceuticals, Clermont-Ferrand, 63100, France)		For routine intracameral injection of 1.0 mg in 0.1 ml at the time of cataract surgery to prevent postoperative endophthalmitis
	Polymyxin B sulphate eye drop (included in combination with other products in some countries)	Bactericidal on cell membrane	G-veR ONLY including *Ps. aeruginosa*
	Polymyxin B/trimethoprim	Trimethoprim blocks synthesis of bacterial nucleic acids and proteins in G+veC	Broad spectrum for treating bacterial conjunctivitis including G+veC and G-veR including *Ps. aeruginosa*
	Propamidine 0.1% eye drops and ointment or Dibromopropamidine 0.15%	Bacteriostatic diamidine against cell membrane	G+veC ONLY. (Only use In combination with PHMB or Chlorhexidine for *Acanthamoeba*)

b) Anti-fungal drugs for ocular use

GROUP	DRUG	ACTION	USE
Imidazole	Clotrimazole eye drops 1%	Inhibits synthesis of ergosterol causing fungus cell membrane to leak—dose dependant whether fungistatic or fungicidal	Drug of choice for *Aspergillus* keratitis, broad spectrum except for *Fusarium*
	Miconazole eye drops 1% (also IV and intra-vitreal)	"	Broad spectrum but *NOT* for *Fusarium*.
	Econazole eye drops 1%	"	Broad spectrum against filamentous fungi especially Fusarium. NOT for Candida sp.
	Ketoconazole eye drops 1%, oral	"	Broad spectrum, give as eye drops and oral. Use as first line treatment until fungus type known
Triazole	Voriconazole eye drops 1%, oral (also IV and intra-vitreal)	Fungicidal	Broad spectrum including Candida sp. and especially effective against Aspergillus sp. Also effective against *Acanthamoeba*
	Fluconazole eye drops 1% (oral, IV)	"	*Candida sp.*, *Cryptococcus sp.* only *NOT* for use against filamentous fungi
	Itraconazole eye drops 1% (oral 200 mg/day)	"	Broad spectrum including *Aspergillus sp.* and *Candida sp.* NOT for *Fusarium*.
Anti-metabolite (Pyrimidine)	5-flucytosine eye drops 1%, oral	Converted into fluorouracil inside fungal cells, inhibiting synthesis of DNA and RNA (fungicidal)	*Candida sp.*, *Cryptococcus sp.* but NOT for use against filamentous fungi
Polyene	Natamycin (Pimaricin) eye drops 5%	Inhibits fungal growth (fungicidal) by interacting with ergosterol in the cell membrane inhibiting transport proteins	*Candida sp.*, *Cryptococcus sp.* and mycelial fungi including *Fusarium sp.* Preferred first line treatment for filamentous fungi **
	Amphotericin B eye drops 0.15/0.3%	Inhibits fungal growth (fungistatic/fungicidal) by binding to ergosterol causing membrane permeability leakage	Effective against a wide range of fungi (*Candida sp.* and mycelium), penetrates deep corneal stroma but can be toxic
	Nystatin eye drops 50,000 U/ml (eye ointment 100,000 U/ml)	Similar mechanism but less active	*Candida sp.*, other yeasts but NOT for use against filamentous fungi
Biguanide (antiseptic)	Chlorhexidine (bis-biguanide) eye drops 0.2%	Leakage of cytoplasmic components and the formation of irreversible precipitates with intracellular ATP and nucleic acids - fungicidal	Use as second line therapy (*Candida* and mycelial fungi including *Fusarium*) */** Also effective against most bacteria—bactericidal at 0.2%. Beware toxicity

*   Arunga S, Tumu Mbarak, Ebong A, Mu J, Kuguminkiriza D, Abeer H. A. Mohamed-Ahmed, et al. Chlorhexidine gluconate 0.2% as a treatment for recalcitrant fungal keratitis in Uganda: a pilot study. BMJ open ophthalmology. 2021 Jul 1;6(1):e000698–8. (https://doi.org/10.1136/bmjophth-2020-000698).

** Hoffman JJ, Yadav R, Sanyam SD, Chaudhary P, Roshan A, Singh SK, et al. Topical Chlorhexidine 0.2% versus Topical Natamycin 5% for the Treatment of Fungal Keratitis in Nepal: A Randomized Controlled Noninferiority Trial. Ophthalmology [Internet]. 2022 May 1 [cited 2022 Oct 11];129(5):530–41. (https://doi.org/10.1016/j.ophtha.2021.12.004).

c) Anti-viral drugs for ocular use

GROUP	DRUG	ACTION	USE
ANTI-VIRAL	Trifluorothymidine (F3T) (Viroptic) 1% eye drops	Fluorinated pyrimidine nucleoside with antiviral activity against herpes simplex virus types 1 and 2	Primary and recurrent epithelial keratitis caused by Herpes simplex virus.
	Aciclovir 3% eye drops, 3% eye ointment, oral	Effective against Herpes simplex and Herpes zoster viruses	Use only for Herpes virus infections. Use by IV route for acute retinal necrosis due to Herpes viruses
	Famciclovir oral	Effective against Herpes simplex and Herpes zoster viruses	High oral doses used for acute retinal necrosis due to Herpes viruses and non-responders
	Ganciclovir 0.15% eye gel, IV and intravitreal	Effective against herpes and cytomegalovirus	Used to treat Herpes infections and CMV retinitis by IV and intra-vitreal routes

d) Anti-parasitic and -protozoal drugs for ocular use

INFECTION	DRUG	ACTION	USE
Onchocerca volvulus Parasitic nematode	Ivermectin 150 µg/kg, taken orally as a single dose every 6–12 months. Repeated treatment is needed to control onchocerciasis to reduce morbidity and lower transmission rates	Kills microfilariae, but *not* adult worms, by binding to chloride channels in nerve and muscle cells leading to an increase in chloride-ion influx, to paralyse the filariae	Alleviates severe itching and reduces inflammation with blindness. Inhibits production of microfilariae by adult female worms for 8 weeks
Loa loa Parasitic nematode	Ivermectin 400 µg/kg, taken orally as a single dose; lower doses are less effective. Careful monitoring is needed. Diethylcarbamazine (DEC) 8–10 mg/kg/day, given orally in three divided doses for 21 days***. For prophylaxis in long-term travellers to endemic areas, give one dose of 300 mg per week	Kills microfilariae, but *not* adult worms, similarly to *Onchocerca volvulus* but has a more rapid filaricidal effect Patients in West Africa can have dual infection with *Onchocerca volvulus* Diethylcarbamazine kills worms and microfilariae, causes bad allergic reactions	Individuals with high *Loa loa* microfilaraemia (over 30,000/mL) given ivermectin can suffer serious adverse events, especially encephalopathy, due to rapid death of microfilariae Use prednisolone to manage allergic reactions
Toxolasma gondii Parasitic protozoa with cysts	Pyrimethamine 100 mg stat, 25 mg/day for 4 to 6 weeks (or Trimethoprim, Atavaquone or Tetracycline) *plus* sulphadiazine 2 g stat oral, 1G qds for 4–6 weeks + folinic acid oral (5–15 mgs daily)	Pyrimethamine and Trimethoprim inhibit dihydrofolate reductase. Sulphonamide inhibits dihydropteroate synthetase Both inhibit folic acid metabolism	Treatment of retinal toxoplasmosis**** In addition, can use intravitreal clindamycin
Toxocara canis Parasitic worm— human is accidental host with systemic larvae (do not become worms)	Ivermectin (single dose refer above) or Albendazole (400 mg bd oral for 4 weeks plus corticosteroids), mebendazole or tiabendazole***** or DEC	Albendazole prevents the larvae and from absorbing glucose, causing them to lose energy and die	Treat if the retinal lesion (second stage larva) is close to the macula Use prednisolone to manage allergy

*** (https://www.cdc.gov/filarial-worms/hcp/clinical-care/loiasis.html)
**** (https://pmc.ncbi.nlm.nih.gov/articles/PMC7961948/)
***** (https://patient.info/doctor/toxocariasis)

e) Anti-Acanthamoeba drugs for ocular use (refer to Chapter 6 for specialist use)

GROUP	DRUG	ACTION	USE
Biguanides	Chlorhexidine (bis-biguanide) eye drops 0.02% Can be given up to a maximum of 0.2% Beware toxicity	Acts on the cytoplasmic membrane causing leakage of cellular components—kills trophozoites and cysts	Acanthamoeba keratitis Also effective against most bacteria—bacteriostatic at 0.02%
	PHMB—Polyhexanide (polyhexamethylene biguanide) eye drops 0.02%. Marketed at 0.08% as Akantior in the EU by Sifi, St Antonio, Sicily, Italy	Acts on the cytoplasmic membrane causing leakage of cellular components—kills trophozoites and cysts	Acanthamoeba keratitis Used commercially as a swimming pool disinfectant
Diamidines	Propamidine (Brolene) eye drops 0.1% Dibromopropamidine eye ointment	Disrupts the cell membrane leading to the leakage of essential amino acids. *Inhibits* trophozoites but does *not* kill cysts Bacteriostatic against *Streptococci*, *Staphylococci* and some Gram-negative bacilli	Used *ONLY* in combination with a biguanide for Acanthamoeba keratitis treatment It is *not* effective as monotherapy
	Hexamidine (eye drops 0.1%)	Similar to propamidine	Similar to propamidine
Azole	Voriconazole eye drops 1%, oral	Inhibits synthesis of ergosterol causing the cell membrane to leak—*kills trophozoites* and *cysts*	Acanthamoeba keratitis Also has a broad antifungal spectrum

f) Drugs for glaucoma

GROUP	DRUG	ACTION	USE
Prostaglandin analogues (eye drops)	Latanoprost 0.005% (1) Tafluprost 0.0015% Travoprost 0.004%(1) Bimatoprost 0.01% and 0.03%	Increases outflow of aqueous humour primarily through the uveoscleral route and less so via the trabecular meshwork, by binding to the prostaglandin F2α (FP) receptor as an agonist	Reduction of ocular pressure
Carbonic anhydrase inhibitors (oral and eye drops)	Acetazolamide (oral 125, 250 and 500 mg) Brinzolamide (eye drops 1%) Dorzolamide (1) (eye drops 2%)	Reduces production of aqueous humour	Reduction of ocular pressure
Beta-blockers	Betaxolol 0.5% Levobunol 0.5% Timolol (0.1%, 0.25%, 0.5%) (1) (2)	Reduces production of aqueous humour	Reduction of ocular pressure
Alpha2 adrenergic receptor agonist	Brimonidine 0.2%(1)	Alpha2-adrenoreceptor agonist. May interfere with prostaglandin synthesis in the ciliary body and increase uveoscleral outflow	Reduction of ocular pressure

(Continued)

GROUP	DRUG	ACTION	USE
Combination of beta-blocker and prostaglandin analogue	*Ganfort* is a combination of Timolol 0.5% and Bimatoprost 0.03%	The combination of these two substances has an additive effect	Reduction of ocular pressure
Combination of beta-blocker and carbonic anhydrase inhibitor	*Dormide-T*(1) is a combination of Timolol 0.5% and Dorzolamide 2%	The combination of these two substances has an additive effect	Reduction of ocular pressure
Combination of beta-blocker and alpha2 agonist	*T-Bridine*(1) is a combination of Timolol 0.5% and Brimonidine 0.2%	The combination of these two substances has an additive effect	Reduction of ocular pressure
Combination of carbonic anhydrase inhibitor and alpha2 agonist	*Simbrinza* is a combination of brinzolamide and brimonidine	The combination of these two substances has an additive effect to reduce the production of aqueous humour	Reduction of ocular pressure

(1) Also available from www.aurolab.com (India).

(2) Timolol is less frequently used as first line therapy for glaucoma management but is used in fixed combinations with other drugs.

Drugs for ocular use produced in India (exported world-wide at affordable cost):

Aurolab (India) https://www.aurolab.com/our-products

DRUG INFORMATION WORLD-WIDE

UK British National Formulary https://bnf.nice.org.uk/

EU National registers of countries in Europe for drug information:
https://www.ema.europa.eu/en/medicines/national-registers-authorised-medicines

European Medicines Agency https://www.ema.europa.eu/en/medicines

Australia https://www.tga.gov.au/products/regulations-all-products/about-australian-register-therapeutic-goods-artg/searching-australian-register-therapeutic-goods-artg

Bangladesh https://medex.com.bd/index.php/brands

Pakistan https://www.dra.gov.pk/publications/national-essential-medicine-lists/—see section 21 for eye products

Saudi Food and Drug Authority https://www.sfda.gov.sa/en/drugs-list

USA FDA https://www.fda.gov/drugs/development-approval-process-drugs/drug-approvals-and-databases

World Health Organization (WHO)

Essential medicines and current list:

https://www.who.int/publications/i/item/B09474

https://www.who.int/groups/expert-committee-on-selection-and-use-of-essential-medicines/essential-medicines-lists

Index

Note: Page numbers in *italics* indicate a figure and page numbers in **bold** indicate a table on the corresponding page.

For Product Safety Concerns and Information please contact our EU
representative GPSR@taylorandfrancis.com
Taylor & Francis Verlag GmbH, Kaufingerstraße 24, 80331 München, Germany